THE 28-DAY ANTIOXIDANT DIET PROGRAM

by

STEVEN C. MASLEY, M.D.

Good Health
& Bon Appetit,

**FEATURING 28 DAYS OF FANTASTIC RECIPES
THAT WILL REVITALIZE YOUR LIFE**

Steven Masley

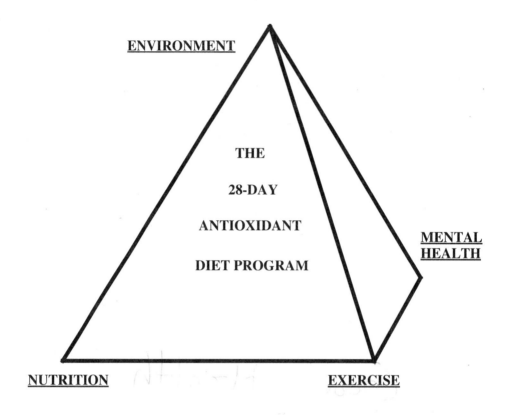

ENVIRONMENT

THE

28-DAY

ANTIOXIDANT

DIET PROGRAM

MENTAL
HEALTH

NUTRITION

EXERCISE

By Steven C. Masley, M.D.

Exclusive Copyright by Steven C. Masley, M.D.

1996 United States Library of Congress

All rights reserved

Manufactured in the United States of America on recycled paper

Printed 1997, by Custom Printing Company

Cover, text, figures, and tables by Steven C. Masley, M.D.

ISBN# 0-9659977-6-6

THIS BOOK IS DEDICATED TO MY WIFE, NICOLE,

AND MY TWO SONS LUCAS AND MARCOS.

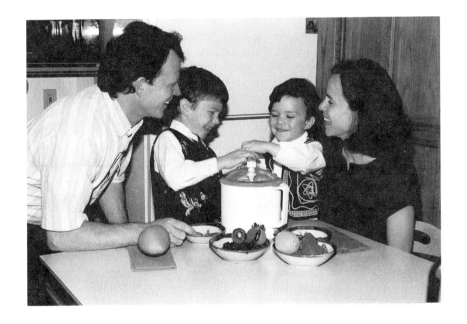

"I am impressed how thoroughly Dr. Masley has researched all the scientific information for his book, and then translated it into easy to understand terms. As a scientist–I am excited, as an educator–I'm inspired! By following his recommendations, readers will find tasty recipes and achieve significant health benefits."

Kirsten Lampi, Ph.D., Assistant Professor of Molecular Biology and Researcher at Oregon's Health Science University

"Steven's book and recipes are so easy to read, understand, and actually cook, I'm sending his book to my mother. It's nice to see a book out there showing that plant-based cuisine just makes sense."

Catherine Geier, the Executive Chef at Café Flora in Seattle, Washington, a restaurant featuring exquisite vegetarian meals

"Dr. Masley's program saved my life. He got me to eat well, quit drinking, and walk daily. This well-being has helped to transform my life. I haven't had angina complaints in years, and I've cut my total cholesterol from the 280's to 179. I haven't cut all the fat from my diet, but I've added all the antioxidant rich foods. I feel great!"

John, an engineer from Olympia, Washington

"I found Dr. Masley's *28-Day Antioxidant Diet Program* authentic, approachable, clear, and motivating. Now I choose antioxidant-rich foods much more often, simply because I know what they are."

Beth Schock, a vintner from Yamhill, Oregon

"I really benefited from reading Dr. Masley's *28-Day Antioxidant Diet Program*. I used to live on fast food for breakfast, lunch, and often dinner. Over the years, I tried dieting, tried eating healthy, but I never really became motivated, and instead felt discouraged. His book has turned around my eating habits, and I think his point system is great! I have found "success" instead of failing a diet. I WIN better health."

Susan Thomas, a TV producer in Salt Lake City

"I found *The 28-Day Antioxidant Diet Program* easy to read and understand. It's loaded with good information and insight on promoting longevity. After reading Dr. Masley's book, I wanted to try all of his tasty, colorful and easy to fix recipes. I found myself with more resolve to eat healthy."

Lu Carlson, a parent and rehabilitation counselor in Olympia, Washington

CONTENTS

FOREWORD

by Gordon Wheat, M.D.
Department of Family Medicine
Committee on Prevention
Group Health Cooperative of Puget Sound

Soon after Dr. Masley joined our medical group, he and his wife, Nicole, had a summer party. Stretched before us were plates of delicious, colorful vegetable curries, fresh homemade chutneys, and home baked breads. It was one of the best vegetarian meals I had eaten in years. Since then, we have shared many meals, all of them nutrition-rich and bursting with flavor.

Nutrition and diet have long been an interest Dr. Masley and I share. We have worked together on committees of physicians on behalf of Group Health Cooperative of Puget Sound, an HMO recognized for its prevention science. Our work has often focused on sifting evidence from research studies in order to make recommendations to prevent heart disease and other debilitating illnesses.

Now Dr. Masley has written The 28-Day Antioxidant Diet Program, the only book available that offers readers cutting-edge nutritional advice, along with healthful, delicious recipes created in Dr. Masley's own kitchen. His recommendations represent the best synthesis of nutrition science that I have seen, written for the lay reader. This is a diet for every generation, from youth to senior citizen, highlighting the latest evidence regarding antioxidants, lipids and other dietary modulators of disease. Dr. Masley's recommendations are based on results of human studies, not animal studies. This alone is quite unique in diet-program literature.

Dr. Masley helps readers make the transition from a high-fat lifestyle by recommending 20% of calories from fat, with a careful selection of fat sources. Evidence is now gathering that this may result in better health than the very-low-fat diet (10% of calories from fat) proposed by Dr. Dean Ornish.

The recipes–all created by Dr. Masley and his wife–reflect a long-standing commitment to creating meals that are health-promoting, flavorful, beautiful, and easy for any busy person to prepare. Readers will actually look forward to serving these dishes to their families!

The 28-Day Antioxidant Diet Program has now become my best resource to help me provide my patients with an effective prescription for a health-promoting lifestyle change.

INTRODUCTION

ABOUT THE AUTHOR

I am a family physician, a husband, and the father of two boys, ages 4 and 7. This book reflects how I've learned to prepare and serve antioxidant-rich foods to my family and friends–with wonderful results. This lifestyle has brought us to an even happier, more loving, and full life. Mealtimes are not only necessary to our lives–they are an experience we anticipate and enjoy. I'd like you to share in this enjoyment, and watch your health improve at the same time!

As a physician/chef, I have come to believe that modern medicine has less effect on our health than our own food choices. Yet, we Americans have unintentionally chosen to eat poorly. Our diets are high in fat and low in grains, legumes, fruits and vegetables. As a result, we struggle with many debilitating illnesses. Heart disease, cancer, and diabetes are three that claim many Americans. In fact, over one-third of Americans will die of heart attacks and strokes. Yet, most of these deaths could be prevented simply by changing one's diet!

As a family physician, I care for patients from birth to death. In the course of my work, I enjoy getting to know my patients and their families, but I become frustrated when I see people I care about lose their health and independence needlessly.

To help my patients maintain their health and vigor, I encourage them to focus on healthful foods and exercise. The satisfaction I've received from encouraging people to live better has pushed me to look in new directions for solid scientific answers to questions about nutrition and exercise.

After sorting through often-conflicting research, I believe the *"gold standard"* for evaluating information comes from controlled, clinical trials of humans. I believe that referring to any other research as "definitive" would be irresponsible–particularly when I'm discussing important health evidence and encouraging readers to change their lives.

"A Passion For Cooking"

Cooking became my passion early in my adult life. In college, I discovered that if I could follow the intricate calculations of physics and chemistry projects, I could also learn to follow a recipe. Because my housemates shared my love of cooking, Saturday nights invariably turned into dinner parties.

Later, when I married, I found a soulmate in the kitchen. My wife, Nicole is a wonderful cook and we continue to share new recipes. Today, when we visit relatives in France, friends in Australia, or family members in Arizona, we cook in their kitchens with local ingredients. We have also spent years working as volunteers in over a dozen countries, including China, Ecuador, France, Guatemala, India, Kenya, and Mexico. There, we were exposed to wonderful foods that continue to influence our cooking.

Like most Americans in the 1950's-1970's, I grew up eating meat, poultry or fish about twice per day. However, I was lucky; my mother and father loved cooking with herbs and spices and taught me to enjoy flavorful food.

My meat-eating days came to an abrupt halt while doing medical volunteer work in India in 1979. For some reason, every time I ate meat, I became very ill. I stopped eating meat for 6 months, and once I came home, I continued to avoid eating meat.

My choice not to eat meat and poultry gradually evolved into a love affair with vegetarian cuisine. I did not make this choice to improve my long-term health. Yet, this diet change has clearly benefited my health and increased my vitality.

While I have not eaten meat or poultry since 1979, I don't call myself a vegetarian. We have fish perhaps once or twice per month, usually at someone's house or in restaurants. We wear leather belts and shoes, and feed our dogs, Tofu and Soya, standard dog food. In our home, we are raising our children as vegetarians and teach them to think of all life as beautiful, and equally important as our own.

Now, I invite you to join my family and a growing number of others who enjoy a new, energy-filled, healthier way of life. I believe that once you've tasted the benefits of this lifestyle, you won't want to turn back!

Good health and bon appétit!

Steven C. Masley, M.D.

AUTHOR'S NOTE

Health is a complex state of physical, emotional, and social well-being. Health represents more than being free from disease. It gives us energy and vitality so that we may function at our highest potential.

This nutritional guide will maximize your health and energy through increasing the amounts of antioxidant-rich foods in your diet. Most diets focus on cutting out foods. I encourage you to <u>ADD</u> colorful, delicious foods to your diet.

By following my program, most of you can expect to lose weight, feel better, and improve your health. You can anticipate reductions in cholesterol levels and improved blood pressure and blood sugar control within two months. Your risk for cancer, strokes, and heart attacks will decrease as well.

SPECIAL NOTE

We as individuals remain genetically unique. No one diet can work for everyone. However, you can learn which dietary changes will maximize your health and energy. Be sure to involve your health care provider in these changes. If you develop any physical complaints following the diet or exercise recommendations, notify your health care provider.

Do not change your diet if you are seriously ill or on medication except under the advice of a medical doctor. Any decision you make involving the treatment of an illness should include the advice of the medical provider of your choice.

ACKNOWLEDGMENTS

First, I want to thank my loving wife, Nicole. When I told her of my desire to reduce my clinic work to half time (and reduce my salary) to pursue writing this book, she supported me fully. She has energetically helped edit this book and assisted me in testing many recipes. Along with Nicole, my boys Lucas and Marcos, have been very helpful in tasting my recipes and offering their suggestions.

My extended family eagerly edited the first version of this manuscript, and provided many appreciated suggestions. Thanks to my sisters, Brooke and Susan, my parents and step-parents, Arpad and Peggy Masley, and Evelyn and Charles Odegaard, and to Nicole's parents, Jean and Joy Vidal.

Many friends have offered practical ideas in creating this book, and I want to thank several of them: Stephen Bray, Pat Carlson, Colette Crosnier, Kelvie Johnson, M.D., Janet LaBranche, Rose Lancaster, Kirsten Lampi, Ph.D, Joseph Pellicer, M.D., and Rachel Wood, M.D.

I am grateful to a variety of co-workers at Group Health Cooperative of Puget Sound, who reviewed the scientific evidence behind this book and challenged my ideas. They include Lois Anderson, R.N., Beverly Green, M.D., Collene Hawes, R.N., Terri Henry, R.D., Megan Hubbard, M.D., Rachel Newmann, R.N., Julia Sokoloff, M.D., Sirkka Waller, MSPH, and Gordon Wheat, M.D.

In particular, I want to thank my agent and editor, Claire Gerus, who has encouraged me and expertly helped make this book more lively and readable.

The medical library staff at Providence St. Peter Hospital has been extremely helpful. They conducted well over 100 topic searches, and obtained over 1,000 medical journal articles to help clarify and answer several critical issues in this manuscript. Thanks to Edean Berglund, Lewis Daniell, Kathy Wagner, and the many volunteers.

I want to thank all the extended staff at Café Flora, a gourmet vegetarian restaurant in Seattle, Washington. They warmly invited me to work in their restaurant featuring elegant fare. In particular, I wish to thank Catherine Geier, their executive chef, for her encouragement and editing.

When I started this project, I viewed the computer as a fancy typewriter. My ability to create documents, figures, and finally a book has grown steadily and I want to thank Eric Hess, Matt Metcalf, Steve Powers, and Anthony Vidal for their technical support.

A special thanks to my many teachers and mentors who have instilled in me "the curiosity to ask why, and the sense to put it together." They include: Vishnu Bhattia, Ph.D. from Washington State University's Honor's Program, John Gayman, M.D. and Michael Stuart, M.D. from Group Health Cooperative in Seattle, Washington, Barry

Weiss, M.D. from the University of Arizona in Tucson, Arizona, and Jeffrey Bland, Ph.D. from HealthComm, Inc. in Gig Harbor, Washington.

Last, I want to thank my patients, who have enabled me to use this health program to treat medical problems daily. Even more important, they have helped me to convert this technical information into everyday words that empower people along a path toward health and vitality. It is my sincere wish that this book will help you reach that same destination.

CHAPTER 1   *THE AMAZING ANTIOXIDANTS*

*T*his book will introduce you to an amazing group of foods rich in "antioxidants"– chemical compounds in fruits, vegetables, and other foods that are vital to your health, vitality and longevity. "Health" means more than simply being free from disease. It is a state of physical, emotional, and mental well-being, a state that's becoming harder to achieve these days, when stress and poor nutrition are at an all-time high. If there was ever a time for antioxidants to come to our rescue and put us back on the road to health, it's now!

Your success on the 28-Day Antioxidant Diet Program will depend on your willingness to change your diet by *adding* more antioxidant-rich foods to your meals. "Wait a minute," you might say. "Did you use the word, adding?"

Yes, and that's one of the delights of this program. Most diets focus on cutting out foods. This book is different–in fact, you'll find that you'll be adding foods to your diet. What a refreshing change for the dieter! In my program, even real chocolate, fat, and red wine are allowed in limited quantities. I will, however, ask that you limit your fat intake, and that you choose olive oil or canola oil over butter and other fats.

To help you create a new lifestyle, I'll provide complete information about how much and what kinds of fats and carbohydrates will benefit you. I'll also show you how daily exercise can revitalize your health and energy.

Later, we'll go shopping, and I'll guide you to healthier food purchases and show you how to store them. At the end of the book, I'll introduce you to a wide range of delicious meals your whole family can enjoy. Most recipes are quick and easy to prepare, and each is full of antioxidant power to boost the immune system, fight aging, and bring you to the peak of health.

By following my *28-Day Antioxidant Diet Program*, most of you can expect to lose weight, feel better, and improve your health. You can anticipate solid reductions in your cholesterol and blood sugar levels, and improve your blood pressure within two months. Your risk for cancer, strokes, and heart attacks will decrease over time, as well.

Of course, we're all genetically unique, and no one diet can work the same for everyone. As you follow the principles of my *28-Day Antioxidant Diet Program*, you'll learn which dietary changes work best for you. Be sure to include your health care provider in any changes you make to your diet and lifestyle, particularly if you have medical problems or take medications.

WHY I CREATED THE 28-DAY ANTIOXIDANT DIET PROGRAM

Nearly 10 years ago, I had a personal experience that made me realize just how powerful our dietary choices can be. In fact, they can make the difference between life and death. I was engaged to a delightful young woman named Nicole. Her mother, Joy, was a funny, happy woman with whom I shared an instant rapport. I was pleased that my future wife had such a terrific mother, and we enjoyed many laughter-filled moments together.

One day while exercising, Joy developed shoulder discomfort and shortness of breath. Uneasy, she went to see a doctor, who put her on a treadmill to check her heart. The results were not good. Joy was scheduled for surgery that same week and at the tender age of 54, my future mother-in-law was about to undergo triple coronary artery bypass surgery.

Our concern turned to relief when she survived the surgery. But her follow-up visits were troubling, revealing persistently high cholesterol levels. Joy was still in danger of re-clogging her arteries.

Like many patients after bypass surgery, she thought the surgery had made her good as new, and initially ignored instituting lifestyle changes to improve her health. I waited patiently as she struggled with what to do next. Later, she asked me for advice, and I designed a diet and exercise program to help her reverse the plaque in her arteries and lower her cholesterol levels. Today, as a result of the program, her cholesterol numbers have plummeted from 390 to 220, and her "ratio" of total cholesterol to HDL has gone down from 8 to 2.5 (an excellent ratio; the average American cholesterol ratio is 5.5).

Joy succeeded because she took the time to change her lifestyle and correct her cholesterol problem. To her delight, her energy level improved so drastically that she now feels better than she did in her youth. Joy's chances for avoiding future heart problems are very promising and I am proud of her.

Through Joy's experience I, too, learned a lesson. I was able to observe how powerful food can be as a healer, and how, when combined with the appropriate exercise regimen, it can promote health. Joy is not unique in her successful quest to vanquish heart disease. I have treated many other patients with a combination of heart-healthy foods called "antioxidants" and exercise to prevent, restore, and improve health.

The program I created for Joy features the same antioxidant-rich, low-fat foods I will share with you on the following pages. It has worked for Joy for ten years, and for hundreds of my patients since then. As a doctor, I've discovered that most patients claim they want to "go on a diet" to achieve some objective, but then slide off the diet wagon soon after the first glimmer of improvement.

To my delight, however, I've found that my patients not only stay on the program, but build it into their lifestyles, and often into those of their families. In my own case, Nicole and I love to create delicious, antioxidant-rich meals. Even our young sons often clamor for second helpings of our red pepper-cauliflower curry with spiced yogurt sauce, or pizza with artichoke hearts, cashews, and garlic.

Let me introduce you to antioxidants, the foods that contain them, and how you can boost your health and lose weight on my easy-to-follow *28-Day Antioxidant Diet Program*.

ANTIOXIDANTS–NATURE'S HEALERS

Have you noticed lately how often you see or hear the words "oxidants," "free radicals," and "antioxidants"? Once found only in health-food stores, antioxidants and books about them can now be found in supermarkets and drugstores. Thanks to medical and scientific studies confirming that these tiny chemical compounds can prevent cell damage leading to fatigue, disease, and aging, antioxidants have earned new respect as compounds that improve health and boost the immune system.

You won't have to know all the intricacies of how antioxidants work in order to benefit from my program. But it will be helpful to understand why the antioxidants in foods are vital to your well-being–and why supplements cannot substitute for natural sources.

The Free Radical Attackers

Oxygen is essential to our lives–without it, our bodies could not function. We humans need oxygen to convert food into energy, just as a car engine uses a spark to convert gasoline into a power source. During this fuel-burning, a car produces exhaust. Similarly, when our bodies burn fuel with oxygen (a process called "oxidation"), we produce "free radicals"–toxic products that, in excess, can cause illness, accelerate aging, and lead to death.

We must also deal with free radicals that infiltrate our bodies from external sources, such as tobacco smoke, smog, pesticides, exhaust, and ultraviolet sunlight. When these internal and external free radicals hit our tissues, they act like small fires spreading through the forest. Free radicals create a chain reaction, attacking fats and proteins, turning them into free radicals as well. These new free radicals attack other chemicals and molecules in our bodies, destroying healthy tissue and threatening our well-being.

Here's what raging free-radicals can do to you:

- Fats in the blood stream can oxidize and turn to plaque, blocking the flow of blood in your arteries, leading to heart attacks and strokes.
- Genetic DNA material can be damaged, making your cells more susceptible to aging and cancer.
- When free radicals attack your eye, they can cause cataracts and macular degeneration, leading to poor eyesight.

A list of additional free radical induced illnesses is shown below in Table 1.

TABLE 1. Illnesses Associated with Free Radical Damage:

Asthma	Parkinson's disease	Arthritis
Crohn's disease	Irritable bowel syndrome	Pancreatitis
Fibromyalgia	Chronic fatigue syndrome	Chronic eczema

On the other hand, oxidation is not all bad. Did you know that white blood cells essentially bleach harmful bacteria to death? Similarly, the liver uses oxidation to convert many toxins, like alcohol, into compounds the kidneys and intestines can excrete. And, when we exercise, oxidation can produce vital energy.

However, because all forms of oxidation generate free radicals, antioxidants are needed to neutralize them. It might seem as if we're in a losing battle. But then our courageous antioxidant team comes to the rescue, extinguishing the free radicals, saving our cells and extending our lifespans.

Natural antioxidants to the rescue

Our lives depend upon photosynthesis: the magical process whereby plants convert sunlight energy into food energy. During this energy conversion, "free radicals" are formed. To protect themselves from these lethal by-products, plants produce "antioxidants," chemical compounds that neutralize free radicals and stop them burning the plants to death.

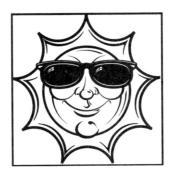

Fortunately, when you eat colorful, antioxidant-rich foods, you'll transfer millions of these life-saving antioxidants into your own body. You'll need all of them to neutralize both the free radicals formed from using oxygen to burn food energy and the added free radicals we accumulate from living in a polluted world.

What Are Antioxidants?

Because antioxidants protect the surface of the plant, we find them in the skin and outer surfaces of grains, beans (legumes), fruits and vegetables. Broccoli and spinach, blueberries, strawberries, grapes and apricots–all are loaded with antioxidants. Many herbs and spices are rich sources of antioxidants as well. Garlic, ginger, parsley, thyme and rosemary not only enhance the flavor in our meals, they improve the health of our cells, thereby increasing our lifespans.

Grains such as brown rice and whole wheat contain antioxidants in their outer husks. Many grains, protected by these husks, can be stored for over a thousand years.

Given water, they will actually sprout and grow! This gives you some idea as to the long-term power antioxidants can have.

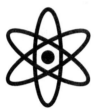

Everything is made of particles called atoms. Each atom is composed of a nucleus with protons and neutrons at its center, and is encircled by electrons. The electrons circle in orbitals around the nucleus, like planets circle our sun. Each stable orbital has 2 electrons. An orbital with only 1 electron is very unstable.

Compounds that have an unpaired, single electron in an orbital are called "free radicals." Free radicals steal electrons from other compounds and make them unstable.

"Antioxidants" can donate an extra stable electron and stabilize a free radical.

Antioxidants work at the cellular level

Our bodies are made of billions of cells. In many ways a cell relates to our body the way a house relates to a city. Our blood vessels transport energy and waste to and from our cells, just as a vehicle moves food to a home and takes away garbage.

Like the walls in a house, the walls in a cell protect it from the outside. The cell walls allow sugar and oxygen to pass through as fuel, but an array of antioxidants block toxic oxidants from entry.

Antioxidants play a critical role in guarding our cell walls from free radical attack. On a cellular level, free radicals start chain reactions within our tissues, damaging one compound after another until the cell's functional capacity is destroyed.

Antioxidants block this process by neutralizing free radicals. Within the cell wall, Vitamin E is often the first antioxidant to defend the cell. Other antioxidants, such as Vitamin C, carotenoids, and flavonoids can neutralize other free radicals, or they can regenerate used Vitamin E back into its active form. These antioxidants become inactive after extinguishing a free radical or after regenerating fellow antioxidants.

Since the antioxidants replenish each other, I visualize free radicals as an outside force pounding and pulling on a chain of interlinked antioxidants. Hence the protective antioxidant chain is only as strong as the weakest link.

As these protective reactions occur, antioxidant stores become depleted. Thus, we must continually replenish our antioxidant reserves through dietary sources. My Antioxidant Diet Program aims to ensure that your antioxidant stores remain intact.

What kinds of antioxidants are there?

There is a vast array of antioxidant compounds. First are the water-soluble antioxidants, such as Vitamin C, which flow through our bloodstream and within our cells scavenging up free radicals. Second are the fat-soluble antioxidants that reside within cell walls and include Vitamin E, carotenoids, and flavonoids.

A third group of antioxidants includes enzymes, nutrient compounds (such as glutathione), and trace elements like zinc that facilitate enzyme reactions. These are chemicals that enhance the life-sustaining chemical reactions in our bodies and neutralize the billions of oxidants produced within us. We need trace elements such as zinc, selenium, copper and magnesium for many of these enzyme reactions to occur.

"Carotenoids" and *"flavonoids"* are specific antioxidant groups you may read or hear about in the media.

Carotenoids, like beta carotene, are antioxidants found in most colorful fruits and vegetables. Carotenoids are actually plant pigments that provide color and protect the plants from the damaging effects of ultraviolet sunlight. Although scientists have identified over 600 types of carotenoids, most health research focuses on five types: beta carotene, alpha-carotene, lutein, zeaxanthin, and lycopene. Cooking does not harm carotenoids, as it does Vitamin C. So, cooked produce retains its antioxidant power.

Flavonoids, like carotenoids, are antioxidant pigments found notably in grape skins, tea leaves, onions, berries, soy products, green leafy veggies and garlic. They also provide the tannic taste in green tea, red wine, and many herbs. There are over 400 flavonoids known in the human diet. At Tufts University in Boston, researchers are studying the antioxidant content of foods, and finding that flavonoids account for a powerful part of the antioxidant activity in fruits and vegetables. Some flavonoids have much greater antioxidant power than Vitamin C or Vitamin E. The deep pigment colors in berries (like blueberries and strawberries), come from flavonoids called "anthocyanins." They appear especially promising in protecting us from oxidation.

Clinical studies in Finland and the Netherlands reveal that eating flavonoid rich foods reduces disease rates. The bottom line remains, *"Eat more colorful fruits, vegetables, herbs, and spices!"* A food chart features foods rich in specific antioxidants on the next page.

TABLE 2. Antioxidant Food Content:

ANTIOXIDANT FOOD CONTENT	Phenols & Flavonoids	Beta-Carotene	Alpha-Carotene	Lyco-pene	Lutein & Zeaxanthin	Vit C	Vit E
Garlic	+++						
Onions	++						
Leeks	+++	+++			+++		
Oranges	++					++++	
Cantaloupe		+++				++++	
Apricot	++	+++				+++	+
Carrot	++	++++	+++				
Broccoli	+++	++			+++	++++	+
Kale	+++	+++			++++	++++	+
Grapefruit, pink	++	+++		+++		++++	
Guava		++		+++			
Mango		+++					+
Beet greens	+++	+++					+
Spinach	+++	++++			++++		
Sweet potato	++	++++					
Yams	++	++++					
Pepper, red	+++	+++				++++	
Pepper, green	++	+			++	++++	
Peach, dried	++	++++					
Peach, raw	++	+					
Strawberries	++++						
Swiss chard	+++	+++					
Tomato, raw	+	++		+++	+		
Tomato paste	++			++++			
Watermelon				+++		+++	
Green tea	++++						
Black tea	++						
Coffee	+						
Red wine	+++						
Blueberries	++++						
Pumpkin	++	+++	+++		+++		
Parsley	+++	++++			++++	++++	+
Almonds							++++
Other nuts							+++
Olive oil							+++
Canola oil							+++

THE PRICE OF UNCONTROLLED OXIDATIVE STRESS: DISEASE

Oxidative Stress

When our antioxidant system is in harmony with our production of free radicals, we enjoy vitality. In contrast, when the number of oxidants overpowers the number of antioxidants, cellular damage occurs. We call that damage "oxidative stress."

Let's look at how cellular damage can arise from an innocent sun tan session. You're blissfully enjoying "the rays," unaware that while you're pleasantly baking, free radicals are being generated in your skin. Later, when you look in the mirror, you see an inflammation, or "sunburn," on your face and body.

Did you know that even sun tanned skin is injured skin? Sun tanning accelerates skin aging and wrinkle formation.

With repeated burning and tanning (injury), free radicals will damage "elastin," the scaffolding that keeps your skin looking youthful. Later, as the structural support declines, wrinkles will form. Each sunning session will repeat the process of damaging the skin cell DNA (the cell's brain). Eventually, this process leads to cell death or skin cancer.

Here is where dietary antioxidants can shift the balance. When you eat carotenoid and flavonoid rich foods, you increase concentrations of these antioxidants in your skin. Just as plant antioxidants protect the surface of a plant from sun damage, they also protect your skin. Carotenoids and flavonoids in the skin can neutralize the free radicals generated by the sun's ultraviolet light.

Sunlight exposure is an example of oxidative stress that affects one organ, the skin. Yet free radical damage occurs in all our tissues continuously.

Aging

A normal cell takes 100,000 "*hits*" from free radicals every day. That's one hit per second! If antioxidants don't protect our cells from this onslaught, those cells will age and eventually die. As we get older, our ability to fight oxidation slows down. In fact, the average person after age 65 suffers more than twice as many daily hits as a 30-year-old. Thus, the elderly need more than double the antioxidant protection.

If you want to slow the physical aging process, I suggest you increase your intake of dietary antioxidants, decrease your exposure to oxidants, and decrease your intake of foods that are easily oxidized. This book will teach you how to do precisely that!

Weaker Immune Function and Frequent Infections

Not only do we need antioxidants to prevent disease, we need them to simply stay healthy. Immune cells are types of white blood cells that fight infections and kill cancer cells. Scientists have found that diets low in antioxidants led to decreased functioning of immune cells, especially in the elderly. However, when antioxidant vitamin supplements (such as Vitamin E) were added to the diet, white blood cell activity and function improved. Similar results will occur when an antioxidant rich diet becomes part of your lifestyle.

Increased Pain and Inflammation

Oxidative stress increases the production of chemical compounds that in excess will inflame and irritate our tissues. Inflammation occurs when our defense cells attack foreign compounds, in essence setting them on fire. If we injure or overuse our joints, tendons, or muscles they become inflamed under free radical attack and turn warm, red, and swollen.

Research shows that people who suffer from inflammatory bowel disease (Crohn's disease and ulcerative colitis) and fibromyalgia show signs of increased oxidative stress in their tissues. Arthritic joints also show signs of excess oxidative stress and inflammation. In Scandinavia, studies show that dietary changes can decrease joint complaints, even in cases of severe rheumatoid arthritis. It's reassuring to know that diet can reduce oxidative stress and ease inflammatory pain.

Accelerated Memory Loss

Dr. Flint Beal, a physician and researcher at Harvard Medical School, recently noted an increase in DNA oxidative damage and oxidative stress in patients with Alzheimer's dementia (an irreversible form of profound memory loss). A growing body of evidence indicates that oxidative stress increases nitric oxide levels in our tissues, including the brain, and that these increased levels are associated with decreased thinking power.

As expected, recent clinical trials have shown antioxidants to slow the progression of Alzheimer's disease, supporting the theory that an antioxidant enriched diet can help prevent this diabling disease.

Increased Fatigue

Oxidative stress increases fatigue. Each cell in our body depends upon a powerplant, called a "mitochondrion," to produce energy. Like a generator, it uses oxygen to burn fuel and generate exhaust loaded with free radicals. These powerplants within cells depend upon an enriched antioxidant system to neutralize all the free radicals formed.

While scientists are far from agreement, there is growing evidence that oxidative stress damages these powerplants leading to chronic fatigue. "Chronic fatigue syndrome" represents an illness with mitochondrial dysfunction and increased oxidative stress. As our powerplant function declines, we age and lose energy and vigor. An antioxidant rich diet aims to maintain powerplant function and slow this aging process.

Detoxification

Your body uses a one-two punch to eliminate toxins that you ingest, like alcohol, pesticides, and poisons. As toxins pass from your intestine to your liver they are first oxidized. For a fraction of a second, these toxins become even more harmful. Fortunately, they are quickly detoxified through a special chemical process. They are thus rendered water soluble, inert, and ready for elimination through the urine and stool.

This detoxification process requires substantial antioxidant backup to protect tissues from damage, and special compounds to detoxify the oxidized toxins. Antioxidant rich foods often contain generous supplies of detoxifying compounds. In particular, onions and garlic, and the cruciferous vegetable family (broccoli, kale, cauliflower, cabbage, and Brussels sprouts) contains rich sources of detoxifying compounds. So you won't be surprised to find these vegetables featured regularly within my recipes.

SUMMARY

The essence of my program is to increase your consumption of foods rich in antioxidants and to encourage your participation in regular physical activity. The dietary bottom line is, "Eat more fruits, vegetables, grains and beans." This diet is found in the world's healthiest populations, and is endorsed by national health organizations. As a result of this program your energy will increase, weight loss will occur, health will improve, and oxidative stress will be reduced.

Now that you better understand the harm caused by increased oxidative stress and the benefits of antioxidants, I want to share with you the many advantages of following my 28-Day Antioxidant Diet Program.

CHAPTER 2   *PUTTING ANTIOXIDANTS TO WORK FOR YOU*

ACHIEVE A DOZEN HEALTH BENEFITS BY FOLLOWING THIS PROGRAM

Naturally, before you enter any new program calling for a change in lifestyle, you'll ask, "Why bother? Will my health improve? Will I feel better?" The majority of people who have tried my 28-Day Antioxidant Diet Program have answered this question with a resounding "YES!"

Many people think that lifestyle changes can't overcome the influences of the environment and their genetic makeup. It may surprise you to learn that choices such as diet, physical activity level, and substance use or abuse (tobacco and alcohol) account for 70% of the causes of death in the United States. In fact, lifestyle is strongly linked to the three big killers–heart attack, strokes, and cancer.

In contrast, genetics and the environment each account for less than 10% of the causes of death.

Knowing that we can tip the odds in our favor by adopting a healthier lifestyle is where this program comes in. If you're willing to make the changes described in this book, you can expect to feel more alert and energetic in two weeks, and begin to see a more toned body within a month. If you opt for a more gradual change in lifestyle, these changes may take a bit longer, but from the first week, you'll notice that you have more vitality. Once you're on your way, you'll experience more benefits than we have space to discuss, so I'll focus on an even dozen you'll receive from following this program.

DECREASED RISK OF HEART ATTACKS AND STROKES

There's good news for fruit and veggie lovers! Clinical trials in Europe suggest that eating more vegetables and fruits can cut your risk of a heart attack in half. And U.S. studies offer more good tidings–they reveal that those who eat three extra servings of vegetables and fruits each day cut their risk of a stroke by 50%!

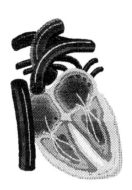

The average American who follows my 28-Day Antioxidant Diet Program will see cholesterol levels fall by about 20%. That all-important ratio of total cholesterol / HDL cholesterol will decrease as well, indicating that your arteries are getting cleaner. (For more cholesterol information, see page 50.)

The way my diet works is simple: the extra antioxidants in your diet (such as from fruits, vegetables, herbs, and legumes) will decrease your oxidation of cholesterol, thus reducing artery-clogging plaque. For those who cut way down on saturated fat, there will be less cholesterol to be oxidized.

Furthermore, a diet rich in green leafy vegetables and certain nuts is high in omega-3 fats, which help prevent artery-blocking clots and further cut your cholesterol level. Garlic, ginger, and other spices that are part of my program also protect against clot formation and reduce your cholesterol level even more.

An unusual feature of my program is that I allow one glass of red wine per day. This decreases clotting tendencies that block arteries, and increases healthy HDL cholesterol levels.

Regular aerobic exercise–another important feature of my program–will improve your circulation and help establish secondary blood supplies within your tissues. This backup supply, enhanced by exercise, can come in handy should you ever develop a circulation problem.

If you already have coronary artery disease (blocked arteries in the heart), you must aggressively take charge of your cholesterol levels. If my diet program does not bring you to your cholesterol target within 3 months, cholesterol-lowering medications should be considered.

Within the heart care team at Group Health Cooperative of Puget Sound, we have set targets for people with known coronary artery disease. People with heart disease should reduce their LDL cholesterol level by at least 30-35%. If the old level is unknown, aim for a LDL cholesterol level below 130. Many patients may need further reductions: either their LDL cholesterol level should be less than 100, (or) their total cholesterol / HDL ratio should be less than 4.0 and their LDL level should be under 130. If you have heart disease, clarify your cholesterol target with your medical provider.

Many people with heart disease can reach these targets by following a lifestyle program. Others will need cholesterol-lowering medication added to it.

Over the years, I've received a variety of thank-you's from patients who have stopped heart disease or strokes in their tracks. Here are two of them.

> *Mr. Kaiser, a minister in Winlock, Washington, says: "I met Dr. Masley several years ago when I was having transient ischemic attacks and was on the verge of a devastating stroke. Multiple studies offered me no surgical solutions. I tried Dr. Masley's program and my stroke warnings stopped. Today, my cholesterol looks great. I feel wonderful. My problem now is that I have so much more energy, I get sore from overdoing my physical activities. I need to start Dr. Masley's weight training activities."*
>
> *Mrs. Vidal in Tucson, Arizona, reports: "A few years ago, I had a heart bypass. I felt better quickly and was very careful to maintain a low-fat, low-cholesterol diet and to walk 3 -5 miles per week. My doctors acted pleased, but my exercise treadmill results remained borderline.*
> *Then I read your book. I immediately began eating more antioxidant-rich fruits and vegetables, with emphasis on the carotenoids and flavonoids. I also decided to add weight-lifting to my exercise routine.*
> *The results have been amazing. Within only two weeks, I felt like a new person! I have so much more energy and not a day passes without some friend commenting on how well I look. My cholesterol ratio shows I am now reversing arterial buildup and my last exercise treadmill test was the best yet. I credit all my health improvements to following the advice in your book.*
> *Thank you from the bottom of my now better heart!"*

REDUCED RISK OF CANCER

If there is one disease that has challenged 20th century Americans, it is cancer. But equally important to finding a cure is preventing it in the first place. Medical research has now confirmed that dietary choices can strongly influence who will develop many forms of cancer. I've designed my *28-Day Antioxidant Program* to help you sharply lower your risk of cancer in the following ways:

- Eating foods rich in antioxidants to lower risk of all cancers.
- Reducing your fat intake and exercising regularly to decrease your risk of breast, colon or prostate cancer.
- Increasing your fiber intake, to decrease colon cancer risk. Whole grains, legumes, fruits, and vegetables improve elimination, removing toxic waste products from our intestines quickly and efficiently. Eating whole grains also helps prevent breast and prostate cancer.
- Adding soy products daily to prevent hormone-related cancers such as breast and prostate cancer.

The table below reflects the relative risk of cancer if you don't eat several servings of fruits and vegetable daily. It may come as a shock, but if you eat only 1-2 servings of vegetables and fruits per day, you have a 2.2 times higher risk of developing lung cancer than someone who eats 5 servings of veggies and fruits per day!

TABLE 3. **Note how the risk of many types of cancer rises if we do not eat vegetables and fruits often. The bottom line is, "Eat lots of veggies and fruits." I recommend seven or more servings daily!**

Site of Cancer	Increased Risk with Poor Produce Intake
Lung	2.2
Larynx	2.3
Mouth and Throat	2
Esophagus	2
Stomach	2.5
Colorectal	1.9
Urinary Bladder	2.1
Pancreas	2.8
Cervix	2
Ovary	1.8
Breast	1.3
Prostate	1.3

We know that certain foods and beverages inhibit the growth of cancer cells. These special foods are emphasized in my recipes and include:

- Cruciferous vegetables (broccoli, kale, cauliflower, cabbage, etc.)
- The onion family (onions, garlic, leeks)
- Soy products (tofu, soy flour, soy milk, and soy products like veggie sausage, veggie burgers, and veggie hot dogs)
- Certain mushrooms (shiitake and oyster mushrooms)
- Green tea

The National Cancer Institute wants the American public to increase fruit and vegetable consumption to 5 or more servings per day, increase grain and legume servings to 6 per day, and cut fat intake to 30% or fewer total calories. These experts believe that their recommendations can help us cut cancer rates by 30%, avoid 160,000 new cases of cancer per year, and save $25 billion in associated cancer therapy costs.

I propose we go even further! That's why my program calls for at least seven servings of vegetables and fruits and 1-2 servings of soy products or beans per day. Choose 5 servings of whole grains per day and drink fluid with these servings. I believe that, by adding these foods and cutting fat intake to under 20% of total calories, we can cut our national cancer rates in half!

PREVENT AND TREAT DIABETES

As you begin to lose weight, improve your selection of starchy foods, and enjoy an exercise routine, you'll find that your blood sugar levels will begin to improve. Here are tips to help reverse or prevent high blood sugar levels:

- Have a serving of beans or soy products at lunch and/or a serving with dinner. They improve your blood sugar control.
- Limit your alcohol intake to 1-2 servings per day or less. Alcohol raises blood sugar levels. Don't drink alcohol if you have uncontrolled diabetes.
- Strive to exercise aerobically for at least 30 minutes every day. If you have diabetes, you'll benefit even more by doubling this to two 30-minute workouts per day, or working-out for 45-60 minutes daily.
- Stabilize your blood sugar levels by eating certain grains, like pasta and bulgur wheat. Green leafy vegetables (tossed salads, spinach, kale, chard), cruciferous vegetables (broccoli, kale, and cabbage), and many other veggies all help control sugar levels and fight diabetes.

People with diabetes (elevated blood sugar levels) need to increase their antioxidant intake because they form more artery-blocking plaque than do non-diabetics with the same cholesterol levels. Diabetics are also at increased risk of oxidation tissue damage, and can suffer from nerve damage, blindness, and kidney failure.

Diabetics who enrich their diets with antioxidants will decrease cholesterol oxidation. A limited amount of monounsaturated fat (from olive oil and canola oil), as outlined in this program, can benefit diabetics, decreasing both cholesterol levels and the oxidation of LDL cholesterol into plaque.

Many diabetics suffer from antioxidant vitamin and mineral deficiencies, including zinc, Vitamin C, Vitamin E, magnesium, chromium, and vanadium. Diabetics oxidize many compounds more rapidly, thus depleting their antioxidant stores more quickly. Diabetes also causes the loss of valuable antioxidants through increased urination. While my program helps control blood sugar levels, you should discuss the option of taking antioxidant supplements with your medical provider. (See "SPECIAL DIABETIC NEEDS" on page 280.)

INCREASED BONE STRENGTH

While calcium balance is a departure from my antioxidant diet theme, it remains a major concern for women. One of the benefits of following this program is enhanced bone health from eating the antioxidant-rich foods on this diet that are often rich in calcium. Non-fat dairy foods add dietary calcium, while remaining antioxidant balance neutral.

With all the controversy regarding the impact of nutrition on bone strength, I agonized over how to enhance calcium balance in women. I reviewed several hundred medical studies to ensure that my Antioxidant Diet Program would maximize bone health.

Good bone health begins by putting calcium into bone early in life and then keeping it there. Depositing calcium in our bones is like putting money into a retirement fund. When we deposit more calcium than is removed, our bank account grows.

Osteoporosis refers to the gradual loss of calcium from bones, resulting in brittle bones and subsequent fractures. This condition afflicts over 23 million Americans. Forty percent of Caucasian women will have fractures of the spine, hip, or forearm after age 50. Men and women from other ethnic groups have lower rates of fractures than Caucasian women, yet many will still suffer from osteoporosis.

We reach our maximum bone strength in our twenties, and then face a gradual loss in bone density and strength after age 30. One of the keys to preventing osteoporosis is to form the maximum possible peak bone mass at an early age. It is critical that teenagers exercise regularly, have adequate calcium intake, limit protein intake, and avoid tobacco products. They have a "once in a lifetime opportunity" to increase bone density. After age thirty, we can slow our loss of calcium, but we cannot normally increase bone strength. (See Figure 2 below.)

Figure 2: Projected Bone Density Loss Figure: Note how bone density rises rapidly from age 10 to 20, and then slowly declines thereafter. Notice the different ages at which women reach the fracture zone, the stage where bones break easily. The variations reflect differences in lifestyle, which include calcium intake, exercise level, salt intake, and meat intake.

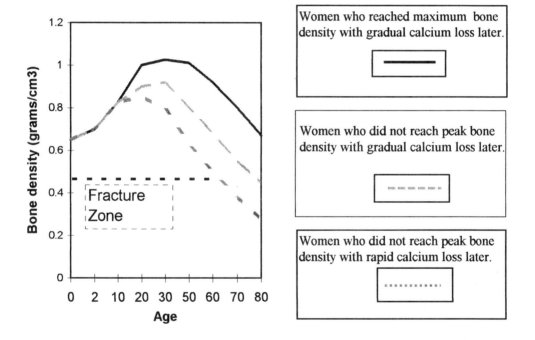

How to strengthen bones

Exercise stimulates our bones to increase their density and grow stronger. Weight bearing exercise, such as walking, and strength training are particularly effective. Strength training includes weight lifting, isometric exercise, elastic band training, and weight machine training. Regardless of our age, inactivity results in our bones releasing calcium and becoming more brittle. We all need at least 30-60 minutes of moderate exercise per day, such as taking a brisk walk or riding a bicycle.

Calcium is essential to bone health. Good sources of calcium include green leafy vegetables, whole grains, and non-fat dairy products. Soy products are another source of calcium, especially for those who are dairy intolerant.

How much calcium do I need?

Too often doctors give the same nutrient recommendation to everyone. Calcium intake is a good example of how needs vary depending upon lifestyle. If you are physically very active, vegetarian, and limit your salt intake–you need between 500 mg to 800 mg per day. If you are inactive, and have a high salt and high animal protein intake (like many Americans), aim for 1,000 mg to 1,200 mg per day.

TABLE 4. **Calcium Food Sources:**

Calcium Sources

Food Item	Calcium content (mg)
Yogurt (8 ounces)	415
Cow's milk (8 ounces)	300
Soy milk (Calcium fortified-8 ounces)	300
Rice milk (Calcium fortified-8 ounces)	300
Figs, dried (10)	269
Cheddar cheese (1 ounce)	204
Oatmeal, instant (1 pkt)	163
Tofu (1/2 cup)	130
Navy beans (1 cup, cooked)	128
Kale, and other greens (1 cup)	94
Garbanzo beans (1 cup)	80
Almonds (1 ounce)	75
Cottage cheese (1/2 cup)	69

Calcium supplements can also slow bone weakening. If your diet has less calcium than you need, consider adding 500 mg to 800 mg of calcium supplements per day. (See Table 4 on page 19) However, if you have a history of iron deficiency anemia or kidney stones, talk with your health provider before taking calcium supplements. These may decrease iron absorption from your intestines and increase the risk of kidney stones.

Stop weakening your bones

Several factors weaken bones and are a result of a western lifestyle. These include eating excess animal protein and drinking beverages with caffeine and phosphates (colas). Tobacco use also causes our bodies to lose calcium.

Since animal protein has a high acid content, our bodies must pull calcium out of our bones to balance the acids we absorb from eating meat, poultry, or fish. Thus the more animal protein we eat, the more calcium we lose. My diet program calls for limiting animal protein intake, like lean meats and poultry, to 2 servings per week or less.

Excess salt intake also increases urinary calcium loss. However, if a woman eats adequate calcium and exercises regularly, she can compensate for a high salt intake. Most women in the United States unfortunately don't follow a lifestyle that favors bone formation, so added salt produces substantial added bone weakening over a lifetime.

Fortunately, my program provides a lifestyle that favors bone formation. If you eat a lot of salt, you can balance that calcium loss with just an extra 150 mg of calcium per day (the amount found in an extra 1/2 cup of milk or 1 serving of oatmeal.)

Both tobacco and caffeine decrease your kidney's ability to retain calcium, resulting in substantial calcium loss. Younger women seem able to compensate for caffeine consumption of 1 to 2 cups of coffee per day with adequate calcium intake. After menopause, women risk increased bone density loss by drinking caffeine.

What about menopause?

Calcium intake, exercise, and dietary protein reductions remain important after menopause, with or without hormone replacement therapy. For women who won't or can't take estrogen, natural plant generated progesterone creams applied daily appear to slow bone density loss.

Most women lose 30% or more of their bone strength and bone mass during the first three years of menopause if they do not take some form of estrogen. Women who have chosen a lifestyle compatible with solid bone health (especially during their teen years), should have substantial bone reserves to cover this loss. Unfortunately, it seems that most western women reaching menopause in the 1990's have failed to choose (or were unaware of) a bone strength enhancing lifestyle over their lifetime and are at increased risk of osteoporosis. Hormone replacement therapy with estrogen and sometimes progesterone can slow the rapid loss in calcium that occurs during menopause.

If a woman chooses hormone replacement therapy, and has her uterus, she needs estrogen and progesterone. If she doesn't have a uterus, she can take estrogen alone. Of the pharmaceutical estrogens available, I prefer to prescribe "Estratabs R," which are esterified estrogens derived from Mexican yam and soybeans. The other popular form of estrogen is "Premarin R," a conjugated estrogen, which comes from pregnant horse urine.

Do I need Vitamin D supplements?

Vitamin D is a hormone that is important to bone health. Vitamin D fortified, non-fat dairy products, and fortified vitamins and cereals are good sources of Vitamin D. People over age 65 often fail to get adequate Vitamin D, so supplements for this age group can help prevent debilitating fractures. For those who don't eat dairy products or fortified cereals, just 15 minutes of exposure to sunlight three times per week will give you sufficient Vitamin D.

Are there other benefits to following a bone strengthening diet?

My diet program does more than reduce the calcium loss in your urine, it cuts down your risk of forming calcium containing kidney stones. Diets high in meat and low in fluid intake will increase your chance of forming kidney stones, which can be very painful.

To prevent kidney stones, which form when bones lose calcium, cut back on the meat, poultry, and fish you eat. Drink at least 2 quarts of fluid per day. If you have a history of calcium containing kidney stones, avoid high calcium sources and calcium supplements.

Summary To Maximize Your Bone Strength:
- Add calcium to your diet. Aim for your recommended need per day.
- Cut down on salt intake.
- Minimize your intake of meat and poultry.
- Exercise at least 30-60 minutes per day. A 30 minute walk or bike ride helps to build stronger bones.

Remember, treat your bones as you would your "retirement fund." Build up your calcium funds early in life, particularly before age 30. Then, keep putting calcium in your "bone bank" to ensure bone health. My diet program will reduce the bone-wasting effects of too much animal protein and sodium, by increasing your selection of low-fat, calcium rich foods.

FEWER INTESTINAL PROBLEMS

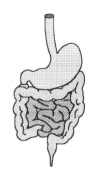

To give you an idea of the importance of your digestive tract, consider its impressive size and functions. If flattened, the human intestinal surface would measure larger than a tennis court. Its role is to screen all the nutrients and fluids that pass across its extensive surface and exclude all the toxins and wastes.

When you consider the complexity of its task, it's not surprising that intestinal   problems are common and mostly due to poor diet. An improper diet stimulates crampy abdominal pain, increases gas formation, aggravates Irritable Bowel Syndrome, worsens constipation, and increases hemorrhoids.

My Antioxidant Diet Program will prevent nearly all of the above, as well as help prevent gallbladder stones from forming. Did you know that vegetarians develop fewer gallstones than people who eat meat regularly? The reason is likely related to a low-fat and low-cholesterol diet.

The most common dietary problems that I see in my office arise from inadequate fiber intake and too little fluid intake. Most people need five servings of whole grains per day, one serving of legumes, and at least five servings of fruits and vegetables. But many people need even more fiber for proper intestinal function. (My program advocates seven or more servings of produce per day.)

If you don't get enough fiber, eat more vegetables (like spinach, broccoli, or carrots), or try more fiber-rich fruits, such as apples, prunes, and oranges. Low-fat bran muffins, whole wheat foods, and brown rice products also help move food along the intestinal tract. Some people also choose to use a wheat fiber supplement, such as "Metamucil," to increase fiber intake.

However, if you normally eat refined grains, which are low-fiber products, it might be a challenge for your body to handle the extra fiber. Adding fiber too rapidly could cause gas or stomach aches. If you are bothered at first, try only 2-3 whole grain servings per day, and increase slowly over a month or two to 5 servings per day.

Rice fiber is easier to digest than fiber from wheat products, bulgur, or corn. If you have problems during the first month with intestinal gas, add more rice meals to your diet. If increasing fiber fails to improve your intestinal problems, you might have a food intolerance. If you have new or severe complaints, contact your medical provider.

Food Intolerances

The most common food intolerance is "lactose intolerance." Lactose is the sugar found in dairy products. You'll need to avoid all dairy sources for at least 3-4 weeks to see if this makes a difference. Yogurt is an exception, as it is essentially lactose free.

"Gluten intolerance" is a rare problem that occurs when the body does not properly digest wheat, barley, or bulgur. If this is your case, use more rice products, including rice flour, rice bread, and rice crackers as substitutes for wheat products. Again, you should feel better within 3-4 weeks of restricting gluten.

Most stomach problems should improve or resolve themselves within a few weeks of my program. If they persist, ask your medical provider to help you find the cause.

DECREASED EYE PROBLEMS

Reduce your risk of cataracts and blindness

Carotenoids and Vitamin C are powerful antioxidants that can lower your risk of cataracts and macular degeneration. Both of these conditions arise from oxidation activities in the eye.

Cataracts

Cataracts are usually caused by the oxidation of proteins in the lens of the eye. The primary purpose of the lens is to focus light on the retina. The retina then converts light into image-producing sight. As the lens becomes more oxidized, less light reaches the retina and sight decreases.

The greater your exposure to oxidative stress, such as smoking, the higher your risk of forming cataracts. If your diet is low in antioxidants, your risk will grow even higher. Increasing your blood levels of Vitamin C, carotenoids, and other antioxidants will help lower your risk of cataract disease.

Macular Degeneration

The retina, which forms visual images in our brain, requires a high density of yellow carotenoid pigments. If these are not present in your diet, your risk of blindness increases. Age-related macular degeneration is the leading cause of blindness late in life.

But a diet high in carotenoids, especially the carotenoids lutein and zeaxanthin that abound in green leafy vegetables like broccoli, kale, greens, and spinach, can decrease your risk of macular degeneration. High blood levels of Vitamin C, Vitamin E, and other carotenoids also help lower your susceptibility to macular degeneration.

Smoking tobacco and a high exposure to ultraviolet light and other known oxidants will increase your risk of macular degeneration.

IMPROVED BLOOD PRESSURE CONTROL

We in the medical profession probably overemphasize the use of drugs to control blood pressure. In fact, treating mildly elevated blood pressure can cause as many problems as it fixes. Some blood pressure medications can worsen cholesterol levels, blood sugar control, potassium levels, and wheezing problems. They can also cause sedation, sexual dysfunction, or depression. The trick is finding a medication that controls blood pressure without causing side effects. Because of these possible problems, average healthy adults with high blood pressure do not usually benefit from medication unless their blood pressure exceeds 150/100.

Even with a blood pressure of 150/100 to 160/105, we would have to treat 70 people for 10 years to prevent a single death related to high blood pressure. However, once blood pressure exceeds 180/110 the benefit of therapy increases markedly. These increases in high blood pressure are associated with rising risks for strokes, heart attacks, heart failure, and kidney failure.

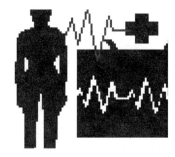

Most people who start drug therapy have untreated blood pressures in the 160/105 range or less. I believe these people will benefit from trying the lifestyle changes I propose in my *28-Day Antioxidant Diet Program*. This provides an excellent opportunity to control blood pressure without medications. Four to eight weeks seems a reasonable time to try this, but always consult with your own doctor who understands your unique medical situation. People with histories of diabetes, heart attacks, previous strokes, heart failure, or kidney disease do need stricter blood pressure control.

Here are some of the special features of my program that will improve your blood pressure:

- You will lose weight on this program. Weight loss can produce the biggest improvement. Most people above their target weight who follow my program should lose 10-20 pounds within 6 months and will keep it off as long as they continue this lifestyle plan.

- You will enjoy plenty of delicious fruits and veggies. Produce-enriched diets such as mine have been shown to drop blood pressure 5-10 points within 2 months. Eating 8-9 servings of vegetables and fruits per day has been proven to drop blood pressure dramatically.
- You will be adding garlic to your diet. Taking garlic (1-2 cloves per day in your diet or with garlic capsules) also drops blood pressure a few points.
- You will be drinking a healthy amount of alcoholic beverages or not drink them at all. Reducing your alcohol intake to 1 glass per day tends to lower blood pressure, especially if you have been drinking more than two drinks per day.
- You will be reaping the benefits of an exercise program that fits your needs. Regular moderate exercise lowers blood pressure.

Eugene from Olympia, Washington, told me, "I felt tired, my blood pressure was too high, and my blood sugar was borderline high. I didn't want to start medications for my blood pressure unless I had to, so I tried Dr. Masley's program. Within six weeks I had lost 10 pounds, my blood pressure was back to normal, and I felt great. I didn't give up all the meat and poultry in my diet, but I did add extra antioxidant rich fruits, vegetables, and grains. I also found time for a 30 minute walk and workout each day, and I'm glad I did. Dr. Masley's program sure works for me."

SUCCESSFUL WEIGHT LOSS

It's hard not to lose weight on my program, and as long as you follow my guidelines, you'll keep the weight off. That's because the 28-Day Antioxidant Program is designed to be low in fat, to guide you to hunger-suppressing foods, and to provide you with regular exercise.

First, as you cut down on your fat intake, you'll be able to eat more food than before and still lose weight! Why??? Because the less fat you eat, the less weight you gain. This diet will provide about 20% of calories from fat, a bit more than Dr. Dean Ornish or Dr. John McDougall propose but less than the American Heart Association's guideline of 30%. And you won't have to count calories or count fat grams to succeed with this program!

Second, I'll help you choose foods that will satisfy your appetite. Carbohydrates (breads, pastas, sweets, and produce) are not all the same. As you'll learn, some carbo-hydrates will increase your blood sugar level and your appetite more than others. I'll teach you to choose the best carbohydrates to suppress hunger.

Third, exercise, an important part of this program, will help speed physical well-being. If you fail to get exercise, your metabolism will drop, and eating less will just make you tired. By combining better nutrition with exercise, you'll have more energy. This creates a positive cycle: you feel better, you eat better, you exercise more.

The goal is to break the old cycle of fatigue, lethargy, and weight gain.

Those of you whose weight is already in the normal range might lose a few pounds too, because the overall fat content of this program is about half that found in the average American diet.

Another benefit of my diet program might be a boost in metabolism, which helps control weight and improve vitality. As Dr. Neil Barnard points out in his book, *Eat Better, Live Longer*, diets high in vegetables, fruits, and grains have been shown in clinical studies to boost thyroid activity and improve weight control.

My program does NOT rely upon cutting calories to lose weight! As I will repeat often in this book, cutting calories to lose weight doesn't work. This "NO-NO" approach to eating causes your fat cells to wait until the "starvation" period is over. Then they "YO-YO" that weight right back on, plus extra. My Antioxidant Diet Program is NOT a quick weight loss program. It is a LIFESTYLE that will keep your weight exactly where it should be.

IMPROVED SEX LIFE

Yes, *food and sex are related*. When you eat healthier meals, you'll improve the romantic side of your life, too.

What happens when you stuff yourself with high fat food? Your belly will swell, and all your energy will be diverted to help digest that load of fat in your stomach. Instead of feeling sexy, you'll feel sleepy. Somehow, eating a big steak dinner and then heading straight to the bedroom just doesn't mix.

What are the best foods to inspire our romantic instincts?

Since good love making requires lots of energy, you'll want clean burning fuel for activity. The best source is grains, fruits, vegetables, and low-fat protein. Stick to light foods rich in complex carbohydrates, such as pasta, veggies, and fruits. A low-fat pasta salad with lots of veggies is great food for romance.

And don't forget your need for fluid to keep your energy level up. Seltzers, tonics, herbal teas, and juices are your best sources of liquid before romance.

What about sex, alcohol, and tobacco?

Because alcohol acts as a sedative, it puts most people to sleep. Men in particular find that alcohol may increase the fantasy element of sex, but puts a real damper on sexual function and performance.

Tobacco use remains one of the leading causes of male impotence. The more you smoke, the more damage you cause to your circulation by oxidizing your arteries. Without good genital blood circulation, you can forget erections. Just think what would happen to teen tobacco use if cigarette packs contained an extra warning that said, "**WARNING: This product may cause impotence!**"

ENHANCED ATHLETIC PERFORMANCE

Food has a strong effect on your ability to exercise. High-fat diets, for example, make you feel lazy. Both saturated fat and polyunsaturated fats make your blood sluggish and sticky, slowing the vital nutrient exchange between your muscle cells and your bloodstream. My Antioxidant Diet Program features special foods (like garlic and certain omega-3 fats) that will maximize the blood flow to your tissues. This program will also stabilize your blood sugar levels, so that even with strenuous exercise, these levels will remain steady.

Some of the world's top athletes attribute their success to vegetarian diets. These athletes include Dave Scott (six-time Iron Man winner), Gayle Oline Kova (marathon champion), Bill Pearl (former Mr. Universe) and Carl Lewis and Edwin Moses (Olympic track stars).

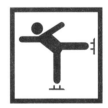

You may be surprised to learn that the ideal protein source for athletic training is not meat; even lean meats contain small amounts of saturated fat that slow you down. Soy and bean sources are likely the best protein sources for athletic activity. They are low in fat, high in protein, help prevent blood sugar levels from dropping during strenuous exercise, and contain omega-3 fats that maximize blood flow to your tissues.

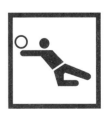

BALANCED MOODS AND EMOTIONS

Depression

Not surprisingly, diet appears to influence feelings of depression and anger. In particular, if we don't eat enough omega-3 fats we're more likely to experience depression. Omega-3 fats are found in seafood, nuts, legumes, and green leafy vegetables, such as spinach and kale.

People with lower levels of omega-3 fats, such as alcoholics and pregnant women, appear to be more susceptible to depression. Alcohol abuse depletes supplies of omega-3 fats, while pregnant women give up omega-3 fats to the growing fetus. Not surprisingly, rates of depression are very high after childbirth.

Studies of communities in Japan with a high omega-3 fat intake showed much lower rates of depression than communities with low intakes. Most of the relationships between diet and mental health are only now being reviewed, yet the connection seems valid.

One odd phenomenon is the increased rate of violent deaths, suicide, and depression in individuals who are trying to decrease their cholesterol intake. In related studies designed to treat people for heart disease, cholesterol levels were reduced, resulting in lower rates of heart attacks. However, increased rates of violent deaths and suicides occurred. The reason? An increased intake of polyunsaturated fat (from sources like margarine) without an increase in omega-3 fats appears to have contributed to mood changes.

You'll note in my program that while I still want you to reduce your intake of saturated fat (butter and fatty meats), we will not replace that with margarine, but with fats found in olive oil, canola oil, and nuts. These are rich in omega-3 fats and healthy monounsaturated fats. (More in "MEET FATS THAT ARE GOOD FOR YOU" on page 55.)

Back in the early 1900's, our dietary intake of omega-3 fats equaled our intake of regular polyunsaturated fats that now come from sources like corn oil, margarine, and grain fed animal meats. Today, however, the average person eats 10 to 25 times more polyunsaturated fat than omega-3 fats. According to researchers at the Laboratory of Membrane Biophysics and Biochemistry in Maryland, these out-of-balance fats can harm our delicate brain biochemistry and increase the incidence of depression and violent behavior. Since omega-3 fats are easily oxidized and destroyed, an antioxidant-rich diet could be of great help to those vulnerable to unstable mental health.

Complex carbohydrates with a mixture of whole grains, fruits, vegetables, and legumes seem the most important things to eat when you feel depressed and stressed. In particular, eat more green leafy vegetables and bean/soy products, as they are rich sources of omega-3 fats. Eating seafood once or twice per week is another way to add omega-3 fats to your diet.

My own personal experience is that depressed people tend to eat poorly. Because they have less energy, they eat worse, do less, and feel worse as they lose more energy. They gradually fall into a state of despair.

They need to create a new cycle: eat better, exercise more, do more, and feel better. If you're in the midst of a depressed cycle, see your mental health professional or your health care provider for help.

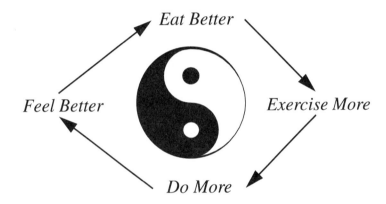

To me, the best part of this program is how energetic I feel when I follow it. Eating well allows me to do so much more, and have more fun. Furthermore, studies show that good nutrition and exercise will boost your energy, memory, and moods.

LOWER HEALTH CARE EXPENSES

The last benefit is that you'll save money. The average person following this program will note improved health, avoid treatments, and cut down on expensive pharmacy prescriptions. And while many nutritional programs these days require extensive vitamin supplements (some cost $50-$300 per month), my program focuses purely on food and exercise.

Many nutritional programs rely on the "supplement du jour," sending the participant running from one health food store to another in search of the newest, most expensive supplement. Few of these "breakthroughs" are based on controlled clinical trials that follow clinical outcomes. Rather, they are based upon someone's well-intentioned "hunch" or theory, or a lab test improvement that may not necessarily improve your long-term health. Not surprisingly, you never seem to find the right combination of supplements.

If you're ready to save TIME, MONEY, AND ENERGY, follow my program and let a balanced diet provide all the nutrients you need for long-term health and fitness.

FIGURE 1. **Diet Program Comparison, the Two Rivers**

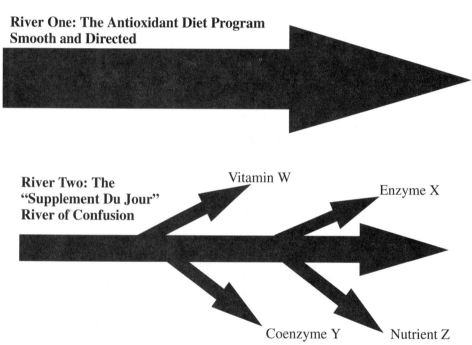

**River One: The Antioxidant Diet Program
Smooth and Directed**

**River Two: The
"Supplement Du Jour"
River of Confusion**

Vitamin W

Enzyme X

Coenzyme Y

Nutrient Z

CHAPTER 3   *THREE HEALTHY ANTIOXIDANT DIETS*

A diet is not just a program to lose weight–it's a recipe to health and vitality. Three of the world's healthiest diets are Mediterranean, Japanese, and Vegetarian. All are rich in antioxidants, fiber, and vitamins, and low in saturated fat. In essence, they rely upon carbohydrates as their primary source of calories. Carbohydrates are compounds found in abundance in vegetables, wheat, rice, corn, beans, and fruits.

Aren't carbohydrates starches? Yes, many are. But I believe starches have unfairly received a lot of bad press. Not all starches cause us to gain weight; rather, we add pounds from the fats we serve with them and the type of starches we choose. Think of some low-fat starches, like pasta, rice, dense breads with whole grains, and tortillas as "good" starches.

John McDougall, a California physician who created The McDougall Health Program, describes carbohydrates as a wonderful energy source. He praises carbohydrates as "foods that offer large quantities of clean burning, high-energy fuel."

Some diet programs label carbohydrates as bad, but their claims can be disputed. Stating that eating rice causes us to gain weight seems ridiculous when you realize that rice eating cultures like Japan and China have some of the slimmest populations in the world. These same cultures also eat large amounts of noodles.

Yet, there remains a "grain of truth" behind the carbo-slander that we will explore in detail in Chapter Four. Before diving into carbohydrate details, however, I want to contrast how different cultures choose different types of carbohydrates.

Compare the diets from three countries: the United States, Greece, and Japan. These countries not only focus on different foods; they emphasize different food groups.

TABLE 5.

Dietary comparison between the United States, Greece, and Japan. Adapted with permission from Kushi et al., Am J Clin Nutr 1995; 61S:1416S-1427S.

Dietary characteristics	United States	Greece	Japan
Fat (% of energy)	39	37	11
Saturated fat (% of energy)	18	8	3
Vegetables (gram/day)	171	191	198
Potatoes (grams/day)	124	170	65
Fruits (grams/day)	233	463	34
Legumes/beans (grams/day)	1	30	91
Breads/ cereals (grams/day)	123	453	481
Meat (grams/day)	273	35	8
Fish (grams/day)	3	39	150
Eggs (grams/day)	40	15	29
Alcohol (grams/day)	6	23	22

In the United States, we eat much more saturated fat and meat, and far fewer legumes, cereals and grains. (See Table 5.) In Greece and Japan, people eat greater amounts of green leafy vegetables, spices, grains, and legumes than we eat in the United States.

In Figure 2 on page 33, note that even when total cholesterol levels are the same, people in the United States have higher rates of heart attacks. I believe the southern Europeans and Japanese are protected by their antioxidant rich diets.

FIGURE 2. : Twenty-five year coronary heart disease death rates per baseline cholesterol, adjusted for cigarette smoking, age, and systolic blood pressure. Adapted with permission from Verschuren et al., JAMA 1995;274:131-136.

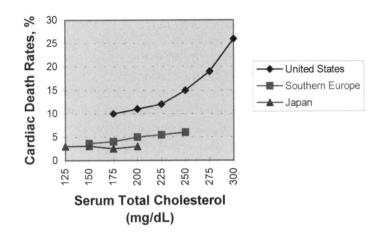

Death Rates at Different Cholesterol Levels

The United States has one of the highest death rates from heart attacks in the world. Japan, despite being one of the wealthiest countries in the world and able to buy foods high in fat and sugar, has a very low death rate from heart attacks. Southern Europeans also have low death rates from heart attacks.

The Japanese and Greeks also have much lower rates of breast, colon, and prostate cancers than found in the United States. These three cancers are more common in the United States than elsewhere in the world.

Studies that compare Americans who eat 30% of their calories from fat with those who eat 40%, have not found a significant difference in cancer rates between these two groups. However, because very few groups eat fewer than 30% of their calories as fat, our ability to study cancer rates and diet in the United States is limited. If we look to other cultures that consume fewer than 20% of their calories from fat (like many Asian countries, including Japan) cancer rates drop. Unfortunately, many factors other than fat intake change too, so it is hard to draw clear conclusions.

I suspect there is a threshold for fat intake, especially saturated and polyunsaturated fat, above which cancer rates increase when you cross it. Since populations that eat less than 20% of their calories as fat have lower cancer rates, it makes sense to choose a diet that limits fat intake to 20% of total calories.

Yet another compelling reason to decrease our fat intake to well below 30% of total calories comes from the diet and lifestyle study performed by Dr. Dean Ornish from the University of California. He showed that the standard American Heart Association dietary recommendations failed to work. Encouraging people to cut down on their cholesterol and saturated fat intake, and limit their intake of fat to 30% of total calories did not stop the progression of coronary artery disease. A year after making this recommended dietary change, patients showed increased plaque formation in their arteries. This diet plan alone didn't work! Thus, limiting total fat intake to 30% of total calories is not enough, especially if you already have coronary artery disease and you choose typical American fat sources. Dr. Ornish's study did show that by cutting fat intake to less that 10% of calories and by eating more grains and produce, a modest reduction in artery plaque occurs.

In contrast to this low-fat mentality, the Greeks have a highly active population with lower rates of heart attacks, despite a much higher fat intake. The Greeks studied were largely farmers who were physically active several hours per day. They also chose healthy fats from olive oil and nuts while avoiding dairy fats and meats. Further, their diet was very rich in antioxidants.

Finally, perhaps the best reason to restrict fat intake relates to weight control. In America, where weight gain and health related problems have reached epidemic proportions, and where fat intake relates strongly to weight gain, we need to address cutting out the fat.

It seems clear to me that for the average, moderately active, health-conscious American, a diet with 30% of calories as fat is excessive and likely dangerous. The trick in "cutting out the fat" is to leave in the fat-soluble antioxidants, like Vitamin E.

THE MEDITERRANEAN DIET

During the 1960's, people in southern France, southern Italy, and the Greek island of Crete were observed to have the healthiest and longest life spans in the western world. They had low rates of cancer, heart attacks and strokes. What made them so special?

When I think of Mediterranean food, I remember the year I spent working in southern Europe, with long evenings eating delicious food by candlelight. There were always great pastas, with aromatic sauces full of garlic, tomatoes, and basil that lingered in my nostrils and flavors that tantalized my taste buds. This would be followed by another elegant vegetable dish, usually made with eggplant, peppers, or artichokes, and served with a hearty whole grain bread. Of course, there was a bold red wine to wash it all down. Dessert was either fresh fruit sliced on a plate, or fresh sorbet, tinted with port or a liqueur. What magnificent meals!

What I didn't know until just recently was that the food was as healthy as it was delicious! Unlike cuisines that depend upon meat and potatoes, Mediterranean cuisine uses a wide variety of grains, vegetables, fruits, legumes, and of course olive oil and red wine. Garlic and herbs hold an equally important position. Altogether, this represents an "antioxidant diet extraordinaire."

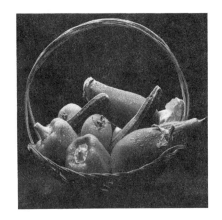

Not only is the traditional Mediterranean diet full of antioxidants, it is very low in saturated fat and meat. The Mediterranean diet is largely a vegetarian diet that occasionally includes meat, more as a condiment than as a staple. Fish appears more often, but still in small portions. Dairy products are limited mostly to yogurt and grated hard cheese.

A Closer Look at Mediterranean Foods

Green leafy vegetables are an important part of every Mediterranean meal. Vivid green salads often accompany a meal, in contrast to the lifeless, colorless iceberg lettuce salads that predominate in the United States.

Whole grains dominate many meals, with a great variety of rice, pasta, and hearty breads. Mediterranean grains, until recently, have not suffered from over-processing and refinement, as have the grain products of North America.

Herbs and spices are used generously in the Mediterranean cuisine. Garlic in particular plays a major role in this cuisine. Olive oil represents over 70% of all fat intake. As we will discuss in detail, olive oil, while still a fat that needs limits, is high in monounsaturated fatty acids (a good type of fat) and low in harmful fats.

TABLE 6. Types of antioxidants in Mediterranean foods

FOOD	TYPE OF ANTIOXIDANT
Whole grains	Vitamin E and Phytoestrogens (Phytoestrogens have beneficial antioxidant and hormonal properties.)
Garlic	Flavonoids, plus anti-cancer compounds
Leafy vegetables	Carotenoids & Vitamin C
Tomatoes	Carotenoids & Vitamin C
Olive oil & Canola oil	Flavonoids & Vitamin E
Red wine	Flavonoids
Fresh fruit	Carotenoids, Flavonoids, & Vitamin C
Spices & Herbs	Carotenoids & Flavonoids
Nuts	Vitamin E
Beans	Ligans & Phytoestrogens

Alcohol is used in moderation, and the predominant form of alcohol consumed is red wine. Although no alcohol is good when used in excess, red wine has many merits. Red wine contains an abundance of antioxidants (flavonoids). And, for the rare occasion you risk contracting diarrhea, even diluted red wine has an ability to kill bacteria and purify drinking water. People with a traditional, healthy Mediterranean diet usually drink alcohol moderately, and only with meals. (I define moderate alcohol intake as 1-2 drinks per day or fewer for men and 1 or fewer drinks per day for women.)

Lastly, Mediterranean desserts typically feature fresh fruit or light sorbets, in contrast with high-fat American versions.

THE JAPANESE DIET

Japanese cooking is an artistic experience, featuring creative presentation and use of color to play up the foods selected.

Rice shapes most Japanese meals. An ever-present bowl of white rice sits on nearly every table. Sake, the national alcoholic beverage, is also made from rice. Alas, the search for the "perfect" bowl of white rice detracts from the quality of nutrition in a Japanese meal; most Japanese rice served is polished, with the outer, antioxidant rich husk removed. Fortunately, other foods featured have high amounts of antioxidants, including green leafy vegetables and soy products.

In fact, soy products provide the backbone of protein in Japan. Tofu, tempeh, miso, and soybeans are served with artistic flair. As we will review repeatedly, soy products benefit our health in many ways.

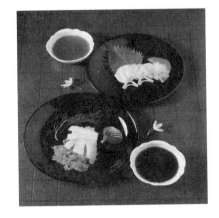

The traditional Japanese diet avoids meat and dairy products, and has almost no saturated fat. It is rare to find dairy products at any meal. Fish serves as a source of protein, and along with soy products, increases the intake of essential omega-3 fats. (I'll review the merits of omega-3 fats throughout this book.) The huge difference in saturated fat intake helps to account for the big contrast in heart attack rates between Japan and the United States. This benefit continues, despite a heavy overuse of tobacco products across Japan.

Of the vegetables consumed in Japan, the Japanese shun potatoes for more green leafy and yellow vegetables loaded with antioxidants. Steamed, green leafy vegetables are popular. Japanese cuisine also benefits from the frequent use of antioxidant rich ginger.

In Japan and throughout the Orient, people also eat sea vegetables. Sea vegetables, or seaweed (like nori), contain both antioxidants and other immune-stimulating compounds. While the average western palate fails to appreciate the taste of seaweed, many westerners do enjoy sushi rolls (rice and condiments rolled in seaweed) and soups flavored with seaweed.

The Japanese also eat mushrooms with medicinal properties. Shiitake, oyster, and maitake mushrooms are commonly seen in Japanese cuisine. These mushrooms inhibit cancer cell growth, stimulate the immune system, and help control cholesterol and blood sugar levels.

While the Japanese and southern Europeans drink more alcohol than we do, they drink it more moderately and traditionally serve alcohol with food. Serving alcohol with food blunts the blood sugar level spike and the surge in alcohol level that occurs with drinking on an empty stomach, thus minimizing the harm caused by alcohol-induced oxidation.

In the United States and in northern European countries, alcohol is consumed between meals. Hence the Japanese and southern Europeans may reduce the harm from drinking alcohol while still benefiting their cholesterol levels from moderate alcohol use. (See "Can drinking alcohol reduce cholesterol levels and heart disease?" on page 54.)

The traditional Japanese beverage of choice is not alcohol, but tea. Green tea, in particular, is packed with beneficial antioxidants. We can learn much about health from the image of a Japanese monk, sitting quietly sipping from a cup of green tea. In Japan, drinking tea is such an important tradition that there is a special ceremony to serve tea to honored guests.

While the merits of a Japanese diet are strong, there are notable drawbacks. In Japan, salt is known as the symbol of "purity." Therefore, the Japanese consume salt (sodium) in large quantities. Soy sauce and miso are loaded with sodium which raises blood pressure. This helps account for the increased rate of strokes in Japan. (See "SALT" on page 72.)

The Japanese diet also uses large quantities of pickled vegetables. Pickled vegetable consumption is associated with an increased rate of stomach and esophageal cancer.

Despite concerns regarding salt and pickled food intake, the Japanese have the longest lifespans in the world. We would prosper nutritionally by incorporating aspects of their diet into our own.

While writing this book, I have read hundreds of articles about traditional Asian diets and the Asian food pyramid. "Traditional" Asian food is repeatedly recommended by national health foundations as a way to cut out the fat and to add more fruits, vegetables, grains, and legumes to the American diet. I am delighted that this trend is growing in popularity in the United States.

Balancing the best of Mediterranean and Japanese diets brings variety, elegance, and vigor to our meals. Now let us look at a third eating style: vegetarian diets.

THE VEGETARIAN DIET

A vegetarian program is another excellent example of an antioxidant diet. If you are ready to make a drastic diet change, it could be the best thing you ever did for your health and vitality.

Vegetarian diets are more popular than they were 10 years ago. Now, almost every restaurant has a variety of veggie meals or low-fat meals on the menu. Most cooks can whip up a variety of vegetarian meals if notified in advance, whereas 10 years ago, many hosts panicked when a vegetarian came for dinner.

The health goal of a vegetarian diet is to limit the intake of saturated fat, and to eat more fruits, vegetables, whole grains, and legumes. In essence, a balanced, low-fat, vegetarian diet represents the ideal antioxidant diet.

What if I'm not ready to become a vegetarian?

Not everybody sees the need, nor is ready to make a major dietary change. If you choose to eat meat and poultry, limit your intake to 2-3 servings per week. If you can't imagine limiting your meat intake to this extent, you can still follow this program. Find extra lean cuts, remove excess fat and skin, and limit your portions to 3-4 ounces (100 grams) per serving. Make sure that when you eat meat, you also include several sources of antioxidants in your meal. These will help prevent the bubbles of fat in your bloodstream from being oxidized into plaque. Try to increase the total number of vegetarian meals you eat per week.

If you choose to eat seafood, limit it to 2 servings per week. Studies have shown that the health of people with coronary heart disease improved by eating 2 servings of fish per week. A diet with more than 2 servings per week does not improve health; rather, it will increase exposure to heavy metals like mercury.

Types of Vegetarian Diets

Not all vegetarian diets are the same. Most vegetarians are "lacto-ovo vegetarians." That means they eat dairy and egg products, but avoid eating meat, poultry, and fish.

"Vegans" go a step further and avoid both dairy products and egg products. Vegan diets depend on grains, vegetables, and legumes for protein. The diet is very high in fiber and vitamins. While a vegan diet represents a healthy dietary choice, some experts are concerned that it provides less than adequate vitamin intake. Health-conscious vegans ensure that they have an adequate intake of Vitamin B-12, zinc, and iron. Some vegans will take vitamin supplements, while others will check themselves regularly on these critical nutrients.

There are a variety of myths about vegetarian diets. We are now going to examine these in detail. By doing so we can discuss how vegetarianism can insure the intake of essential minerals and vitamins. Many hard core meat-eaters also worry about not having meat at every meal; hopefully, this section will put those concerns at ease and encourage them to eat more vegetarian meals.

ELEVEN MYTHS OF A VEGETARIAN DIET

Myth #1

Protein: "You can't get complete protein without meat."

You receive plenty of protein from grains, vegetables, and legumes. Even vegans, who avoid dairy products and eggs, get plenty of protein.

Back in the 1970's, it was believed that it was hard to put amino acids together to form "complete protein." However, there is no evidence to substantiate this theory, nor are any specific amino acid deficiencies regularly found in vegetarians. By eating a variety of grains, vegetables, legumes, and fruits over several days, you receive adequate protein. As long as you eat a variety of foods, you do not need to try to combine amino acids at each meal.

The World Health Organization recommends that protein should represent at least 5% of our total caloric intake. By following this diet program you will consume around 15% of your calories as protein, which is plenty for healthy individuals.

Myth #2

Fat: "Vegetarian diets are always low in fat."

This is not true. Vegetarians too often add extra cheese, milk, and eggs to assure that they get enough protein and can end up with too much protein and fat in their diets. A vegetarian diet can also be high in fatty oils from frying food. Just choosing a vegetarian meal alone will not guarantee it will be low in fat; you have to choose to cut out the fat.

Myth #3

"My child's growth will be stunted on a vegetarian diet."

Many well-monitored scientific studies have shown that children on vegetarian diets grow as well as those who eat a mixture of meats and vegetables. Scientists have also found no difference in IQ levels between vegetarian and non-vegetarian children.

Many of the growth studies were performed on Seventh-Day Adventist families in southern California. This religious group advocates a lacto-ovo vegetarian diet. In one large study with Seventh Day Adventist children and ethnically similar non-vegetarian children, the children on a vegetarian diet were slightly taller.

Myth #4

"You can't get enough iron on a vegetarian diet."

Iron is vital for producing blood cells. Without enough iron we can become anemic with fatigue and a low blood count. This is especially true for women with regular menstrual periods and for growing children. Yet, high iron levels in humans are associated with higher rates of heart attacks and colon cancer. Iron is believed to be a pro-oxidant, increasing the formation of free radicals. In excess, iron is also thought to contribute to oxidative stress in the brain leading to neurodegenerative disease. These include: Alzheimer's dementia, multiple sclerosis, and Parkinson's disease (tremor and rigidity).

We have a variety of iron sources available to us–some more healthful than others. "Heme iron" is the easiest to digest and absorb and comes from animal products. But we absorb heme iron whether we need more iron or not, which can lead to iron overload, increased oxidative stress, and rarely, liver damage.

"Non-heme iron" is not absorbed as well as heme iron, yet is abundant in whole grains, legumes (beans and soy products), and green, leafy vegetables. A clear advantage of non-heme iron is our ability to regulate its absorption depending upon our needs. An anemic person needing iron will absorb much more non-heme iron than someone with normal iron levels. Because Vitamin C improves the absorption of non-heme iron, eating green, leafy vegetables with our beans and legumes will increase our intake and absorption of iron.

Most studies show that vegetarian groups, including women, have no more problems with anemia than do those who eat meat. It's especially important for women who menstruate and for growing children to eat plant foods rich in iron and Vitamin C. Cooking with cast iron pans increases your non-heme iron intake, too. Pregnant women and growing children should have routine blood samples drawn to screen for anemia and iron deficiency as determined by your medical provider.

Myth #5

"Vegetarians don't get enough zinc."

Zinc intake is important for everyone, but especially for vegetarians. While zinc deficiency is rare in vegetarians, they do have lower zinc levels than omnivores. Dairy products, especially yogurt, contain moderate amounts of zinc. Those who do not eat dairy products (vegans), have lower zinc levels than lacto-ovo vegetarians.

Zinc deficiency can cause decreased appetite, stunted growth, poor wound healing, and a lowered immune response. We also need zinc for proper antioxidant enzyme action.

Good vegetarian sources of zinc include legumes, nuts and seeds, yogurt, cheese, wheat germ, yeast extract, miso, and peas. Vegetarians with a balance of grains, legumes, nuts and seeds, and vegetables reach the RDA (Recommended Daily Allowance) for zinc. Semi-vegetarians who occasionally eat seafood, especially oysters, may exceed the RDA. Because high-fiber diets decrease zinc absorption, it is even more important for vegetarians to ensure that they are getting enough. There is no good evidence that more zinc than what the RDA specifies is needed, but zinc's effects upon immune function and antioxidant balance will be worth following.

Zinc Content Table:

Food Group	Zinc Content (in mg)
Oysters, Atlantic (6 med)	76.4
"Total" cereal (3/4 cup)	15.0
"Product 19" cereal (1 cup)	15.0
Oysters, Pacific (6 med)	14.13
Wheat germ (1/4 cup)	4.73
Ground beef, lean (3 oz)	4.37
Pumpkin seeds (2 ozs.)	4.24
Crab (3 oz., cooked)	3.58
Swiss cheese, (3 oz.)	3.33
Cashews (2 oz.)	3.18
"Cheerios" cereal (1 cup)	4.00
Lentils (1 cup, boiled)	2.50
Yogurt, low-fat (8 oz.)	2.20
Blackeyed peas (1 cup)	2.20
Walnuts (2 oz.)	1.94
Mozzarella cheese, (3 oz.)	1.89
Kidney beans (1 cup, boiled)	1.89
Pinto beans (1 cup, boiled)	1.85
Clam chowder, (1 cup)	1.68
Almonds (2 oz.)	1.66
Chicken, thigh (1)	1.46
Mussels (3 oz.)	1.36
Tofu (1/2 cup)	1.00
Swordfish (3 oz.)	0.97
Milk, low fat (8 oz.)	0.95
Spaghetti, enriched (1 cup, cooked)	0.70

Many foods are supplemented with zinc, such as "Total" and "Product 19" cereals. One serving per day contains 100% of the RDA (recommended dietary allowance).

While the minimal US RDA of zinc is 12 mg per day for men and women, the optimal daily allowance may be more, 15-25 mg per day. At home, I don't take zinc supplements, but the boys and I eat zinc-fortified cereal a few times per week.

TABLE 7.

Recommended zinc intakes by various national groups. The British recommendation is based on meeting the nutritional needs of 97% of the healthy population. The American and Australian recommendations were judged to meet the needs of all healthy people.

	BRITISH RNI in mg	US RDA in mg	AUSTRALIAN RDI in mg
AGE			
Infant	3 to 5	5	3 to 6
Child	5 to 7	10	4.5 to 9
Teen Male	9 to 9.5	15	12
Female	7 to 9	15	12
Adult Male	9.5	12	12
Female	7	12	12

Diabetics in particular should consider zinc supplements (10-15 mg extra per day), as they tend to lose zinc in their urine. If you have diabetes, check with your medical provider. (See "NUTRIENT SUPPLEMENTS" on page 268.)

Myth #6

"If you don't eat enough dairy products, you won't get enough Vitamin B-12."

Vitamin B-12 is essential for many cellular functions. The first signs of this deficiency include memory problems, anemia, nerve pain, and sensory loss.

It's true that Vitamin B-12 is abundant in animal and dairy products, and that vegetables do not contain Vitamin B-12. However, bacteria in our own intestines produce Vitamin B-12, and may provide an important source of this vitamin for their vegan hosts. Vegans rarely develop B-12 deficiency but if they do, it can cause serious, irreversible neurologic harm. Anemia and irreversible memory loss can also develop from Vitamin B-12 deficiency.

Many foods are supplemented with Vitamin B-12, including breakfast cereals, cow and often soy milk. If you do not eat any form of animal products regularly, either take some form of supplement, or have an annual blood test to monitor your Vitamin B-12 level.

On rare occasions when either the stomach or small intestine is diseased, the body may not be able to absorb Vitamin B-12. Even non-vegetarians can develop these diseases. In these cases, medical providers commonly prescribe monthly B-12 injections; but many of these same patients do well with oral megadoses of 1000 ug (micrograms) taken daily. In you have questions, check with your medical provider.

Myth #7

"You'll be worn out if you don't eat meat."

Not true! In fact, the opposite may be true. Dense, complex carbohydrates represent the ideal food source for sports, providing a slow release of sugars that keep blood sugar levels even. "Carbos" require little energy to digest, leaving you ready for exercise.

In contrast, meat and fat are hard to digest, shunting blood from your muscles to your intestinal tract for hours, and reducing the blood supply to your extremities and brain. The saturated fat in animal products makes your platelets stick together, further slowing blood flow through the tiny capillaries in muscle tissue.

Many famous long distance athletes are vegetarians, like six-time Iron Man winner, Dave Scott. The Hawaiian Iron Man competition is likely the world's most grueling sport: swim 2.4 miles, bike 112 miles, and run 26.2 miles. You need incredible endurance for this and a vegetarian, complex-carbohydrate diet is the ultimate sports diet.

Myth #8

"You can't build muscle without beef."

The beef industry would like you to believe this so you'll continue to buy meat. But, this statement is not true.

Several of the world's top sprinters and track superstars follow a vegetarian diet: Carl Lewis, and Edwin Moses are Olympic track stars. Further, Bill Pearl, a former Mr. Universe body builder, is a vegetarian.

You do not need to eat meat or poultry to be strong. You do need a balanced diet, preferably one that is low in saturated fat.

Myth # 9

"You'll be hungry all the time if all you eat is 'rabbit food'."

The truth is a vegetarian diet can be extremely varied and satisfying. There are an infinite number of grains, spices, flavors, vegetables, legumes, and nut and seeds to use. You are limited only by your imagination.

Eating some foods (such as air-filled breads, potatoes, and candies) will add to your hunger. But my program features solid foods such as pasta, beans, wild rice, and many vegetables and fruits that will satisfy your hunger.

Myth # 10

"Vegetables can't build brain cells, can they?"

On the contrary! It's amazing how much more creative people can become when they change to a vegetarian diet. They also report faster comprehension. I can't explain this increased sense of alertness, but many of my patients report a clearer mind following a vegetarian diet.

One reason may be that plant foods activate thyroid function and increase metabolism. Another explanation might be that antioxidant rich foods slow brain aging. Since "dementia" (permanent memory loss) is related to brain damage caused by oxidative stress, it seems likely that an antioxidant rich diet could slow brain aging.

Consider that the following great minds followed a vegetarian diet:

Albert Einstein	George Bernard Shaw	Pythagoras
Albert Schweitzer	Benjamin Franklin	Voltaire
Thomas Jefferson	Socrates	Ghandi
Leonardo da Vinci	Leo Tolstoy	Plato
Thomas Edison	Sir Isaac Newton	Daniel
Charles Darwin	H.G. Wells	

Said Ben Franklin, "My refusing to eat flesh occasioned an inconvenience, and I was frequently chided for my singularity, but, with this lighter repast, I made the greater progress from greater clearness of head and quicker comprehension."

A growing body of evidence suggests that oxidative stress increases nitric oxide (NO) levels, a chemical known to affect brain neurotransmitters and worsen cognitive function. Stated another way, an inadequate intake of antioxidants may worsen thinking power, and in an extreme case, could result in what has been called "brain fog." Perhaps what these great minds of history had in common was really a diet that was rich in antioxidants, and consequently lower than normal levels of cerebral nitric oxide.

Myth # 11

"It is hard to cook vegetarian food."

Hey, how long does it take to cook broccoli? On the other hand, meat, poultry, and fish do take considerable time to cook. With meat, you need to worry about bacteria, disease, and hygiene, as well as cooking techniques.

Realistically, beans and grains do take some time. However, beans can be cooked once a week and stored in the refrigerator. Or, you can buy canned or frozen precooked beans. Grains take between 10-25 minutes, usually the time you'll need to chop up veggies, set the table, and throw things together.

It's a matter of adapting a new attitude toward cooking. See it as fun, rather than a chore. Get excited about choosing new foods in the store. Get creative in deciding how these foods can fit together to form a delicious meal. The actual food preparation is easy once you get the hang of it.

CHAPTER 4   *BALANCED DIET, BALANCED HEALTH*

*F*ood can be divided into three groups: protein, fat, and carbohydrates. We need all three of these food groups to live healthy, active lives. We also need to keep the portions of these food groups in balance.

In this chapter I'll discuss these food groups and present information that will help you to lower your cholesterol and blood sugar levels, while helping you to control your appetite and weight.

PROTEIN

Protein is essential in our diets–it provides the amino acid building blocks for our bodies. There isn't much danger that we'll eat too little protein–in fact, the average American (even the average vegetarian) eats nearly twice the recommended daily protein requirement.

However, unlike eating excess fat or carbohydrates, eating excess protein strains your kidneys and liver. Since you can't convert excess protein into fat, your liver and kidneys must work overtime to excrete the extra amount.

What are the best sources of protein?

Soy protein and beans represent the ideal protein. Not only do they provide protein without extra fat but they contain a vast variety of health enhancing antioxidant compounds. Eating legumes also lowers cholesterol and blood sugar levels. Many carbohydrate rich foods (such as brown rice, whole grain products, and vegetables) contain substantial amounts of protein and valuable nutrients.

Egg whites and non-fat dairy products provide an excellent source of protein, but they fail to provide all the *extra* nutritional and antioxidant benefits of legumes.

Seafood provides a good supply of protein and other health benefits (such as omega-3 fats that we will review later). However, since seafood often contains trace amounts of chemicals and heavy metals (like PCB's and mercury,) this potential contamination restricts you from eating seafood daily. If you eat seafood, many authorities recommend eating no more than one to two servings per week.

Lean meats (such as broiled, skinless chicken breast) provide lower fat (about 20% of calories from fat), but much of the fat is harmful, saturated fat. Although chicken is a very common protein source, it also fails to provide the antioxidants found in legumes.

My *28-Day Antioxidant Diet Program* features the best types of protein for you.

Do competitive sports influence protein needs?

Repeated studies show that competitive athletes do require some extra protein. Unfortunately, many elite athletes overestimate the need for dietary protein and under-estimate their need for dietary carbohydrates and fluid replacement, which are essential to athletic performance.

The average person needs about 2 ounces of protein per day.[1] Dr. Peter Lemon, a national leader in exercise nutrition research over the last 10 years at Kent State University, has evaluated protein needs in many levels of athletes. Heavy resistance training athletes (weight lifters, and those who are actively building muscle mass)

---

1. To calculate protein needs for an average person, multiply your weight in kilograms by 0.8 grams of protein. Hence a 70 kilogram (154 pound) person needs: 0.8 x 70 = 56 grams of protein daily. A resistance training athlete needs 1.7 grams per kilogram of weight daily, and an endurance training athlete needs 1.3 grams per kilogram of body weight daily. (An ounce of protein = 28 grams; 2 ounces = 56 grams. One kilogram = 2.2 pounds.)

require the most protein, about 5 ounces daily or about twice the recommended intake for the average person. Endurance training exercisers (long distance runners) require 3-4 ounces of protein daily.

What surprised me was that these athletes meet their protein needs with only 10-15% of their total calories from protein. Since these elite training athletes eat more food, a lot more, they get more protein eating the same foods as you and me.

Many athletes exceed 15-20% of their calories as protein, often in the form of expensive protein powders and elixirs. Yet, this added protein strains their kidneys and liver without any known performance benefit. I agree with the majority of national sports organizations that continue to recommend a diet with 10-15% of total calories from protein.

TABLE 8. Protein Comparison Table

HIGH QUALITY, LOW-FAT PROTEIN SOURCE

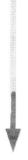

1 Soy products
   (soy-veggie burgers, soy milk, tofu, etc.)
2 Beans
   (lentils, black beans, garbanzos, etc.)
3 Egg whites
4 Non-fat dairy
5 Seafood
6 Low-fat poultry and meats
7 High-fat red meat
8 Regular dairy
   (Whole milk, and regular cheese)

POOR QUALITY, HIGH-FAT PROTEIN SOURCE

FATS

The chemical group known as "fats" is essential in our diets. Fats store energy and contain important vitamins and building blocks for our tissues.

So, why should you avoid fats? They are high in calories. One gram of fat has more than twice the calories of one gram of protein or one gram of carbohydrate. Furthermore, when we eat excess fat, we store it directly as fat. When we eat excess carbohydrates, our bodies convert their energy into fat, thus losing nearly 20% of the calories in the conversion. Hence, not only do fats contain more calories than carbohydrates and protein by weight, but we gain more weight from eating fat even when it has the same quantity of calories. It's a no-win situation!

Fortunately, our preference for fat is an acquired one. It's also one we can lose. If you've switched from whole milk to non-fat milk, you probably noticed that it tasted watery at first; and not totally pleasant. But after continued use, whole milk seemed too rich and fatty. You can decrease your fat intake and still love the taste of your food!

To emphasize the connection between fats and disease, consider that next year more than 500,000 Americans will suffer their first symptoms of heart disease. Over one third of these people will die before reaching a hospital. Cutting fats and eating more antioxidant rich foods would, over time, prevent the vast majority of these deaths.

The 28-Day Antioxidant Diet Program offers you the best fats in a healthy proportion similar to the world's healthiest diets: Mediterranean, Japanese and Vegetarian.

CLEARING UP THE CONFUSION ABOUT CHOLESTEROL

It's everywhere–the "C" word–but, how many of us really understand what "cholesterol" means? There are self-tests in drug stores that measure it but don't tell us the full story. Health professionals send us to the lab to measure it, but don't always fully explain the results. Even our family members want to know, "What is your cholesterol?" This section will explain what you need to understand.

The good and the bad news about cholesterol

In proper amounts, cholesterol is essential to our bodies. It functions like the plastic sheath wrapped around electric wires, coating our body's nerves and improving message relays. It also helps make hormones such as testosterone and estrogen. Since it is important, our bodies produce it, whether we eat it or not. The bad news, however, is that too much cholesterol clogs up our arteries which can lead to heart attacks and strokes. Heart disease is the #1 cause of death in America for both men and women. When blood can't get through to the heart tissue because of clogged arteries, heart tissue dies causing a heart attack. Similarly, a stroke is caused by a blocked artery to the brain.

Lipids

Often when a doctor discusses blood fats, you'll hear the term "lipids." Lipids are fats in the blood stream. Both cholesterol and triglycerides are types of lipids. Together they are the total cholesterol that is measured in our blood.

FIGURE 3. An artery with cholesterol plaque blocking blood flow.

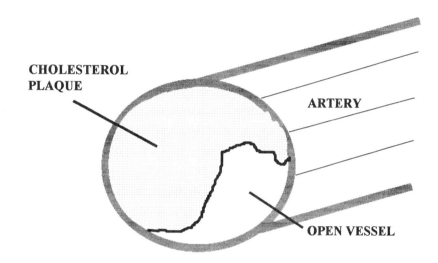

What is "good" cholesterol and "bad" cholesterol?

There are basically two types of cholesterol. "Bad" cholesterol (LDL) is a type of cholesterol that can clog up our arteries. "Good" cholesterol (HDL) is a type of cholesterol that cleans them out.

Imagine a city and its garbage. We put our trash cans along the side of the road and garbage trucks pick it up. If there aren't enough garbage trucks, the trash overflows, clogs up our streets and slows down traffic. "Bad" cholesterol (LDL cholesterol) acts like garbage cans leaking trash and blocking our arteries. Unfortunately, LDL cholesterol often represents the major portion of our total cholesterol.

The "good guys" (HDL cholesterol) act like that garbage truck cleaning up excess cholesterol. We need to keep the ratio of bad cholesterol to good cholesterol in balance. The bigger our fleet of garbage trucks, the cleaner will be our streets! Likewise, the more HDL cholesterol we have, the cleaner our arteries.

Another way to distinguish HDL from LDL is to think of **H**DL cholesterol as **H**ealthy, and **L**DL cholesterol as **L**ethal.

FIGURE 4. Oxidation converts LDL cholesterol into plaque, while HDL cholesterol collects cholesterol and transports it back to the liver.

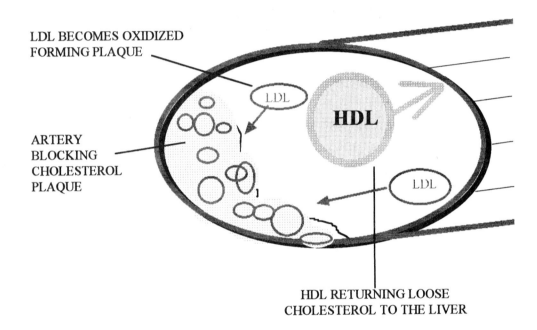

LDL BECOMES OXIDIZED
FORMING PLAQUE

ARTERY
BLOCKING
CHOLESTEROL
PLAQUE

HDL RETURNING LOOSE
CHOLESTEROL TO THE LIVER

What should my cholesterol level be?

After a blood draw to check cholesterol, we usually look at your total cholesterol level and your total cholesterol/HDL ratio. To calculate your ratio, take your total cholesterol level and divide it by your HDL. The average cholesterol level for an American is 210 with a ratio of 5 to 6. The average American will likely have problems with strokes and heart attacks during his/her lifetime. Therefore, an average level may not be a good thing. The higher your cholesterol level, the greater becomes your risk of heart attacks and strokes.

When your ratio is greater than 4.5-5.0, you build cholesterol plaque that over decades plugs your arteries. People who have dropped their ratios to less than 3.5 can absorb the plaque so that their arteries flow smoothly again (more garbage trucks than trash). A good cholesterol reading is less than 180, with a ratio less than 4.5. People with a cholesterol level under 160, or those who have a ratio under 3.5, almost never develop coronary artery disease.

To dissolve existing arterial plaque, lipid levels need drop so low that your body suffers from a cholesterol scarcity. Since, your body needs cholesterol as a building block, when blood cholesterol levels drop, your body steals cholesterol from plaque. This reduces your risk of heart disease.

How can I decrease my bad cholesterol?

It's simple. You can decrease your cholesterol level by eating less saturated fat. Eating saturated fat is like smoking cigarettes–both cause heart attacks and strokes. The most harmful saturated fats are found in meats, poultry, and margarine. Many dairy products, like 2% milk and butter, are also high in harmful fats. If you eat less of these foods, your cholesterol drops. Non-fat dairy products appear to do no harm.

The average American consumes 40% of calories as fat. A diet that limits fat intake to only 20% of total calories will not only lower your cholesterol and decrease your risks of a stroke or heart attack; it will decrease your risk of many cancers as well.

If your cholesterol is still high, see your health care provider to exclude factors, such as thyroid problems, diabetes, or some medications which affect cholesterol levels.

Losing weight will also decrease your cholesterol. The easiest way for you to lose weight is to exercise daily and to cut the fat in your diet. Eating too much fat makes you fat. In particular, saturated fat causes weight gain. In her book *FOOD*, Susan Powter uses nearly 200 pages to depict food fat as Public Enemy # 1. Well done Susan! If you are not convinced to cut your fat intake after reading this book, read her book next.

If you have a history of coronary heart disease or a history of strokes, you should immediately reduce your fat intake.[1] The first step is to reduce lipid levels with **lifestyle** changes. If you have coronary artery disease, you need to reach lipid level targets set by you and your medical provider. If you don't reach your target, the second step involves adding medications that further reduce your lipid levels. (If you only decreased your fat intake from 40% of calories to 30%, you have NOT really tried Step 1.)

---

1. Dr. Dean Ornish, a cardiologist at the University of California started a program for treating heart disease. He advocates eating no more than 10% of calories from fat. If you have heart disease, consider reading his book, *Reversing Heart Disease*.

Foods that decrease cholesterol levels

Garlic, onions, and leeks decrease your bad cholesterol and improve your total cholesterol/HDL ratio by 10%. You should eat them every day. Even one to two cloves of garlic per day can drop your total cholesterol by 10%. If you are concerned about "garlic breath," try garlic capsules sold in health stores or try eating garlic daily for a month. Many people find that over time their bodies adjust to the garlic, and body odors decrease or resolve.

Soluble fiber, the kind found in oat flour, vegetables, and fruits can lower cholesterol 10 to 20%. Each serving of oat products eaten daily (1 bowl of oatmeal or 1 oat bran muffin) drops your cholesterol level 3%, so several servings per day are needed for a significant drop. Insoluble fiber (wheat bran) impacts cholesterol levels only minimally.

Soy products and legumes can decrease cholesterol levels over 10%, so include a serving daily. These include tofu, beans, miso broth, and soy products like veggie burgers, soy pepperoni, and soy hot dogs. (More on soy products in Chapter Five)

Choose olive oil or canola oil when you use oils or fat. Eating these types of oils will decrease your LDL cholesterol levels and total cholesterol levels too.

How do I increase my good HDL cholesterol?

Aerobic exercise will increase good HDL cholesterol in most of us. When we exercise more than 20-30 minutes at a time, we exhaust our liver's supply of sugar stores, and our bodies start to burn fat. HDL cholesterol draws the loose cholesterol from our arteries and sends it back to the liver to be burned as fuel and excreted.

What would it take for you to exercise 30-60 minutes every day? How about a brisk walk at lunch time, a 30 minute walk to work, or a 30 minute walk before or after work? Or you might enroll in an aerobics class 3-4 times per week. Other options include: take the kids for a bike ride or take the dog for a walk. If you can't carry on a conversation while you exercise, you are pushing yourself too hard.

Always talk with your health care provider about any current health problems before starting an exercise program.

Eating the right foods also increases HDL. Raw onions and garlic contain chemicals that increase your HDL levels. An onion a day can keep the doctor away; hopefully it won't drive other people away, too!

Can drinking alcohol reduce cholesterol levels and heart disease?

Alcohol in small amounts can increase your HDL cholesterol levels. One drink of any kind of alcohol a day for women and 1 to 2 drinks per day for men improves the total cholesterol/HDL ratio and is linked to a longer life. Unfortunately, if you drink more alcohol than this amount, the effect can be detrimental to your health and can lead to alcohol abuse. Excess alcohol consumption (more than 2 drinks per day) is associated with cancer, liver disease, stomach ulcers, death, drunk driving, and the destruction of families and jobs. Think of it as a potentially toxic medication: a little may be good, too much is poison. If you are unable to limit yourself to 1-2 drinks per day, you should NOT drink alcohol at all.

Like all forms of alcohol, red wine increases HDL cholesterol levels. But unlike others, it decreases oxidation, including blocking oxidation of LDL cholesterol. If you drink alcohol, red wine in limited quantities "appears" to be preferred for health benefits. (See "ALCOHOL" on page 119.)

MEET FATS THAT ARE GOOD FOR YOU

In this section, I'll explain why you should choose some fats over others. For some readers, this grouping may seem simplistic, but my goal is to make this information as accessible as possible.

TABLE 9. Good Fats:

Fat Type	Food Sources
Monounsaturated Fats	Canola oil, olive oil, avocados, hazelnuts, almonds, cashews
Omega-3 Fats	Canola oil, green leafy vegetables, nuts, soy products, seafood, flax seeds and flax oil

TABLE 10. Bad Fats

Fat Type	Food Sources
Polyunsaturated Fats	Corn oil, peanut oil, grain oils, margarines, processed foods
Saturated Fats	Animal fats, dairy fats, palm oils, coconut oil
Trans Fats	Margarines, processed foods

MAKE FRIENDS WITH MONOUNSATURATED FATS!

In small quantities, olive oil and canola oil (monounsaturated fats) may be good for us. Near the Mediterranean Sea, some of the world's healthiest populations use canola and olive oil. Cooking with these oils can decrease your cholesterol level and improve your ratio of total cholesterol to HDL.

Monounsaturated fats provide an excellent source of Vitamin E. They also contain a vast array of antioxidants that remain essential to your health. Monounsaturated fats have been proven to decrease the oxidation of cholesterol in your blood stream.

In Crete, a Greek island, physically active people have excellent health into old age while eating almost 40% of their calories from fat, mostly from olive oil. They are also physically active for several hours each day. The evidence that a diet rich in olive oil can be found in one of the world's healthiest populations testifies to its record of safety when used in moderation. It also suggests that, if you exercise or work actively for   several hours per day, you can eat more "good fat" and remain in good health.[1]

A well-controlled study in France has shown that changing from a diet with mild saturated and polyunsaturated fats (30% of calories from fat) to a monounsaturated fat diet decreases the rate of deaths in people with heart disease. What impressed me when I first read this study was that this simple change in **type of fat** decreased death rates in people with known heart disease by **70%**! They noted this without reducing the quantity of fat. The same study group also had similar reductions in rates of heart failure, strokes, sudden death, and blood clot formation.

EAT MORE OMEGA-3 FATS

Omega-3 fats (also called omega-3 fatty acids or n-3 fatty acids) became popular in the 1980's after scientists noted that Eskimos seldom developed coronary artery disease, despite their high meat and fat diet. Omega-3 fats hit the lay press "big time" in the late 1980's when people started taking fish oil supplements for a variety of conditions, especially for treating heart disease. Public interest declined after studies failed to show that fish oil pills prevented coronary artery disease, even though direct dietary sources continue to show success.[2]

Dietary omega-3 fatty acids come from plant and seafood sources. These tiny, carbon-chained compounds benefit our health in many important ways. They:

- Improve cholesterol levels by decreasing LDL levels
- Decrease the stickiness of your blood, thereby reducing blood clots that cause heart attacks and strokes

---

1. Don't use this information as a health excuse to eat more than 20% of your calories from fat unless you are also willing to exercise for more than an hour every day.
2. This highlights for me a critical point. *The public, guided by the media, searches for "a magic bullet in the form of a pill," when the real secret to health and vitality lies in a nutritious diet.*

- Regulate inflammation in your joints and muscles, decreasing joint pain even from rheumatoid arthritis
- Improve rashes from psoriasis and chronic eczema
- Control intestinal flares from inflammatory bowel disease (such as Crohn's disease)

Seafood provides a rich source of omega-3 fats. Several studies have indicated that people with coronary heart disease decrease their risk of death after a heart attack by eating fish 1-2 times per week. However, eating more than 2 servings of fish per week has actually been associated with increased heart attacks and with increased tissue levels of mercury.

For healthy people, researchers worldwide have not found a consistent benefit to eating fish. It is unclear why people with heart disease seem to benefit and healthy people do not.

In a recent study of 43,757 healthy American health professionals, eating plant sources of omega-3 fats provided strong protection against developing coronary artery disease. In fact, adding plant sources of omega-3 fats was more important in preventing death from heart disease than was cutting the consumption of saturated fat or total fat! Seafood intake failed to provide any benefit.

Most research to date has concentrated only on omega-3 fats from fish. Yet legumes, nuts, and green leafy vegetables (such as herbs, spinach, and greens) are an excellent alternative source of omega-3 fats and should be a big part of your diet.

Before urbanization of human civilization over the last 2,000 years, our intake of vegetable sources of omega-3 fatty acids was 10 to 30 times what it is now. Green herbs and green leafy vegetables (like spinach, Swiss chard, kale, and many green weeds) provided much of our body's nutrition. We need to return to the diet our bodies were designed for if we want to enjoy excellent health and abundant energy.

Omega-3 Fat Summary

An easy way to balance your healthy intake of all these complicated fats is follow two simple steps. The result can be a healthy, nutritious and tasty diet.

First, choose canola or olive oil when you cook with fat, and choose processed foods that are made with these types of oils (like breads, pasta, or ready-made foods). This adds omega-3 fats and limits your intake of unwanted fats.

Second, you also need to eat more green leafy vegetables, beans, and soy products, boosting your omega-3 fat intake. Not only do these plant based foods contain rich sources of omega-3 fats, but they are loaded with antioxidants, cholesterol lowering agents, and compounds that prevent cancer. Seafood can provide another rich source of dietary omega-3 fats.

FATS WORTH LEAVING BEHIND

Yes, I promised to emphasize "adding" foods in this book and I've tried to follow that trend. Yet, often when you make food choices, you must pick one food over another. I've given you reasons why you should pick monounsaturated and omega-3 fats when you add fat to your diet. Now, let me digress for a moment and explain why you should "dump" those other fats before they dump you into a state of poor health.

AVOID EATING POLYUNSATURATED FATS

We require tiny amounts of polyunsaturated fats in our diets. Fortunately, even a limited consumption of canola and olive oil combined with whole grain products, vegetables, and fruits supply all the essential polyunsaturated fats we need.

Polyunsaturated fats come from corn oil, safflower oil, peanut oil, fats in animal meats, and other seed and grain oils.

During the 1980's, we were encouraged to consume polyunsaturated fats because their intake was noted to decrease cholesterol levels and our total cholesterol/HDL ratio. However, we have since discovered that there are disadvantages to their use.

Dietary polyunsaturated fats (PUFAs) are undesirable because:

- They lack a long-term safety record.
- In humans, increased PUFA intake is related to higher rates of melanoma (fatal skin cancer).
- Eating them may weaken your immune system.
- They increase LDL cholesterol oxidation, clogging your arteries.
- A diet high in PUFAs is associated with increased rates of sudden death and irregular heart rhythms.
- They make your platelets sticky, increasing your chance of clots blocking your circulation.
- Eaten in excess they may increase inflammation, which worsens arthritis and muscular pains.
- They can aggravate problems like Crohn's disease and eczema.
- Eaten in excess, they may aggravate depression and intensify anger.

With all these concerns in mind, I recommend you choose fats rich in monounsaturated oils and omega-3 fats in place of polyunsaturated oils.

SHUN SATURATED FATS

Saturated fats are bad news. Eating them causes you to gain weight and increase your LDL cholesterol levels. Yet, they can do even more harm.

Under normal circumstances, platelets are blood cells that help your blood clot. Saturated fats make your blood clot even more easily. If your arteries are narrowed, these clots can become stuck and block your blood flow, leading to a heart attack or a stroke. Even a small narrowing in an artery can be blocked by a large clot. Saturated fats are high in animal products like meat, poultry, butter, cream, 2% and whole milk, and many cheeses.

Some vegetable sources (like coconut products, palm oils, chocolate, and some margarines) are also high in saturated fat. However, many vegetable sources of saturated fat have a less negative impact on your cholesterol levels than do animal fats. In particular, eating chocolate increases your cholesterol levels far less than does eating butter or beef.

Patients often ask me if they should use butter or margarine. I always respond, "Neither!" Choose olive oil or canola oil, or jams and marmalades instead.

Adding more vegetables, fruits, whole grains and legumes to your diet will benefit you tremendously. But you'll benefit even more by avoiding saturated fat such as butter, cream, whole milk, 2% milk, beef, and other fatty meats.

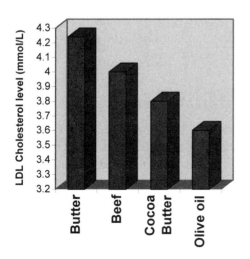

Type of Dietary Fat

TABLE 11. This data comes from a study where men were fed 40% of their calories as fat in liquid formula diets. The type of dietary fat influenced LDL cholesterol levels. Notice in this table how butter and beef fat increase bad LDL cholesterol levels more than either cocoa butter or olive oil. *Adapted with permission from Denke MA et al. Am J Clin Nutr 1991;54:1036-1040.*

BYPASS TRANS-FATTY ACIDS (**The invisible saturated fats in our food supply**)

Chemists designed trans-fatty acids (trans-fats) to make oils solid at room temperature. Voilà, margarine was created, as well as a new threat to your heart. Margarine with trans-fats increases LDL cholesterol levels, worsens your total cholesterol/HDL ratio, and decreases your HDL levels.

Trans-fats and saturated fats can also block the formation of beneficial omega-3 fats. So, not only are these bad fats terrible for your cholesterol levels, but eating them chips away at your health and increases pain and inflammation.

Food Label Warning

More bad news about trans-fats is that food producers don't have to identify them in the "Food Facts" section on food labels. They are hidden within the total fat category, when they should be included with the saturated fat total.

For example, if a slice of bread has 2 grams of fat and no saturated fat, the fat could be from olive oil or canola oil and be excessive, but generally OK. However, if 70% of that fat came from trans fats, I'd want to know, and I wouldn't buy that loaf of bread. With the current labels, it's hard to tell unless I actually subtract the monounsaturated and polyunsaturated fat from the total fat to see what's left–something most people won't do. The solution is to not buy foods with significant fat unless you are sure that most of the fat comes from monounsaturated fat!

In response to public concern, margarine manufacturers are changing their formulations. Now, a few margarines are appearing that contain mostly monounsaturated fat, made with canola oil. Someday they might make them without trans-fats.

HOW DO ANTIOXIDANTS AND OXIDANTS AFFECT FAT?

Oxidants, like tobacco, convert cholesterol into plaque, a hardened substance that forms inside the lining of our arteries and blocks blood flow. Antioxidants prevent fat from being oxidized and can slow or reverse this plaque forming process. Good examples of foods containing antioxidants include broccoli, kale, tomatoes, berries, oranges, peppers, melons, legumes, and whole grains like whole wheat and brown rice.

Diets rich in antioxidants protect the outer walls of LDL from oxidation (See Figure 5 on page 61). Diets that use monounsaturated fat (MUFA) in place of polyunsaturated fat further decrease the oxidation of LDL cholesterol into plaque.

Imagine yourself floating through your own blood stream, drifting with tiny fat bubbles. The LDL fat bubbles float along, constantly under attack by free radicals. You watch Vitamin E and monounsaturated fats (MUFAs) on the outer surface of the LDL bubble extinguishing free radicals. Carotenoids, flavonoids, and Vitamin C then regenerate the Vitamin E back to an active, protective form. As long as your antioxidant support holds, your blood vessels should remain free of plaque.

FIGURE 5. Antioxidants in the outer LDL cholesterol membrane protect against free radical attack, protecting the LDL cholesterol from oxidation.

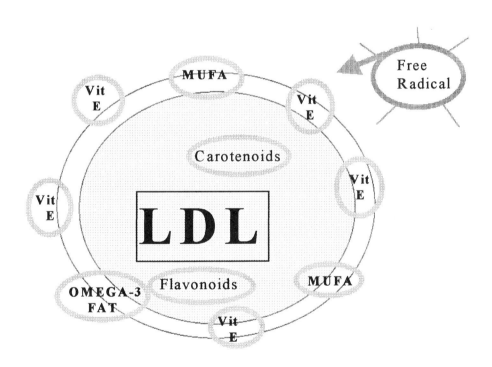

Our typical Western diet fails to protect LDL cholesterol from the free radicals that attack its outer wall. To form plaque, local white blood cells engulf the damaged LDL-free radical. Then, the white blood cells, stuffed with oxidized fat, die and form artery clogging plaque.

Summary on cholesterol levels and fats

We can eat better *and* enjoy delicious food! It won't just improve our cholesterol levels; it will also make us feel better and live longer.

- Concentrate on eating a minimum of 7 servings of vegetables and fruits.
- Colorful foods make meals more attractive and healthier. Choose colorful, antioxidant rich fruits and vegetables (like tomatoes, peppers, broccoli, oranges, and melon) when shopping and cooking. Repeated studies show that eating *green leafy vegetables* helps prevent heart disease and plaque formation.
- Cut way down on the fat you eat. Very low-fat diets are almost as effective at reducing cholesterol as are cholesterol lowering medications.
- When you choose fat for cooking, use monounsaturated fats like olive or canola oil in limited quantities. Avoid saturated fats, polyunsaturated fats, and trans-fats.
- Eat garlic, soy products, soluble fiber and beans every day to reduce cholesterol levels.
- Garlic, minimal alcohol consumption, and monounsaturated cooking oils decrease platelet stickiness and blood clot formation in our arteries.
- For most people, regular aerobic exercise, minimal alcohol consumption, and garlic increase HDL cholesterol levels.
- Fruits and vegetables, garlic, red wine and monounsaturated cooking oils decrease the oxidation of LDL cholesterol.

Notice how bad fat choices affect your health.

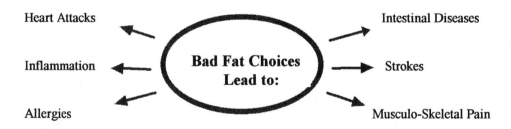

Heart Attacks

Inflammation

Allergies

Bad Fat Choices Lead to:

Intestinal Diseases

Strokes

Musculo-Skeletal Pain

CARBOHYDRATES

Carbohydrates furnish a clean form of energy that we can burn immediately. In addition to providing high performance energy, carbohydrates supply the vast majority of nutrients and antioxidants in our diet. Examples of carbohydrates include vegetables, fruits, beans, pasta, rice, breads, alcohol and other plant products.

SURGES IN BLOOD SUGAR LEVELS AFFECT WEIGHT CONTROL

After carbohydrate rich foods are eaten, they are broken down into simple sugars in our digestive tract. But not all carbohydrates break down equally. Glucose, the simplest form of carbohydrate, is absorbed directly into the blood stream. When we eat 2 ounces (50 grams) of table sugar, our blood sugar level will rise and drop rapidly. When we eat 2 ounces of pasta–a dense, more complex, carbohydrate–it takes longer to break it down into a simple sugar, and our blood glucose level rises more slowly. In contrast to eating sugar, pasta provides a sustained source of energy.

To estimate your rise in blood sugar level after a meal, scientists have created an index, called a *"glycemic index."* [1]

Measuring Surges in Blood Sugar Levels

Recently, researchers started using bread as a standard to compare rises in blood sugar levels with other carbohydrates and have given bread an arbitrary glycemic index of 100. After eating an equal quantity of either green lentils or bread, lentils produce only 36% of the blood sugar rise as does bread. So, green lentils have a glycemic index of 36. Likewise, eating white macaroni produces only 67% of the blood sugar rise as does eating bread, so it has a glycemic index of 67.

From these numbers, you would expect eating bread to cause a higher rise in blood sugar levels than would eating lentils, and that is what you find. (See the table below.) And, as you will see, you'll control your appetite, weight, and blood sugar level better

---

1. In the word glycemic, *glyc* refers to sugar level and *emia* or *emic* refers to blood. Thus, a glycemic index refers to the rise in blood sugar level after the food is ingested.

by choosing foods with a <u>low</u> glycemic index. (See Table 13 on page 65 to compare indexes of different carbohydrate foods.)

TABLE 12. **Notice the dramatic difference in blood sugar levels after eating 50 grams of white bread versus 50 grams of lentils. After eating bread, your blood sugar level increases rapidly and then plummets. In contrast after eating lentils, it remains steady.** *Adapted with permission from Jenkins, DJA et al., BMJ 1980;281:14-17.*

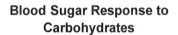

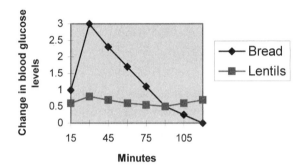

How does a diet with a high sugar surge make us gain weight?

When we eat foods with a high glycemic index, our blood sugar levels rise rapidly and our bodies produce insulin to control this rise. Insulin pushes glucose out of the blood stream and into cells, turning that sugar into fat. When insulin levels rise in our blood stream, they also make us hungry. Insulin stimulates hunger to help prevent a big drop in blood glucose levels.

So, eating foods with a high glycemic index makes many people constantly hungry. Further, with high insulin levels, the calories consumed are immediately stored away as fat. The result is that many people gain weight by eating high glycemic index foods.

High insulin levels increase the risk of developing diabetes, heart disease, high cholesterol levels, and high blood pressure.

How do different foods and meals affect blood sugar control?

You may find some surprises in Table 13 on page 65. Maltose, a chief component in beer, has an <u>huge</u> glycemic index, (GI=152). This score explains why the term "beer belly" is associated with beer. Compare this to orange juice, with a GI of 71.

TABLE 13. GLYCEMIC INDEX FOOD TABLE: After eating foods with lower glycemic numbers, your blood sugar level rises less, and you control your hunger and weight better. (Note that canned foods have higher numbers because of their sugar content.)

FOOD	GLYCEMIC INDEX	FOOD	GLYCEMIC INDEX
BREADS		**LEGUMES**	
Rye (pumpernickel)	68	Dhal (Indian lentils)	12
Rye (wholemeal)	89	Peanuts	15
Rye (crispbread)	95	Soy beans	20
Wheat (white)	100	Lentils (green, dried)	36
Wheat (whole meal)	100	Lentils (red, dried)	38
PASTA		Kidney beans (dried)	43
Macaroni (white)	64	Chick peas (dried)	47
Spaghetti (brown)	61	Green peas (canned)	50
Spaghetti (white)	67	Chick peas (canned)	60
CEREAL GRAINS		Pinto beans (dried)	60
Barley	36	Baked beans (canned)	70
Rye kernels	47	Kidney beans (canned)	74
Bulgur	65	**FRUIT**	
Buckwheat	78	Apple	52
Sweet corn	80	Orange	59
Rice (brown)	81	Orange juice	71
Rice (polished)	81	Banana	84
BREAKFAST CEREALS		Raisins	93
All Bran	74	**SUGARS**	
Porridge oats	89	Fructose (fruit)	26
Muesli	96	Lactose (milk)	57
Shredded wheat	97	Honey	126
Puffed wheat	110	Glucose (lab sugar)	138
Cornflakes	121	Maltose (beer)	152
Puffed rice	132	**DAIRY PRODUCTS**	
ROOT VEGETABLES		Whole milk	44
Sweet Potato (baked)	70	Non-fat milk	46
Yam (baked)	74	Yogurt	52
Potato (new, white, boiled)	80	Ice cream	69
Potato (mashed)	98	**SNACK FOODS**	
Potato (baked)	116	Potato chips (High fat)	77
Potato (instant)	120	Corn chips	99

Now, let's compare different ethnic meals (See Table 14 on page 67). Each of these meals contain equal amounts of protein, fat, and carbohydrate. The difference is in the type of carbohydrate used. Examples include a Western meal with potatoes, an Italian meal with spaghetti, a Greek meal with lentils and a little bread, a Chinese meal with rice, and a Lebanese meal with mostly bread and a little lentils.

As you can see in the next table, eating lentils and spaghetti helps to control sugar elevations. In this same study, insulin output was also controlled with eating glycemic foods. Note that in the typical Western, potato diet, after the blood sugar level peaks, it drops below normal. (Some people complain of dizziness, fatigue or anxiety when blood sugar levels drop low.)

This doesn't mean you should never eat potatoes again. We sometimes add potatoes to soups, or occasionally have them as a side dish. However, you should avoid using potatoes as a staple in your diet if you have trouble controlling your weight or your blood sugar level.

Potatoes have had their day. They frequently saved Europe from famines, providing a reliable source of calories that stored well over the winter. As a good source of Vitamin C, they helped eliminate scurvy, which occurred during the winter months in northern Europe. It is said Europe gained more economically from the potato trade with America than it gained from all the gold and silver ever mined and shipped.

But now, at the turn of the 21st Century, we face not famine and scurvy, but an epidemic of obesity and deficiencies in antioxidants due to an addiction to "processed food." Nationally, health would improve if we used potatoes less often, concentrating instead on colorful vegetables, low-glycemic grain products, and beans.

One of my concerns about most ultra low-fat diets is that they don't emphasize the importance of choosing the best carbohydrates. You eliminate all fatty foods and eat more complex carbohydrates, but some people then risk elevating their blood sugar and insulin levels in exchange for cutting cholesterol levels.

As this book reveals, not all foods are created equal. Just as some fats are better than others, some carbohydrates are better too. My *28-Day Antioxidant Diet Program* makes that distinction!

Why do some carbohydrates raise blood sugar levels more than others?

Compare the spaghetti meal with the bread meal in Table 14 on page 67. Pasta is denser because pasta contains less air. Pasta's greater density slows down its transformation into simple sugars in our intestines, and the delay prevents a rapid release into the blood stream. That is largely why pasta has a lower glycemic index.

TABLE 14. Compare meals with different sources of carbohydrates. Eating lentils and spaghetti improves blood sugar control. The Western, potato based diet is the one most likely to cause increased blood sugar levels and elevated insulin levels. *Figure adapted with permission from Chew, et al. Am J Clin Nutr 1995;47:53-56.*

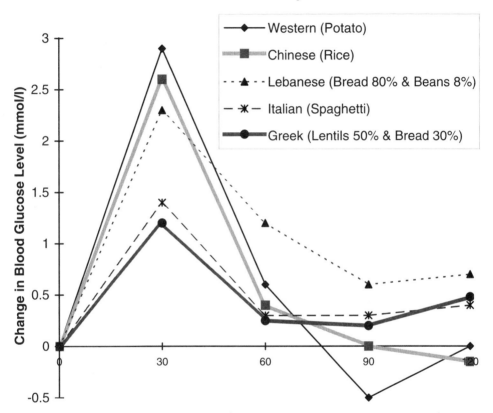

The type of fiber can also influence how quickly a carbohydrate is digested. Various strains of rice have different fiber content and different glycemic indexes. Barley has a much lower glycemic index than rice, although their density is similar. So, you can't gauge foods on their density alone.

Did you notice that whole wheat bread and white bread have the same glycemic index? But, compare pumpernickel bread (GI=68) with whole wheat bread (GI=100). Pumpernickel bread has whole grains mixed in with the flour so it is denser. Look for breads and cereals that are whole grain, not just whole meal.

My wife and I bought a bread maker with a timer for under $100. Suddenly, we were eating great whole grain bread. It's denser (hence, it has a lower glycemic index), it tastes better than packaged breads, and it fills the house with a wonderful, yeasty fragrance while it's baking. We can even set the timer, so the bread is warm and aromatic when we wake up in the morning.

If you eat a lot of bread, I urge you to consider buying a bread maker. You can add whole grains to the flour that match your own taste preferences.

"Refined grains" (highly processed) used in white bread and those in whole wheat bread have nearly the same density and the same glycemic index. The same is true for whole wheat pasta and refined white flour pasta. Yet, the whole grain products still have more fiber, antioxidants, and vitamins than the bleached flour products, so they are much better for you, even if their glycemic index is the same.

What happens to the glycemic index when we process foods?

Take an apple, for example. When you mash an apple and turn it into applesauce, eating the applesauce rather than the whole apple sends sugar from your intestines into your blood stream more quickly and it increases insulin production, too.

Similarly, compare the glycemic index of boiled potatoes (GI=80), with mashed potatoes (GI=98), and with instant potatoes (GI=120). By mashing, grinding, and pulverizing food, we predigest it and increase the surge in blood sugar level and insulin production after eating refined foods.

How do protein and fat affect surges in blood sugar levels?

Both fat and protein slow digestion and nutrient absorption, decreasing the surge in blood sugar level after a meal. But, since our goal is to cut down on our fat intake, we need to find another way to lower a meal's glycemic index. Notice that non-fat milk has a glycemic index of 46, while whole milk has a glycemic index of 44. The increase in fat slows slightly the absorption of sugars into the blood, but this is a tiny drop in glycemic index (2 points) at the cost of a huge increase in fat content (5% fat to 35% fat).

There are several reasons why adding extra protein is not the first step in controlling a meal's glycemic index. First, excess protein strains the liver and kidneys. Second, foods high in protein are often high in fat. It would not be wise to rely on common sources of protein (like fatty meats) to lower a meal's glycemic index. However, eating a moderate quantity of protein (non-fat dairy, skinless poultry, legumes, or seafood) does decrease a meal's glycemic index slightly.

Legumes are likely the ideal protein source as they have a low glycemic index, are low in fat, and add many antioxidants and nutrients to your diet. Soy protein is also rich in an amino acid, called "arginine," that helps control blood sugar levels even more. I believe that people who have trouble controlling blood sugar levels (such as diabetics) should consume two servings of soy products daily (veggie-soy burgers, soy sausage, tofu, soy flour, soy milk, veggie-soy hot dogs, etc.).

Some people will show a clear rise in blood sugar levels if they add refined carbohydrates to their diet. But they don't have to eat more protein to offset this. Eating low glycemic carbohydrates can prevent most of this sugar rise.

In fact, in a study published in 1997 on over 60,000 American nurses, researchers at Harvard's School of Public Health showed that total carbohydrate intake was NOT related to the risk of developing diabetes. Rather, eating highly refined, high glycemic foods increased rates of diabetes. As expected, eating non-refined carbohydrates (with a low glycemic index) reduced rates of acquiring diabetes.

How do low glycemic index foods affect cholesterol levels?

Insulin also stimulates the liver to produce more LDL cholesterol, which contributes to plaque formation in your arteries. Long periods of increased insulin secretion increase your risk of developing diabetes, heart disease, strokes, high blood pressure, and obesity.

Studies that substituted low glycemic foods for high glycemic foods decreased LDL cholesterol and the total cholesterol/HDL ratio. I believe that eating low glycemic foods maintains cleaner arteries.

Glycemic index summary

Foods that cause your blood sugar level to surge increase insulin production. Increased insulin stimulates fat formation and an increased appetite. To control your appetite, concentrate on eating carbohydrates like beans, pasta, fruits, and green leafy vegetables. Choose unprocessed foods over refined foods daily.

Let me share how one of my patients benefited from putting an understanding of glycemic indexes to work for her.

Mary, a 45-year-old school teacher, had tried nearly every diet in the book. Despite this and to her despair, her weight had slowly crept up and now exceeded 200 pounds. Recently, she was following a low-fat diet approach, but found that she was constantly hungry and eating all the time.

She had toast with jam and coffee for breakfast, and a sandwich with non-fat cheese, carrot sticks, non-fat potato chips, and apple juice for lunch. For an afternoon snack, she would have non-fat chips and apple juice. And for dinner, she usually had potatoes with either skinless chicken or fish with a salad and one light beer, and non-fat popcorn or pretzels for dessert.

Mary certainly had cut down on her fat intake, but all her meals and snacks struck me as being very likely to stimulate hunger and cause weight gain. Why? Because many of her food choices produced a surge in her blood sugar level.

I encouraged her to stay with the low-fat approach, but to add foods with a low glycemic index. She was thrilled with this information on glycemic indexes, and plunged into a diet featuring cooked oatmeal with non-fat milk and fruit for breakfast. Sandwiches were now made with pumpernickel bread with tomato and soy pepperoni, or she had leftover pasta dishes with vegetables, tomato and bean sauces.

Now, Mary rarely needed to eat snacks at mid-afternoon, but if she did have non-fat chips, she scooped deeply into non-fat, spicy bean dips. For dinner, she enjoyed pasta, bulgur wheat, barley, or rice with many types of vegetables and tofu or non-fat cheese, and she ate bean side dishes 3-4 nights per week. She gave up potatoes and regular bread and ate more salads or side vegetable dishes. Lastly, for dessert she had frozen yogurt or soy milk mixed with fruit in the blender.

The first thing Mary noticed was that she wasn't hungry all the time. The second was that without cutting calories, she was comfortable eating less, and she lost weight. For Mary, adding foods (namely pasta, vegetables, fruits, and beans) helped to control her appetite.

As you read through this book, you'll observe that low-glycemic index foods are often loaded with antioxidants. Next, when we talk about fiber, you'll see the same trend: low-glycemic index, low-fat, abundant fiber, and meals packed with antioxidants. Our goal is to use the best foods daily, make them simple to prepare, and delicious to eat!

FIBER

Fiber is good for us because high fiber foods are packed with antioxidants. People who follow high fiber diets have lower heart attack rates, lower cancer rates, and fewer intestinal problems. We should strive for more fiber daily.

A good example of a high fiber food is a pinto bean. It even *looks* tough. Stab it with a knife and you hardly pierce the skin. Fiber is one of the factors that make it dense. When cooked into soft, refried beans, fortunately the fiber remains. Our digestive tracts are slow to break down the bean's dense, strongly-joined carbohydrates into simple sugars for absorption. Not surprisingly, beans have a low glycemic index.

In contrast, let's look at a slice of fluffy, store-bought bread. We can easily tear it into shreds or roll it into a tiny ball. Our digestive tract turns this low-density carbohydrate into sugar in a hurry, hence the higher glycemic index.

While fiber doesn't always increase the glycemic index, it does add essential minerals, vitamins, and antioxidants to our diet. Even though fluffy, whole wheat bread has the same glycemic index as fluffy, white bread, it's clearly more nutritious.

Rice bran, wheat bran, rye bran, and oat bran have their own special biochemical properties and advantages. Adding a *variety* of fibers to your diet can improve your health greatly.

Generally, fiber comes in two *forms*, "*soluble*" and "*insoluble*." Soluble fiber dissolves in fluid. Insoluble fiber does not. We do best by eating a balance of soluble and insoluble fiber every day.

Soluble Fiber

We find soluble fiber in beans, soy products, fruits, and leafy vegetables. Barley, oat bran and oat products are other excellent sources of soluble fiber.

Soluble fiber contains a vast array of nutrients. It can also:

- Lower cholesterol levels
- Lower blood sugar levels
- Aid digestion and elimination

Insoluble fiber

Wheat products, especially wheat bran, are good sources of insoluble fiber.

When our diet is deficient in insoluble fiber, we develop abdominal cramps and other intestinal problems. Constipation is very common when insoluble fiber and fluid intake are inadequate.

Unlike soluble fiber, insoluble fiber does not reduce cholesterol levels. But it does help our digestion. Insoluble fiber absorbs water in our intestines and swells like a sponge creating loose, soft stools, and decreasing the work-load of excreting food from our intestines.

Many patients enter my office wondering why they have problems with constipation, even though they eat lots of fiber. About half of them underestimate how much fiber they need (needs vary from 30-40 grams per day). The other half don't drink enough fluids. Since coffee, colas, and alcohol increase urination, they do not help hydrate our intestines. You need fluid and insoluble fiber to help move the digestive process along. Be sure to drink at least 2-3 liters (quarts) of fluid per day; don't count coffee, caffeinated black teas, colas, or alcohol.

SALT

Many medical providers overemphasize cutting salt from the diet. A limited quantity of dietary salt is essential to our lives. Salt helps us retain a healthy amount of fluid, which we use to regulate our blood pressure. It also impacts the electrical impulses across cell walls. Because of its physiological importance, our taste buds reward us when we use it sparingly.

Sodium

If you use regular table salt, you are using sodium salt. If you eat too much sodium, your kidneys retain extra water to maintain a steady salt concentration and must then work overtime to excrete this extra fluid and sodium.

Over 24 hours, most people take approximately 1/3 of their salt with dinner, 1/3 with lunch and drinks, and 1/3 with breakfast and snacks. Packaged snacks, such as chips and dips, can be loaded with sodium. If your snack serving size exceeds 500 mg of sodium or your dinner exceeds 1,000 mg per serving, start choosing foods with less sodium.

One-third of us note a significant rise in blood pressure if we eat too much sodium; some of us are more sensitive to salt than others. Not everybody has to worry about salt intake and blood pressure problems, yet increased sodium intake raises everyone's blood pressure at least a little. People with high blood pressure problems should talk with their health care providers to learn if they are salt-sensitive.

People with heart failure, diabetes, osteoporosis or kidney disease should avoid added salt entirely.

When we eat too much sodium, our kidneys excrete more salt, and we lose calcium in our urine. High sodium intake therefore leads to calcium loss from our bones, one of the factors that contributes to osteoporosis.

Because women have more frequent debilitating bone fractures than men, they need to reduce their sodium intake or increase their calcium intake at an early age to prevent debilitating fractures in later life.

The first step in reducing salt intake is to find another taste to replace it, such as garlic, chili, or herbs. (I find that a squirt of lemon satisfies my desire for salt.) Second, read the labels on food packages; processed food is loaded with sodium salts. Finally, stop automatically adding salt to food while cooking.

When I first tested my recipes on friends, I used no salt, and several of my dinner guests asked for the salt shaker. So, in later meals, I compromised by using small amounts of salt in my cooking and recipes. The standard salt quota for people with heart disease and high blood pressure is 2 grams of sodium per day. By limiting sodium intake to 2-3 grams per day, you can also help prevent bone weakening.

BALANCED HEALTH SUMMARY: USING PIE CHARTS

Having looked at protein, fat, and carbohydrates in detail, let's see how we should put them together in our diet.

I personally hate trying to count calories, and won't ask you to count calories in this book. A calorie is a unit of energy. It gives us a way to measure how much energy we consume and expend. When we consider which foods to eat, we can divide our daily intake to decide how much energy should come from protein, fat, and carbohydrates.

Our need for protein varies throughout our lives, yet we receive ample to build and repair our bodies from eating 10-15% of calories from protein. You will hear claims of "improved health" or "enhanced weight loss" on high protein diets, but there is NO evidence from clinical trials that high protein diets bring any *long-term* benefits.

Although some fat intake is essential, I believe we do best by limiting it to between 15% and 20% of our total calories. Compared to ultra-low-fat diets, this offers us an opportunity to increase our variety of food choices and cooking styles. Just remember, "if we add more fat, it should be high in antioxidants and low in harmful fats." Good fat sources include nuts, soy products, avocados, olive oil, canola oil, and possibly seafood.

After protein and fat, carbohydrates provide the rest of our energy. Complex carbohydrates, such as whole grains, legumes, vegetables and fruits, should furnish at least 60-65% of our energy needs. These rich carbohydrate sources provide most of the antioxidants, nutrients and vitamins in our diet. The pie charts below represent two approaches to calorie intake.

FIGURE 6. **The Typical, Nutrient Inadequate, American Diet, 1997**

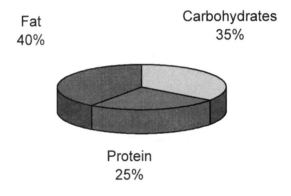

Fat
40%

Carbohydrates
35%

Protein
25%

As of 1997, the average American was eating more than 38% of calories from fat, and more than 20% of their calories from protein. No wonder lifespans in the United States fail to improve, despite all the miracles of modern medicine! My *28-Day Antioxidant Diet* offers increased calories from carbohydrates. As our carbohydrate intake increases, so does our intake of antioxidants, vitamins, and nutrients–improving the quality of our lives.

FIGURE 7. The 28-Day Antioxidant Diet

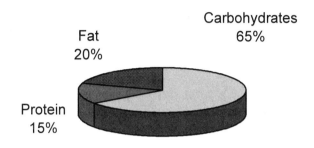

Fat
20%

Carbohydrates
65%

Protein
15%

"BUT HOW DOES IT TASTE?"

Let's face it, while the fat, protein and carbohydrate content of foods are important, what we really want to know is, *"How does it taste?"* Bitter, sweet, sour, pungent, and salty are primary tastes, and they drive our food preferences. Knowing this, I've put as much work, research, and time into creating the recipes in this book as I have expended researching and writing the text. I know that for this program to work for you, the food has to taste terrific–and it does.

In Chapter 10, I feature dishes that are low in fat, yet full of exciting flavors. Anyone can make unhealthy but flavorful food out of white flour, butter, sugar and a few spices. What I find exciting is creating delicious meals out of "healthy" food using the principles outlined in this book. Now, let's find out how we can build a healthier food pyramid, for longer lives and disease-free living.

CHAPTER 5   *BUILDING A*
HEALTHIER
FOOD
PYRAMID

In the early 1990's, the U.S. Department of Agriculture created a new food pyramid to guide American diets. I suspect the new pyramid was designed because irrefutable proof showed the former "basic food groups" guide to be unhealthy. Unfortunately, it appears a great deal of politicking and marketing of specific food products was included in the making of this new pyramid.

The new food pyramid improves over the old system by emphasizing grains, vegetables, and fruits. However, I am disappointed that the American beef, poultry, and dairy industries were able to include their foods prominently in the revised food pyramid, not out of a concern for American's health, but out of a concern for their own economic health.

What we need is a food pyramid based on healthy, tasty foods. I would like to propose the following:

BUILDING A NEW ANTIOXIDANT FOOD PYRAMID

Below are my suggestions for a new food pyramid:
- Choose fruits and vegetables (7-10 servings daily), especially colorful and green leafy ones, such as broccoli, spinach, and peppers. Limit potatoes.
- Aim to eat beans and soy products daily.
- Choose whole grains: whole grain pasta, rice, amaranth, bulgur, and corn.
- Use monounsaturated fats; they should provide > 60% of total fat intake.
- Limit total fat to less than 20% of calories.
- Keep saturated fat less than 5% of total calories.
- Make protein about 15% of total calories (.8 to 1.0 grams per kilo).
- Limit alcohol intake to 1 drink per day for women and 1 to 2 drinks per day for men. Red wine is preferred.
- Fish is not encouraged, but is optional. (Meat and poultry are not recommended. If you choose to eat meat and poultry, keep the serving size small, 3 ounce servings, and limited to 2-3 times per week.)

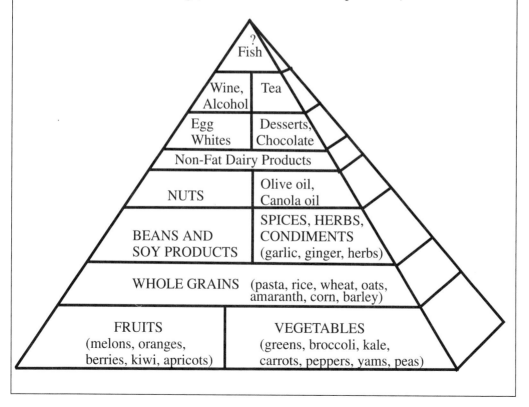

FRUITS AND VEGETABLES

If you decided to change only one thing in your diet I urge you to, "Eat more fruits and vegetables." Fruits and vegetables provide most of the antioxidants our bodies require for healthy living.

Many of my patients tell me they don't like fruits and vegetables. But after we go through a list, they discover there are several that they do enjoy. We have hundreds of choices in the produce section of our supermarkets. Search for something green, red, and yellow or orange to eat every day.

"What is a serving of produce?" I'm often asked. One produce serving equals any of the following:

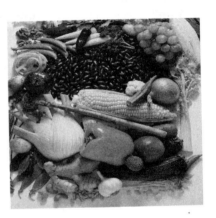

- 3/4 cup of juice (juice counts as 1 serving per day)
- 1 piece of medium-size fruit
- 1 medium-size carrot, artichoke, or potato
- 1/2 cup fruits or vegetables, fresh or cooked (such as berries, peas)
- 1 cup leafy greens

We should eat *at least* seven servings per day of fruits and vegetables. To put it another way, one third of the food we eat should be fruits and vegetables. (See Table 15 on page 79 to learn how you can eat seven servings of produce per day.)

FRUITS

Fruits provide us with a valuable source of fiber, Vitamin C, folic acid, and antioxidants (especially carotenoids and flavonoids). Most fruits also provide sustained energy, which help control blood sugar levels.

Fruits make easy, appealing, and delicious desserts as well as great snacks during the day–just toss them into a lunch bag or add them to cereal. They are also easy to buy, store, and eat–we don't even have to cook them! Flavonoid packed blueberries and strawberries go well in cereal. There is hardly a worthy excuse *not* to eat more fruit.

TABLE 15. How to eat 7 servings of fruits and vegetables daily!	
Breakfast (1 serving):	1 glass of juice, or, 1 piece of fruit
Lunch (3 servings):	1 cup of veggies with lunch (usually leftovers heated in the microwave, or veggie sticks with lunch) 1 serving of fruit after lunch or as an afternoon snack
Dinner: (3 servings)	1 cup of veggies with dinner, or 1/2 cup veggies and 1 cup of salad, plus 1 serving of fruit with or for dessert

Dried fruits are a welcome snack at home or on a hike, and provide many of the nutrients found in fresh fruit. Drying fruit is a fun family activity. Home dried fruit is tastier and cheaper than commercially dried fruit. Just buy fruit in season.

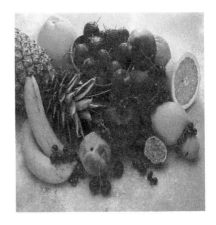

I usually buy 5-6 crates of fruit per year to dry: apricots, pears, cherries, plums, and peaches are my favorites. Sometimes we will dry bananas, apples, or pineapple, too. I dry them, stuff them in zip-lock bags, and put them in the freezer. Dried fruit can be a welcome addition to curries, or mixed in with frozen yogurt.

Fruit juices

Juices can be rich in Vitamin C, carotenoids, flavonoids, and folic acid. But choose those that are 100% juice and avoid those with added sugars. Drink a glass of juice in the morning with breakfast, or during the day with food as a snack. You can count one serving of juice toward your goal of two to three fruit servings per day.

TABLE 16. Dr. Masley's Fruit Choices:
These are my favorite fruits based upon antioxidant content including: Vitamin C, carotenoid, flavonoid, fiber, and folic acid. All the fruits on this list are good for you. Some have more antioxidant activity than others.

Find items you like and eat them often.

Fruits	Dr. Masley's Scores
Blueberries	100
Strawberries	86
Oranges	86
Plums	72
Cantaloupe	72
Grapes, red	72
Papaya	72
Mango	68
Grapefruit, pink	65
Kiwi	65
Apricots	54
Cherries	54
Raspberries	54
Blackberries	54
Watermelon	41
Peaches	41
Pears	32
Apples	32
Bananas	18

Many juices combine apple or pear juice with more nutritious juices. Although these juices are better than sodas, they aren't nearly as nutritious as citrus, grape, and vegetable juices. Be aware that apple, grape, and pear juice have a high glycemic index, so your blood sugar level surges if you drink them without food.

Juicing vegetables and fruits at home is easy if you have a juicing machine. The only disadvantage is in the loss of fiber. However, if you already eat seven or more servings of fruits and vegetables daily and five servings of whole grains–you get plenty of fiber, so enjoy one to two glasses of juice per day.

When the fiber is removed from produce, you get more of some nutrients, but you also get a quicker blood sugar rise when drinking these types of juices than you get from eating whole fruits and vegetables. If you drink small amounts at a time, or enjoy them with food, the blood sugar rise is moderated.

TABLE 17. **Dr. Masley's Juice Scores:**
Dr. Masley's total score reflects antioxidant content including: **Vitamin C, carotenoid, flavonoid, and folic acid.**

Juice Type	Dr. Masley's Scores
Orange Juice	100
Grape Juice, red	96
Pink Grapefruit Juice	68
Tomato Juice	64
Carrot Juice	50
Apricot Juice	46
Pineapple Juice	41
Apple Juice	10

VEGETABLES ARE FOR YOU–HERE'S WHY

I adore vegetables. Vegetables (along with grains) are likely the most important foods we eat. Many, especially green leafy ones, provide all the essential vitamins and minerals that our bodies need: Vitamin C, folic acid, soluble and insoluble fiber, zinc, calcium, and antioxidants including carotenoids and flavonoids. Vegetables are also usually low in fat.

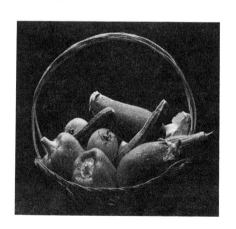

Dinner is the easiest time to eat two servings of vegetables. Check the recipe section in this book for some delicious vegetable dishes.

Carrots, broccoli, cauliflower, and bell peppers also make great snacks. Enjoy them with low-fat dips or sauces, or, steam them and toss with a vinaigrette salad dressing. Grated vegetables are terrific for salads for lunch or dinner.

And now, a final word on America's favorite vegetable–French fries. These are high in fat, have a high glycemic index, and are low in calcium, Vitamin C and folic acid. Eating them raises cholesterol levels and adds unwanted inches to your waistline. Let's change our preferences to <u>real</u> vegetables that will heal us!

Special Healing Vegetables:

Some vegetables have special health promoting properties. In particular, look at the six groups listed below. They fight cancers, and are loaded with antioxidants and nutrients. I've included many recipes at the end of the book featuring these particular vegetables. Your health will improve by including them in your diet regularly.

Broccoli, kale, cauliflower, Brussel sprouts, and cabbage

This group of vegetables, known as *"brassicas"* or *"Cruciferae,"* is very nutritious. They grow well in cold climates and appear in our vegetable produce section year round but especially in the winter months. They contain antioxidants called "indoles," which are proven to decrease cancer rates when eaten regularly. This group is also very rich in carotenoids, vitamin C, calcium, and flavonoids.

Crucifers contain enzymes that activate the nutrients in these vegetables. You can eat these vegetables raw, steamed, or lightly sautéed. Be careful not to overcook them, since they lose their valuable enzymes.

Indoles remain active for a couple of days in our tissues, so you need only eat a serving or two of vegetables from this group 3-4 times per week. If eaten several times per day, these vegetables can suppress thyroid activity. However, this is usually only a problem for people who drink freshly juiced vegetables, like cabbage juice, daily.

Some people complain of intestinal gas problems after eating these vegetables. Try eating small servings, 1/8 to 1/4 cup daily. In time, your intestines may learn to digest them better.

To be honest, I only recently started cooking with kale. I had never bought kale in the grocery store until I started researching this book. Learning to cook with this delightful vegetable has been a pleasant surprise. It has an attractive lace-like edge, and comes in purple and green. It goes well in soups, stir-fries, and rice dishes. It takes longer to cook than other greens like spinach, so plan to cook it almost as long as you would broccoli (three to five minutes).

Greens (spinach, beet greens, Swiss chard, mustard greens, collard greens)

Green leafy vegetables are an important source of many vitamins and antioxidants. They also provide a valuable source of omega-3 fats.

You can do many things with them. Add them to a soup three to four minutes before serving, or chop and add to a stir-fry one to two minutes before serving. Steam them, or sauté them in garlic with a dash of balsamic vinegar for three to four minutes as a side dish. Chop and mix in a casserole before you put it in the oven.

TABLE 18. **Dr. Masley's vegetable scores**:

Essentially all the vegetables in this table are good for you (except French fries because of their high fat content). Concentrate on eating a few of the best daily. Scores come from flavonoid, carotenoid, Vitamin C, and absorbable calcium content. Plus an added factor for cancer fighting properties.

VEGETABLES	Dr. Masley's Score
Kale	100
Broccoli	96
Red Bell Pepper	92
Yams	88
Peas	88
Snow Peas	88
Beet Root	88
Beet Leaves	84
Green Bell Pepper	84
Pursalane	84
Sweet Potato	84
Swiss Chard	**84**
Tomatoes	84
Spinach	80
Leeks	80
Artichoke	80
Pumpkin	72
Onions	71
Cauliflower	71
Red Cabbage	63
Carrots	59
Green Beans	59
Romaine Lettuce	59
Zucchini	55
Celery	55
Eggplant	38
Cucumbers	38
Iceberg Lettuce	36
Potatoes	35
Radish	33
French Fries	8

Sweet potatoes and yams

These colorful root vegetables are full of antioxidants and nutrients. They cause less of a blood sugar rise than regular potatoes, too. You can dice them and put them in stir-fries, or pop them in the microwave and serve them as a side dish. They also add a pleasant sweetness to desserts. Yams cook in less time than sweet potatoes, and are slightly less fibrous.

When baking muffins, breads, and cakes, I've explored ways to cut out the fat without losing the moisture. I've discovered when baking that if I microwave and mash a yam and add it to the batter with the wet ingredients, the result is delicious, moist, and low-fat. Try my chocolate cake recipe as an example.

Leeks, garlic, and onions

We already reviewed garlic. Leeks and onions belong to the same family and have several of the same beneficial properties– they fight cancer, lower cholesterol levels, reduce blood pressure, stimulate the immune system, and are loaded with antioxidants. Leeks are milder than onions and garlic, and have a higher carotenoid content.

Onions are a popular vegetable. Some people complain of bad breath or intestinal gas if they eat raw onions. However, you can avoid this by sautéing them lightly until they turn slightly yellow. Then use them in recipes as directed. If you still have problems, carry Beano ᴿ, an over-the-counter enzyme that helps prevent gas.

Leeks are excellent for people who can't tolerate onions and garlic. The flavor is milder and leeks rarely cause intestinal complaints. While leeks are more expensive than onions, they are easy to grow in your own garden year round.

To store leeks, first discard the tiny roots at the bottom and tough green tops. To cook, slice them from the root end towards the tops lengthwise. The first 1-2 inches of green color are tender, but quickly turn tough. So, toss the remaining tops into the compost bin or use them in stock. Rinse the chopped leeks well, as they often have sand between their layers.

Peppers (red, green, orange, yellow)

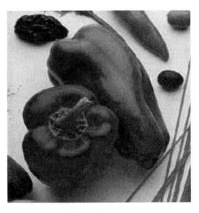

Peppers are a wonderful addition to meals. They are packed with carotenoids, Vitamin C, and folic acid. You can sauté them, stuff them with rice or bulgur and bake them, add them to soups, or slice them as snacks. The trick is not to overcook them, as this destroys some of their valuable nutrients. Peppers are delicious in salads.

Peppers freeze very well. We try to buy a few crates in the summer when they are inexpensive, slice them and freeze them in zip-lock bags. You can roast them in the oven, peel off the skin and have frozen roasted peppers on hand for dishes, too. Green peppers are inexpensive and available year round.

Tomatoes

Tomatoes are juicy, luscious "fruits" that hold an important place in western cuisine. While technically a fruit, we use them as vegetables are good for us as they are rich in carotenoids, Vitamin C, and absorbable calcium.

While the habit of eating tomatoes started in South America, it later became extremely popular in Italy. Today, we can easily find dried tomatoes, canned tomatoes (stewed, puréed, tomato sauce, tomato paste), and we can buy fresh tomatoes year round.

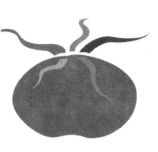

Tomato sauce complements many rice, pasta, and vegetable dishes. The flavor goes well with garlic, Herbes de Provence, and olive oil. Non-fat or very-low-fat tomato sauces provide moisture to dishes without making them fattening. We will use tomatoes in many of the dishes in the recipe section.

MUSHROOMS

During my youth, my family and I gathered Chanterelle mushrooms in the forests around our home. To this day, we look forward to the first rainy weekend in late August or September heralding mushroom season. If you ever cook batches of Chanterelles (*Cantharellus cibarius*), your home will be filled with a musty, earthy fragrance that will awaken your taste buds.

Mushrooms carry a certain mystique. While some varieties are poisonous, others hold beneficial medicinal properties. I do **not** encourage the novice mushroom lover to hunt for wild mushrooms. It's too difficult to distinguish good from bad varieties.

The Japanese and Chinese have cultivated and gathered Shiitake mushrooms (*Lentinus edodes*) for 2,000 years. This variety is delicious, and brings a rich flavor to soups and stir-fries. Shiitakes contain anti-tumor and blood pressure lowering properties. In laboratory testing, they inhibit the growth of breast cancer cells and stimulate immune cells. Many grocery stores carry fresh or dried Shiitake mushrooms in either the produce or Oriental food sections.

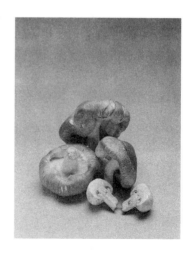

Oyster mushrooms (*Pleurotus ostreatus*) are another delicious variety with a milder flavor than Shiitakes. Scientific studies show that oyster mushrooms provide antioxidant, anti-tumor, and immune system stimulating properties. Extracts from oyster mushrooms also improve cholesterol and blood sugar levels.

The common, button mushrooms have been cultivated for mass production for over 200 years, starting in France. Unfortunately, they provide no known medicinal properties. Oyster, Shiitake, and other Oriental mushrooms are clearly more expensive than button mushrooms, but their richer flavor and healing properties make them worth the cost.

How to Cook Mushrooms

Mushrooms are mostly water and shrink greatly with cooking. To cook them, sauté them in a pan with a sprinkle of salt. Avoid stewing a long time or they toughen.

To use dried mushrooms, place them in a bowl, add hot water, and allow them to soak for 30 minutes. Filter or screen the fluid to avoid any sand or grit. Save the remaining liquid for soups and stocks; it is rich and delicious.

GRAINS

The coating on a grain helps it last 1,000 years. If we are ever to understand the process of immortality, we need to grasp how antioxidants help seeds and grains survive for this length of time.

We are only beginning to understand the benefits of eating whole grains. The outer layers of a grain (wheat bran, rye bran, etc.) contain most of their antioxidant value. An important part of the bran layer, or outer husk, contains fibers called "ligans." Many plant ligans have antioxidant, anticarcinogenic, and antimicrobial activity. These properties help to protect grains from disease. Once they are absorbed by our bodies, they can improve our health too.

Of the three layers of grains, the tiny aleuronic layer (part of the bran) contains the highest concentration of ligans. In fact, whole grain fiber appears to lower rates of hormone-induced cancers. People who eat ample ligans (like some areas in Finland, where whole rye sourdough bread is consumed in large quantities) have low rates of prostate and breast cancer.

Dr. Adlercreutz, a physician and biochemist in Helsinki, Finland, has shown that ligans from rye products, once modified by normal intestinal bacteria, can inhibit breast cancer cell growth. He also reports that ligans from soy products decrease breast and prostate cancer growth.

In order to become active, the ligans in whole grain products require modification by normal intestinal bacteria. Therefore, people who frequently take antibiotics–which lower the number of normal intestinal bacteria–produce lower levels of health-promoting ligans. After antibiotic use, live yogurt consumption might help reactivate them.

FIGURE 8. A grain.

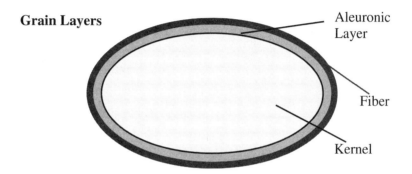

Grain Layers

Aleuronic Layer

Fiber

Kernel

Plan to have five servings of whole, non-refined grains per day. Apart from their health benefits, grain products are popular because they taste good and help define the rest of the meal. Look how they can shape a meal:

- rice and stir fry
- pasta and spaghetti sauce
- bread and soup
- breakfast cereal and milk

Ethnic foods offer us an even greater variety from which to choose.

- Chinese: noodles, rice, or won tons
- Mexican: rice, or tortillas and beans
- Italian: pasta, pizza
- French: bread, pasta
- Middle Eastern: bulgur and chick peas (garbanzo beans)

Whenever I consider what kind of grain I want to complement my meal, I consider which spices, sauces, types of vegetables, and protein will work best for the meal I have in mind. There is no limit to my choices–or yours! Let your imagination be your guide.

SELECTING THE "RIGHT" GRAIN

Quality grains can bring a meal to new heights: whether it's pasta, whole wheat tortillas, wild rice–all form the substance of a meal. Grains vary in nutritional value. Table 19 on page 88 scores their nutritional value for you.

Grain Type	Dr. Masley's Score
Amaranth	100
Wild rice	64
Whole wheat pasta	60
Rye bread	56
Pumpernickel bread	52
Bulgur wheat	52
Whole wheat	48
Brown rice	44
Corn bread	36
White pasta	32
White Rice	28
White bread	28

TABLE 19. **Dr. Masley's Grain Scores:** **They were calculated by grading and combining their antioxidant content, fiber content, zinc, calcium, glycemic index and folic acid content.**

(I would have used amaranth in recipes often, but I couldn't find it easily in many local stores. Look for it in your area.)

Rice

Rice is the most popular food grain in the world and one of the oldest. Rice production in southeast Asia started 7,000 years ago.

Rice is divided into two categories. The first refers to *how the rice is processed:* into white rice and brown rice. The second refers to the *type of rice*: long grain rice, short grain rice, and wild rice. Wild rice is botanically different from regular rice, but I will group them together here for simplicity.

We create white or "polished" rice by removing the outer husk on the rice kernel. The rice husk contains most of the antioxidants and many of the nutrients in each grain. Nonetheless, polished rice can be served with other foods to form an antioxidant and nutrient rich meal. I don't expect connoisseurs of the "perfect bowl of polished rice" to substitute brown rice in every recipe; however, I hope that the white rice connoisseur will learn to enjoy brown rice and gradually choose it more often.

In our home, we use different types of rice with different ethnic meals. Basmati rice (or less expensive Texmati rice) is perfect with many Indian curry dishes. For most Oriental dishes, it'll be a toss-up between brown short kernel rice and polished short kernel sticky rice. Stuffed peppers and casseroles go beautifully with either brown short kernel rice or wild rice. When we cook Mexican food, we usually serve it with brown rice.

Wild rice brings a nutty, chewy flavor to many meals. It is very nutritious and high in protein, nutrients, and zinc. It takes much longer to cook, up to an hour, so we usually cook enough for several meals and store the rest in the refrigerator to be used over the week.

Rice stores very well, so keep several types on hand sealed in a container in the pantry. When you cook rice, cook extra. It refrigerators well over a few days and you can use it with stir-fries for a quick meal later.

Wheat

Wheat is the most common grain in crackers, breads, cereals, and pastas in the western diet. Unfortunately, most of today's wheat products are "highly refined," which means they have lost most of their antioxidants and many of their nutrients when food producers removed the outer husk.

I admit it's difficult to substitute whole wheat for the light, airy white flour of a fragrant, fresh baguette (a French loaf of bread with a crispy crust). Yet, we can learn to enjoy whole grain breads and use whole grain products more often. Start by substituting 100% whole grain bread for the average sliced white bread sandwich.

Here's a word of caution when buying multi-grain breads. Look at the ingredients: they often contain 70-80% enriched flour, which means white bread flour. If the first ingredient is enriched flour, look for another loaf. Choose a loaf that has the first two to three ingredients as whole wheat, whole rye, or whole oat flour. Also avoid loaves that use caramel coloring to make white flour bread look like whole grain flour.

I'm pleased to report that whole wheat pastas are gaining in popularity and are more available in supermarkets. Look for them in the bulk foods section.

Bulgur Wheat and Couscous

Bulgur wheat (also called cracked wheat) comes from the middle east, where wheat is boiled and redried. Bulgur wheat is quick and easy to prepare. Many cooks use it to make *tabbouleh* (a delicious Middle Eastern salad), but you can also substitute it for rice in many casserole dishes.

Bulgur wheat has a chewy texture and soaks up a miso flavor nicely. It serves up very well with greens, parsley, tomatoes, nuts, and peppers–with a generous squeeze of lemon or lime juice just drizzled over it. My entire family enjoys it and bulgur appears on our table often.

Couscous is another form of wheat, and is a staple grain in northern Africa. It goes well with many spicy bean and vegetable dishes and, like bulgur, can be used in salads.

Buckwheat (Kasha)

Buckwheat is gluten free (for those with gluten intolerance) and can be cooked as a grain or used as a flour. Roasted buckwheat, called "kasha," is served with winter vegetables to make a popular Russian dish.

Oats

Most people limit oats in the diet to oatmeal. Oatmeal, combined with non-fat milk or yogurt, almond slices, and fresh or frozen fruit makes a great breakfast. However, oat flour also combines well with wheat flour in breads and crackers. Since oat fiber is rich in soluble fiber, people with high cholesterol levels should eat more oat products.

Oat bran muffins can be delicious. Watch out for the ones you buy in stores as they are often loaded with fat. When making oat muffins, to keep them moist, add lots of fruit in place of fat. Applesauce, blueberries, cranberries, bananas, raisins, or dried apricots and dates are welcome additions to home-made oat flour or oat bran muffins.

Barley

Barley is a great grain to add to soups. Similar to oats, it is nutritious and loaded with soluble fiber. Barley lowers blood sugar and cholesterol levels. In our home, we also serve it like rice with stir fried vegetables or with curry dishes.

Rye

Rye is an important grain in eastern and northern Europe. In particular, it can be used to make sourdough rye bread, which is delicious and packed with antioxidants. The addition of sourdough is tasty and may help convert cancer-fighting ligan fiber to its active form. Sourdough contains an acidophilus (yogurt like) bacteria.

Rye crisp, my preferred cracker, is usually very low in fat and very tasty. It's excellent with dips and low-fat spreads.

Amaranth and Quinoa

Amaranth is a small grain from ancient Central America and was important to the Aztecs and other populations of the altiplano, in what is now the highlands of Mexico. It is very high in many nutrients and protein. Amaranth flour is becoming trendy in health food stores. Try cooking amaranth with a mixture of grains in Mexican dishes.

Unfortunately, it is not as easy to find as other grains. Hence the recipe section at the back of this book rarely calls for amaranth. If you find it in your area, I encourage you to cook with it often.

TABLE 20. Grain Cooking Table:

GRAIN TYPE	Water-to-Grain Ratio	Cooking Time
Brown Rice	2 1/2 cups water to 1 cup rice	35-45 minutes
Basmati Rice	2 1/2 cups water to 1 cup rice	20-25 minutes
Polished Oriental Rice	2 cups water to to 1 cup rice	20-25 minutes
Fluffy White Rice	2 cups water to 1 cup rice	15-30 minutes
Wild Rice	4 cups water to 1 cup rice	45-60 minutes
Bulgur Wheat	1 1/4 cups water to 1 cup bulgur	15-20 minutes
Buckwheat (Kasha)	2 cups water to 1 cup buckwheat	20 minutes
Amaranth	3 cups water to 1 cup amaranth	20-30 minutes
Quinoa	2 cups water to 1 cup quinoa	20-30 minutes
Couscous	2 cups water to 1 cup couscous	5-8 minutes
Barley	3-4 cups water to 1 cup barley	15-25 minutes

The Incas of the Andes relied on quinoa as their staple grain. Quinoa, like amaranth, is highly nutritious and high in protein. Like amaranth, it is hard to find in stores.

Use either amaranth or quinoa when you need a small, delicate appearing grain for bean dishes or when stuffing vegetables.

GRAIN PRODUCTS

Grain products create the foundation for a meal. People often ask, "What is a grain product serving?" One serving equals any of the following:

- 1 slice of whole grain bread
- 1/2 cup of rice, pasta, or cooked cereal
- 3/4 cup of dry cereal

Some people shy away from grains because they worry about weight gain. Whole grains are not fattening. However, any grain product covered with fat can become fattening. And remember, dense grain products (such as pasta, barley, bulgur wheat, and pumpernickel bread) control blood sugar levels, hunger, and weight gain. So, think of new ways to use the best grain products daily.

Pasta

"Pasta!" The word speaks for itself. It's delicious, it's diverse, it's healthful and it comes in hundreds of shapes and colors. Whenever I want to make a quick meal for the family, it's pasta to the rescue! Wheat, the primary ingredient in pasta, is often mixed with small amounts of basil, tomatoes, and spinach to add color and subtle changes in flavor.

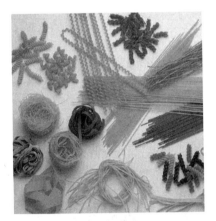

My family eats variations of pasta three to four times per week. Sometimes we make fresh pasta, or for convenience we choose typical dried pasta noodles. We serve it with vegetables and garlic, spicy stir-fry dishes, tomato sauces, or in casseroles, like eggplant lasagna.

Not only is pasta nutritious, but because of its high density it provides sustained energy. It won't make you FAT unless you pile on the fat. Avoid pasta with rich creamy sauces; they ruin the nutritional value of pasta and add inches to your waist line.

Tortillas

We eat lots of tortillas in our house for three reasons. The first reason belongs to my wife, Nicole. Although she has American and French parents, she was born and raised in Mexico. She loves tortillas; she even makes them from scratch. Second, tortillas make quick, nutritious, and easy meals. Third, our boys love them; just add some non-fat refried beans, salsa, and some non-fat cheese and in five to ten minutes everybody's happy.

Be sure to look for whole wheat or corn tortillas; then check out the ingredients, because the fat content of tortillas varies greatly. Skip those brands that have more than 20% of calories from fat or those that use excess saturated fat, such as lard.

Bread

There are three things I want to say about bread:

1. Buy whole grain breads. Whole grain bread is far more nutritious.

2. Check out the fiber content and the percent of calories from fat on the food label on the back. Fat content varies widely and some breads are startlingly high in fat.

3. Develop a preference for dense breads, such as pumpernickel.

As I noted, if you eat bread regularly, consider buying a bread machine. You can make delicious, dense, low-fat bread with a minimal fuss.

Crackers and Chips

Buyers beware–this is a BIG source of fat in the typical American diet. Don't trust the front label; "lower fat" is relative. Lower than what? Calculate the percent of calories from fat in the food table on the back of the box; it should be under 20% fat. (To discover how to calculate the percent of calories from fat, see "LEARNING THE TRUTH ABOUT FOOD LABELS" on page 156.)

Look for whole grain products. If you can't find low-fat options, consider using pita bread or whole wheat tortillas to dip into those low-fat dips. Rye crisp crackers are great "dippers"–they're nutritious, low in fat, and very tasty.

LEGUMES, BEANS, AND SOY PRODUCTS

"Beans, beans, the musical fruit. The more you eat, the more you toot."

Beans will improve your energy and health; I want you to eat more beans! They decrease elevated blood sugars, reduce high cholesterol, improve hormonal problems, and decrease cancer rates. Yet some people can't think about beans without thinking about gas. Yes, beans can produce intestinal gas, so let's deal with this problem first.

Gas

Beans contain some sugars that our intestinal enzymes can't digest. Intestinal bacteria then ferment those undigested sugars, producing gas.

People who eat beans daily report producing less gas from eating beans than people who eat beans rarely. One reason may be that the intestines learn to digest some of the fiber and sugars by producing more enzymes. Another possibility is that with time, people who eat beans regularly become less bothered by gas.

TABLE 21. Beans rated by gas production. Some beans produce more gas than others.

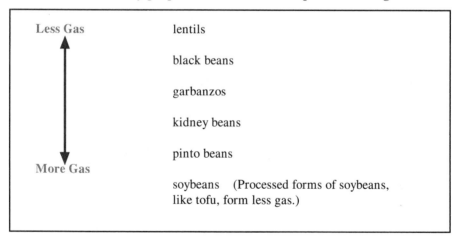

Less Gas	lentils
	black beans
	garbanzos
	kidney beans
	pinto beans
More Gas	soybeans (Processed forms of soybeans, like tofu, form less gas.)

Many of the foods in any healthy diet produce increased gas: legumes, broccoli, cabbage, onions, and garlic, to name of few. But having some gas may, in fact, be related to excellent health. Some researchers have even proposed that hydrogen gas produced in the intestines acts as an antioxidant, extinguishing intestinal free radicals.

Here are some hints to decrease gas production:

- Eat beans daily. Start with a couple of tablespoons per day and increase over time up to 1/4 to 1/2 cup of cooked beans daily.
- Rinse beans before cooking them, or rinse them out of the can.
- Try products like Beano, an enzyme sold in health food stores. Put a few drops in your food; it contains digestive enzymes that will help digest beans and decrease gas.
- Cook beans with herbs like pigweed, ragweed, or epazote. It cuts down on gas production.
- Choose beans like lentils, or soy products like tofu, that produce less gas.
- Mash beans into "refried" versions, or into hummus.
- Try eating peppers with your beans. They're reported to decrease intestinal gas and they taste great with beans.

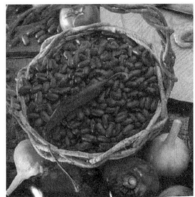

Why eat beans?

There are so many reasons why we should eat beans, I'm tempted to ask instead, "*Why shouldn't we?*" Here are just a few reasons why beans are friendly:

1. Daily servings of beans decrease lipid and cholesterol levels. Multiple scientific studies show that beans reduce bad LDL cholesterol levels and increase good HDL cholesterol levels. In simple words, eating beans helps to decrease your chances of heart attacks and strokes.

2. Beans have a low glycemic index. Adding beans will help to control your blood sugar levels after meals and decrease excess insulin production. Eating more beans makes you feel full, and helps you lose weight.

3. Soybeans contain high levels of *phytoestrogens* (plant estrogens that block some of the harmful effects from animal produced hormones). Soybeans appear to decrease the cancer-causing effects of estrogens on women's tissues. This helps explain why women who eat more soy products have lower rates of breast cancer. This makes sense, as high estrogen stimulation increases breast cancer rates.

4. All beans supply us with fiber and antioxidants. They are also low in fat. Therefore, beans help to decrease cancer rates.

6. Beans are a bargain. Even canned beans cost little. Dried beans that you soak and cook cost even less. Help your budget and your waistline–eat more beans!

How to add beans to your daily diet

Since beans are great for your health, I recommend you eat 1/4-1/2 cup of cooked beans per day. Keep cooked beans in the refrigerator and add them to meals. Our refrigerator at home always has a Tupperware container filled with beans. We spoon them into salads, soups, stir-fry dishes, or casseroles every day.

Keep different types of beans on hand. Store cooked lentils for soups or side dishes. Choose mashed garbanzos or refried beans for spreads on sandwiches rather than mayonnaise, butter, or margarine. Non-fat refried beans and low-fat hummus (mashed garbanzo beans) are delicious, especially with tomato, lettuce, sprouts, and whatever else you need to make a great sandwich.

Try soy products as another source of legumes. Soy hot dogs are a lot tastier than they used to be. Other forms of veggie hot dogs vary in quality and taste, so shop around. They make for easy snacks for children or adults.

You can find veggie burgers in most stores and even in some fast-food restaurants. They're usually made with soy protein or a combination of beans, nuts and grains. A veggie burger sandwich with tomato, lettuce, and mustard, and a piece of fruit makes an easy, nutritious lunch. You can also buy soy sausages and patties for breakfast, and even soy pepperoni, which my boys love in sandwiches.

TABLE 22. Dr. Masley's Bean Scores: **Bean scores were calculated by rating and scoring beans for antioxidant content, fiber content, less gas production, zinc content, and iron content.**

BEAN TYPE	Dr. Masley's Score
Soy bean products	100
Lentils	86
Refried beans	69
Black beans	65
Garbanzo beans	65
Split peas	57
Kidney beans	57
Pinto beans	57

To cook dried beans, start by soaking them overnight. Soak one part beans to five parts water. In the morning, pour out the water and rinse well. Then, bring to a boil and simmer with the water quantities listed in the next table.

TABLE 23. **Dried Bean Cooking Tips:**

Bean Type	Water to Bean Ratio	Cooking Time
Black beans	4 to 1	2 Hours
Black-eyed peas	3 to 1	1 Hour
Garbanzo beans	4 to 1	3 Hours
Kidney beans	4 to 1	1-2 Hours
Lentils	3 to 1	30-60 Minutes
Pinto beans	4 to 1	2-3 Hours
Soy beans	4 to 1	2-3 Hours
Split peas	3 to 1	45-60 Minutes

SOY PRODUCTS

Soybeans are a special type of legume. The Chinese and Japanese have used soy products for thousands of years as a staple in their diet. Some of the health benefits of a Japanese diet relate to eating soy products daily.

Soybeans provide an excellent form of low-fat protein. They are high in calcium and are a good source of fiber. Soy oil, however, is 70% saturated and polyunsaturated fat, and should be restricted until we know more about it's long-term health impact on us.

As we noted previously, soy products are very effective in improving blood sugar and LDL cholesterol levels. People with diabetes or high cholesterol levels in particular should use more soy products in their diet.

Japanese researchers note that soy products reduce cholesterol oxidation in our blood vessels by about 50%. Since soy products are a staple in the Japanese diet, this provides yet another explanation why the Japanese enjoy the world's greatest longevity rates.

During clinical studies in Australia, soy products significantly reduced hot flashes in women after menopause. That's because soy products contain phytoestrogens (plant like estrogens) that work with our tissue estrogen receptors. Phytoestrogens may inhibit some of the harmful actions of human estrogens.

Usually, you need at least two ounces of soy products per day to decrease hot flash symptoms. Fermented soy products lose some of their phytoestrogen activity. Therefore, soy flour has the highest phytoestrogen activity, and tofu and miso have less. Unlike hormone replacement therapy, it is not known if the phytoestrogens in soy products help prevent calcium loss from bones.

Benefits from Eating Soy Products

- Decreases cholesterol levels.
- Decreases rates of breast cancer.
- Improves blood sugar levels and helps control insulin production.
- Decreases hot flashes when used daily.
- Decreases rates of death from prostate cancer.
- Influences vaginal cells after menopause to return to a more premenopausal state.
- Contains many antioxidants.

Of interest, while Japanese men have a lower death rate from prostate cancer, they have the same occurrence rate of prostate cancer as American men. It appears that soy products specifically <u>inhibit</u> the growth of prostate cancer cells.

There are even reports that a diet rich in soy products and low in animal fats slows hair loss (balding) in men. I haven't found any well controlled studies to support this yet, but it is an intriguing idea.

I've had a stream of male patients who return thanking me for turning them on to eating soy products daily for several reasons:

- They curb their hunger.
- They note better blood sugar and cholesterol levels.
- They can take control and decrease their chance of suffering from prostate cancer.

Tofu

Tofu (also called bean curd) is an extremely versatile source of protein and vitamins, and has been a staple of the Oriental diet for over 1,000 years. It is made from soybeans, and looks at a glance like cheese.

Yet, despite its proven health benefits, many westerners cringe at the thought of eating plain tofu–it's fairly tasteless. The trick lies in knowing what to do with it. Tofu absorbs the flavors around it like a sponge, so you can blend it with other ingredients to form a dip or spread. Or you can toss it in the blender with fruit to make a shake, marinate it with spices and sauté for a stir-fry, or drop it into a soup to soak up multiple flavors. Tofu's strength comes from its versatility.

The most common mistake people make when buying tofu is to put it directly in the refrigerator in its package. One week later, untouched, people note that it has turned sour. Tofu needs the water changed to remain fresh. Open the package and rinse the tofu. Then place it in the refrigerator in a container immersed with fresh water. Change the water daily or every other day until you use it.

Tofu's fat content varies considerably, from 35% to 65% of calories from fat. Fortunately, tofu fat provides a rich source of healthy omega-3 fats. Usually a dish contains only a small amount of tofu, combined with rice or noodles and vegetables so that the overall calorie content of a meal remains easily under 20% fat.

I prefer flavored tofu to plain tofu, and it marinates extremely well. Usually I rinse the tofu with cold water, cut it in half, and put it in two Tupperware containers. The first I flavor with Mediterranean spices: balsamic vinegar, Italian herbs (Thyme, oregano, basil, sage), and of course, crushed garlic. Then I add a little water until the tofu is completely immersed and put it in the refrigerator. I will use this in a pasta-veggie meal later.

In the second container, I add garlic, ginger, soy sauce, and rice vinegar and save it for a stir-fry. If I want something spicy hot, I'll also add chile, tabasco sauce, or chile paste; tofu absorbs chile flavors nicely. Now I have tasty, flavored tofu, ready to be put into a dish at the last minute. Just keep it in the refrigerator. The vinegars help preserve the tofu from spoiling and turning sour. If you don't use it within two days, consider changing the marinade and water.

Products that contain soybeans:

- Miso (a soup broth, beware of the salt content)
- Tofu
- Soy flour
- Textured soy products, like soy hot dogs, soy bologna, soy veggie burgers, and soy sausage.

HERBS, SPICES, AND CONDIMENTS

A healthy meal needn't be bland–in fact, the tastier it is, the more incentive we'll have for making it again. That's one reason why spices have a definite role in my recipes. We might cut out certain fats in our meals, but we can add spices and condiments to flavor our foods. Herbs and spices are not always hot; mint and cilantro can cool off a hot tongue.

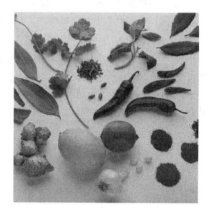

Spices, even dried ones, are loaded with antioxidants and vitamins; they are terrific for us. Spices lose both their flavors and their nutrient values if left exposed to light, so place your spices in a drawer or cabinet away from heat and light. Often a rack or lazy-susan, sorted alphabetically, helps you to sort your spices so you can quickly find them.

GARLIC

Garlic is a modern-day wonder food with ancient origins. The Egyptians used garlic for 5,000 years. It was more than an important food source–it was used to treat a variety of illnesses when the pyramids were being built. Later, Hippocrates and the ancient Greeks hailed garlic as a wonder drug for many ailments.

Today, we find garlic both in the medicine cabinet and in the kitchen. It's no coincidence that garlic figures prominently in French, Italian, Greek, Mexican, Thai, Indian, and Chinese cooking.

Health Benefits of Garlic

Eating garlic increases HDL cholesterol levels and decreases LDL cholesterol levels. Garlic's antioxidant activity can also reduce the oxidation of LDL cholesterol into plaque. The result–cleaner arteries.

Garlic also helps prevent our blood platelets from sticking together. When platelets clump, they form clots that block blood flow, leading to strokes and heart attacks. Garlic's anti-clotting factor helps keep our arterial blood flow open.

Garlic is now being studied for its cancer-fighting benefits. How it works is still unclear, but a variety of laboratory studies reveal that garlic oil decreases tumor growth in human tissues. Garlic also seems to improve the immune response, which can fight infections and deter cancer cells from spreading.

Raw garlic has properties that fight infections and kill bacteria. Cooking garlic neutralizes its infection-controlling properties, but cooked garlic still benefits the lipid, antioxidant, and platelet activities.

Cooking with garlic

When shopping for garlic, be sure it feels firm to the touch. When cooking with garlic, break the cloves apart, place a clove under a flat wooden spoon, or carefully under the flat blade of a knife, and pound with force. After being pounded, the skin peels off easily.

Dice it finely, or pass it through a garlic press. When sautéing with oil, be careful not to overcook. Like an onion, you want it to soften and turn golden but not brown. Garlic sautés well with ginger, herbs, tomatoes, and veggies.

To bake, put a whole head of garlic in the oven. Later pop out the juicy cloves from their skins and use as a spread, or blend the garlic into a soup or a sauce. Roasted garlic is delightful and has a sweeter flavor than when sautéed.

A few people complain of smelly fingers after chopping garlic. If so, rinse them with a dash of lemon juice, or use a garlic press.

One suggestion for using fresh garlic daily is to add one clove of garlic per person to your salad dressing. Garlic adds a wonderful zesty flavor to salads. Raw garlic goes great in dips. You can even buy convenient, pre-diced garlic in a jar, ready to spoon on your food. Use prepared garlic while it is fresh, as I find the flavor goes bad quickly.

Garlic odor and gas

Just watch out for the quantity of garlic you use. Use less garlic if you are sensitive. If you don't like to eat garlic, you can get the same lipid and platelet benefits by taking garlic capsules daily. Look for them in a pharmacy or health food store.

If people notice an odor about you after eating garlic, you probably don't eat it often enough. I believe that odor problems come from eating garlic infrequently. There are many reports that your body will increase the digestive enzymes that process garlic if it's eaten more regularly.

Start with 1/4 clove of garlic per day, cooked lightly with meals. Slowly increase that to 1/2 clove per day the second week, 3/4 of a clove per person per day the third week, and then try one clove of garlic daily for a month. Usually, there will be no odor problems at the end of that time. If it persists, you can accept the aroma, or take garlic capsules instead. I personally enjoy crushing, peeling, and serving 4-6 cloves of garlic with almost every meal I cook for my family of four.

Use good judgment when serving garlic to guests. Not everybody can tolerate 2-3 cloves of garlic in his or her meal without developing significant intestinal gas. In particular, fresh, uncooked garlic can induce intestinal gas for non-garlic eaters. When I use uncooked garlic in a vinaigrette dressing or a dip, I either cut the usual amount of garlic in half, or I sauté the garlic lightly first, and then toss it in. This decreases the chance of an intestinal surprise.

GINGER

Ginger adds a zesty, citrus flavor to food and it goes very well with Indian curries, Oriental stir-fries, desserts, and marmalades. Not only does ginger improve the flavor of many foods, but it is good for us. Two thousand years ago, the Chinese made ginger a staple in their health repertoire. Today we are continuing to learn how ginger can spice up our meals and improve our health.

Health benefits of ginger

We've recently learned that ginger contains several potent antioxidants. Like garlic, this spice decreases platelet stickiness and helps prevent unwanted blood clot formation. These heart-friendly features of ginger should encourage people (especially those with heart or cholesterol problems) to use a teaspoon of ginger in their food daily.

Ginger also decreases nausea and vomiting, whether the cause is the flu, seasickness, pregnancy, or medication upsets. Try an infusion (tea) with 1-2 teaspoons of crushed ginger root brewed in near-boiling water once or twice per day.

Ginger can also relieve joint pain and arthritis. Used regularly over weeks, it provides anti-inflammatory activity and helps relieve arthritis-induced joint pain and even cases of rheumatoid arthritis.

In contrast to most anti-inflammatory medications, ginger does not increase the risk of stomach ulcers. In fact, people use ginger to treat stomach ulcers. This appears to be a great boon for people who have both arthritis problems and stomach ulcers!

Cooking with ginger

For Indian and Oriental dishes, I like to peel off the skin and dice 1-2 teaspoons of ginger to serve 4 people. I slice the ginger root into match-stick shapes and then cut them in half lengthwise.

At home, we often add ginger to tea. Dice one teaspoon of ginger root or pass it through a garlic press and add to 2-4 cups of hot water. Let it brew or add tea bags or other herbs and spices.

Some people find that ginger root dries when refrigerated. If you put it in a jar with sherry or white wine, its flavor will last for months. You can also freeze ginger and grate it when needed.

LEMON AND LIME

Lemon and lime juice add great flavor to a variety of dishes, from guacamole dip, to steamed broccoli, to bulgur wheat and rice casseroles. I use them interchangeably in recipes, depending on what we have on hand. Lemon juice is slightly less tart and sweeter. My wife prefers lime juice for its tartness. We buy a dozen lemons or limes every couple of weeks and we invariably run out.

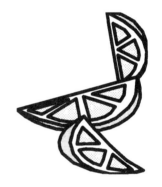

Lemon and lime juices are packed with Vitamin C and are good sources of folic acid. Cooking reduces Vitamin C content, so add your juice just before serving.

Many dishes call for lemon or lime peel. Wash them well before grating, and whenever possible, try to buy organic produce if you are using citrus peel as pesticides can be concentrated in the peel.

HERBS

Green herbs are an essential part of flavoring a dish. Most popular cuisines (whether Mexican, French, Chinese, Italian, or Indian) use herbs to accentuate the flavors in recipes

Green herbs add another important source of antioxidants to our diet and are often rich in Vitamin C and omega-3 fats. Rosemary, in particular, provides rich sources of antioxidants. Try to sprinkle herbs, fresh or dried, on your food daily.

"Herbes de Provence" (thyme, oregano, rosemary, sage, basil)

These are similar to Fine Herbs and Italian Herbs. This is my favorite mixture of herbs and comes in a dried or fresh combination.

I sprinkle this combination on most French, Italian, Mexican, or Greek meals I make. These herbs sauté very well with garlic and the combined aromas make a welcoming fragrance for arriving guests. In the recipe section, I call for Italian Herbs in place of Herbes de Provence only because they are easier to find in grocery stores.

At home, we grow these herbs in the garden, and I love snipping fresh twigs into my basket while something simmers in the kitchen. My wife's cousin in Paris always has a few pots of thyme and oregano growing on the window sill of her kitchen, which provide tasty garnishes and flavors for her meals.

Cilantro (Fresh Green Coriander)

This leafy herb has a tangy flavor and adds a welcome rich green color to sauces and grain dishes. We keep it in a sealed Tupperware container flat with a little water in the refrigerator, and by changing the water every few days, it can easily last a week. Cilantro goes particularly well with Indian, Chinese, and Mexican dishes.

Parsley

Parsley is a versatile herb and can be used in an assortment of dishes and salads. Alas, too often it is pushed to the edge of a plate and treated like an inedible garnish. But parsley should be a featured attraction on the dinner plate. It's full of antioxidants, including Vitamin C, several carotenoids, and flavonoids. You can mix it in with your food, or squeeze lemon or lime juice on it and sprinkle it into a salad.

Parsley is wonderful with tomatoes, garlic, basil, and a splash of fine olive oil. Or you can combine it with cooked bulgur wheat, tomatoes, and lime juice. When you cook with parsley, dice it fine and add it no more than two minutes before serving, or it will lose both its flavor and nutritional value.

OTHER FLAVORS

Mustard

Mustard is a tasty, low-fat spice that adds a rich tartness to food. It's usually spread on sandwiches–a superior alternative to using fatty mayonnaise, butter or margarine.

Mustard goes well in salad dressings, dips, and marinades. Often 1/2 to one teaspoon of mustard will give a non-fat vinaigrette salad dressing a creamy texture.

Vinegar

Although vinegar can be used for a variety of purposes, it is woefully under-utilized in our American cuisine. Vinegar can add a wonderful tartness and flavor to salads and steamed vegetables. It can also serve as an oil-free substitute when stir-frying vegetables.

Most salad dressings are 1/3 vinegar and 2/3 oil. My own formula for a pasta or vegetable salad dressing is very low in oil, but delicious and healthy.

> *I combine two tablespoons (Tbs) of vinegar (usually balsamic), one Tbs lemon juice, one Tbs wine, and one Tbs extra virgin olive oil with a teaspoon of mustard, a dash of dried herbs, and a dash of soy sauce. This recipe cuts out most of the fat, and to me, enhances the dressing's overall flavor.*

I found that in a tossed green salad, with limited calories and delicate flavors, even that much oil seems excessive, so I took out the oil completely. The mustard provides some creamy texture, and if you want more, add some non-fat yogurt. Try it–you might add it to your list of favorite dressings!

CURRY SPICES

So far, we've flavored food with garlic, ginger, and herbs. Then, we mixed in mustard dressings, lemon and lime juices, and vinegars. Now it's time to add spice to our food. Who says that without fat, food can't taste great?

Spice provides balance, depth of flavor, and punch to the taste of our food. There are hundreds of spices, but I'd like to concentrate on curry spices.

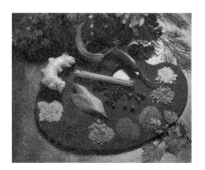

Curry spices offer a blend of exotic, antioxidant rich spices that once combined, form the foundation for a spicy stew. Curry powder combines a variety of ground spices including coriander, cumin, turmeric, cardamom, ginger, anise, cinnamon, cloves, nutmeg, and chile. In my home, we make curry dishes 3-4 times per month and combine ingredients to create the taste we want. However, if you rarely make curries, you are better off buying a pre-made mixture of curry powder.

With a curry dish, we usually serve a dhal dish (lentils), raita (a yogurt dish with onions and cucumber), a fruit chutney, and a grain choice (usually rice or chapatis; we often substitute whole wheat tortillas for chapatis). Each component has its purpose: chutneys add a sweet-and-sour flavor, the raita provides a mouth saving retreat if you bite into something hot, and the onions, cucumbers and yogurt all help neutralize the fires from hot chiles.

A curry dinner with all the trimmings provides a feast for company, especially as they are rarely prepared in most homes. Serve it with tea. For dessert, offer freshly made frozen yogurt with mango or berries.

Chile & Cayenne

These hot peppers flavor food for much of the world. Not only are chiles flavorful, they are used medicinally in many countries. Hot chile peppers open sinus and respiratory passages. Hot mustards do the same. For a cold with congestion and drainage, try a hot spicy curry, spicy Mexican food, or a Thai meal. Suddenly, you can breathe again! Chile spice once or twice a day is good for people with chronic allergies. The spice stimulates your respiratory passages to "water," which clears out mucous. Try it the next time you have a cold.

If your stomach is sensitive to chile spices, avoid them. A word of caution; Be careful handling chiles during their preparation. Do not touch chiles and then touch delicate skin areas, especially around the face; this could cause a painful skin irritation. For extra hot chiles, wear gloves to protect your skin.

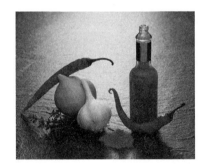

Paprika is a flavorful pepper, but is not spicy hot. If you want the flavor of peppers without the chile burn, use paprika instead. Many eastern Mediterranean dishes depend upon this mild flavor. You can also use it in curries in place of hot peppers.

NUTS AND SEEDS

In small quantities, nuts and seeds can enhance the appearance and taste of a meal. They are also a good source of fiber, zinc, Vitamin E, omega-3 fats, and calcium.

However, nuts and seeds are loaded with fat. Many nuts contain 85% to 95% of their calories as fat. The next time you reach for a handful of nuts, remember that their fat content is equivalent to several tablespoons of oil.

Chestnuts

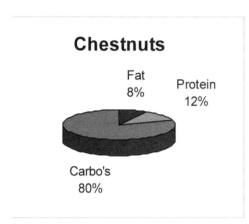

Chestnuts, on the other hand, are a great food source. Of the nuts, only chestnuts are low in fat, with 8% of their calories as fat. I have wonderful memories of walking home from work in Geneva, Switzerland, munching from a bag of sidewalk roasted chestnuts. At the time, I had no idea what a great food source they were. Chestnuts contain the good balance of calories for a meal, with fat under 10%, protein 10-15%, and the rest complex carbohydrates.

You can make great nut roasts and desserts with chestnuts. Look for them in late fall and early winter. The quality varies greatly in stores, so choose your chestnuts carefully. Pick firm nuts, and beware of any mold growing on the shell.

Other Nuts

Since most nuts are very high in fat, the nut scores reflect which nuts are low in saturated and polyunsaturated fat. If you use nuts, serve them with other foods to reduce the percentage of calories from fat.

Chopped cashew nuts, pecans, macadamia nuts, and hazelnuts can be an attractive and healthy addition to many dishes if used in small quantities, such as one to two tablespoons per person. Avoid eating nuts by the handful if you are concerned with calories or weight gain because of their high caloric value. Sometimes I lightly sauté or heat nuts in the microwave just to warm them and serve them as hors d'oeuvres along with veggies or sushi rice rolls. I limit the quantity to two tablespoons per person; just enough to bring out their warm, hearty flavor.

For the normal weight person, nuts can provide a healthy snack. Studies that assess nut intake have repeatedly noted that a greater dietary intake of nuts is associated with improved lipid levels and with decreased death rates and heart attack rates. Most diet programs restrict any use of nuts because they are high in fat. Yet, nuts provide a rich source of omega-3 fats, monounsaturated fats, and Vitamin E–all of which are good for you. So, although nuts are high in fat, it should not surprise you that eating nuts seems to prevent heart problems, and that I encourage you to have a limited quantity of nuts daily.

Almonds

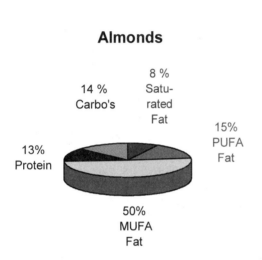

In Dr. Kushi's study on over 34,000 women, eating more nuts was associated with a 40% reduction in the risk of dying from coronary heart disease. Similarly, Dr. Frazer found in a study on over 31,000 Adventists in California that eating more nuts was associated with a 50% reduction in the risk of a heart attack or a death related to coronary heart disease.

Slivered almonds taste great sprinkled over dishes, and give a dish elegance. If you limit the garnish to one tablespoon per serving, you won't add lots of fat. Almonds also contain a rich source of Vitamin E, a potent antioxidant. Part of the polyunsaturated fat (PUFA) content in almonds is represented by good omega-3 fats.

Look at Table 24 for my favorite nuts. The best nuts contain a higher percentage of monounsaturated fat and omega-3 fat, less polyunsaturated fat, and far less saturated fat. This leaves peanuts, the most popular nut in the United States, rated lower. (Technically, peanuts are legumes rather than true nuts, but I've included them with nuts because we use them as such in the kitchen.)

Nut butters fall in the same order, with almond butter, hazelnut butter, and cashew butter on top. Not only are these good for you, but they taste fantastic with toast in the morning, or as a snack. Because of their high fat content, I limit their intake in my own diet to one teaspoon per serving on a piece of toast.

Nuts and Seeds	Dr. Masley's Scores
Chestnuts	100
Almonds	78
Hazel Nuts	75
Cashews	73
Sesame Seeds	68
Pecans	65
Pumpkin and Squash Seeds	65
Sunflower Seeds	62
Walnuts	59
Macadamia Nuts	59
Brazil Nuts	59
Peanuts	56
Pine Nuts	43
Coconut	30

TABLE 24. **Dr. Masley's Nut Scores:** Nut scores reflect total fat content, the type of fat content (monounsaturated fat and omega-3 fat is preferred), plus calcium and zinc content. A higher score reflects healthier nut choices.

FATS AND OILS

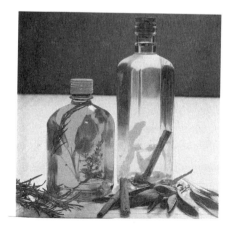

MONOUNSATURATED OILS

Canola and olive oil are high in monounsaturated fats. These oils are not entirely monounsaturated, yet they are as healthy as we can get. Remember, monounsaturated fats decrease bad LDL cholesterol and prevent LDL cholesterol from oxidizing into plaque in our arteries. Populations (such as those in Southern Europe) that use them as their primary source of oil have been blessed with good health. However, I believe we still need to limit our use of good oils to a maximum of 20% of total calories. Fat has lots of calories, so eating even good fat can result in weight gain.

Medical terms for monounsaturated oils can be tricky. Oleic acid is the most common scientific term for monounsaturated fat. You may see these terms exchanged in both the lay media and in medical journals. Monounsaturated fatty acids are commonly abbreviated as MUFAs.

When I look at the type of fat and oil in food, I look at their quantity of bad fat and good fat. That's what you see in the following pie charts for different oils. The combined polyunsaturated fat, saturated fat, and trans fat together should be less than 40%. (You only find trans fats in processed foods like margarines, not in natural oils such as olive oil or peanut oil.) The higher the amount of bad fats, the faster you should run from it.

Canola Oil

Canola oil comes from rapeseed. It contains mostly monounsaturated fat and a small amount of alpha linolenic acid (an omega-3 fatty acid). Omega-3 fatty acids help prevent blood clots, decrease LDL cholesterol levels, and may decrease sudden death heart problems. In contrast to olive oil, canola oil has a much milder taste and can be used for baking, or in dishes in which you do not want the taste of olive oil.

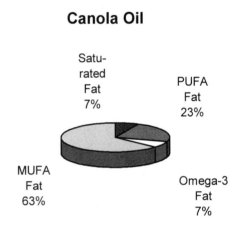

My wife and I use canola oil to make Japanese, Chinese and Thai stir-fries. We also bake with it. New margarines feature canola oil, and soon may be produced without harmful trans fats. Canola oil doesn't burn and oxidize as quickly as other oils at higher temperatures, so it's a good choice for stir-fries. Always avoid burning oil when you cook. Not only will you ruin the flavor, but you'll oxidize the oil, generating free radicals that can adversely affect your health.

Combined Saturated fat + Polyunsaturated fat = 30%. (Hence, it's mostly good fat.)

Olive Oil

Olive oil is wonderful, offering a variety of flavors, colors, and quality. Best of all, it's heart-healthy. Olive oil has the highest percentage (75%) of monounsaturated fat.

Not only does it help decrease your harmful LDL cholesterol levels; it helps prevent LDL cholesterol from being oxidized, as well.

Olive oil producers make olive oil by squeezing olives. The first squeeze produces extra virgin olive oil, the second squeeze, virgin olive oil, and the last squeezes, regular olive oil. During the final presses, they heat the olives to extract their remaining oil. The character of the oil in later presses is altered by the heat.

The extra virgin oils seem to have a lighter, richer taste. It's easier to tell the difference when olive oil is used in a salad dressing. The salads in the recipe section of this book contain a maximum of 1/4 olive oil; go for the extra virgin oil–since you are saving on quantity you can afford to splurge on quality!

Because it is a fat, I use virgin olive oil sparingly to sauté garlic and veggies. I limit the quantity to a teaspoon or less per person per serving. I have a second extra virgin bottle for salad dressings.

Buy all oils, but olive oil especially, in small containers and keep in a cool, dark cupboard. If you buy oil in bulk, refrigerate, as oils oxidize and turn rancid with time. Oil will solidify in the refrig-erator, but will re-liquefy once warmed to room temperature.

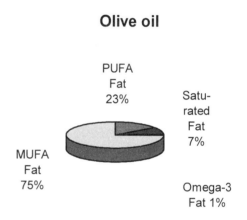

Olive oil

PUFA Fat 23%

Satu-rated Fat 7%

MUFA Fat 75%

Omega-3 Fat 1%

Different regions of the world produce different types of olive oils. Try a variety from Italy, Greece, France, Spain, and now California to discover your favorites.

Combined Saturated fat + Polyunsaturated fat = 30%. (Hence, it's mostly good fat)

POLYUNSATURATED FATS AND OILS

We produce polyunsaturated fats by processing grain and legume products like corn, soybeans, and peanuts. Trans fats act like saturated fats (butter, lard) and are added to polyunsaturated oils to make them soft and spreadable at room temperature.

For the many reasons outlined on pages in the Fat section, we should limit food sources that are high in polyunsaturated fats–especially when we can use olive oil and canola oil in their place. We should also avoid spreads that contain trans fats.

The following pie charts display mostly polyunsaturated fats. Notice that their combined saturated fat and polyunsaturated fat content is always greater than 40%.

Soybean Oil

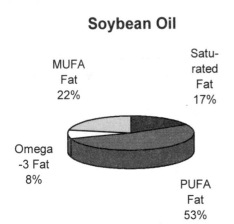

MUFA Fat 22%

Satu-rated Fat 17%

Omega -3 Fat 8%

PUFA Fat 53%

Soybean Oil

In time we may learn that soybean oil, because of its omega-3 fat content, improves health. However for now, because of soybean's high polyunsaturated fat content, I recommend avoiding it.

Combined saturated fat + polyunsaturated fat (PUFA) = 70%. (Too much bad fat)

Peanut Oil

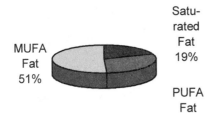

MUFA Fat 51%

Satu-rated Fat 19%

PUFA Fat 30%

Peanut Oil

Of the polyunsaturated oils, peanut oil has the most monounsaturated fat. It should be avoided because it still contains 49% saturated and polyunsaturated fat and no omega-3 fat.

Combined saturated fat + polyunsaturated fat (PUFA) = 49% (Too much bad fat)

Corn Oil

Corn oil contains 82% saturated and polyunsaturated fat. <u>Avoid corn oil whenever possible.</u>

Combined saturated fat + polyunsaturated fat (PUFA) = 82%.

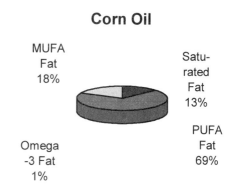

Corn Oil

MUFA Fat 18%

Saturated Fat 13%

Omega-3 Fat 1%

PUFA Fat 69%

SATURATED FAT

Saturated fats abound in animal fats. Pork, chicken, and beef have similar fat percentages, and yes, even chicken fat is high in saturated fat! Many dairy products have more saturated fat than meat.

Remember, eating saturated fat adds an enormous quantity of unhealthy calories to our diet, causes us to gain weight. It increases our blood levels of LDL cholesterol and decreases our blood levels of HDL cholesterol, forming plaque in our vessels. Further, it makes our blood sticky and sluggish, forming clots that can block the blood flow in our arteries.

Beef Fat

MUFA Fat 45%

Saturated Fat 49%

Omega-3 Fat 3%

PUFA Fat 3%

Regular moderate exercise, 5-10 hours per week, counters some of the negative impacts of eating saturated fat. However, even if you do exercise daily, I recommend that you limit your saturated fat intake greatly.

DAIRY PRODUCTS

Dairy products provide essential nutrition to infants. Yet in all the animal kingdom, only humans continue to use milk after infancy. Although dairy products, especially ice cream and fatty cheeses, are popular worldwide, they can also be harmful.

THE PROBLEM WITH DAIRY FATS

Fat

Clearly, high fat dairy products can do us harm. Even "2% milk" has more than 35% of total energy as fat. Unlike olive and canola oil, MOST DAIRY FAT IS 66% SATURATED FAT. Dairy products supply much of the saturated fat in American diets.

Did you know that the dairy industry has bypassed the normal food labeling process, with the help of Congress? It counts fat by weight, not by percent of calories. Since most of the weight in milk is water, this results in a deceptively low percentage. A look at Tables 25 and 26 will probably surprise, if not shock you!

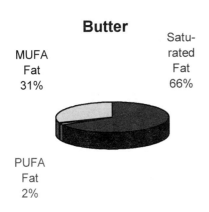

Butter

MUFA Fat 31%

Satu-rated Fat 66%

PUFA Fat 2%

If we must use dairy products, we should use those products with less than 20% of calories from fat.

Really "low fat" dairy products include non-fat and skim dairy products. Cheeses made from 1% milk contain around 20-23% of their calories from fat. Fortunately, many other non-fat and "truly low-fat" cheeses are appearing in the grocery store. Of course, you can sprinkle one teaspoon to one tablespoon of grated cheese on top of a dish without making the meal high-fat. Regular parmesan is delicious and easy to grate. Or, buy non-fat parmesan grated cheese or a low-fat cheese to grate over your meal.

A warning on baking non-fat cheeses: These don't melt as well at high temperatures. Therefore, sprinkle on less cheese, bake for less time, and reduce the heat by 25-50 degrees when baking dishes with non-fat cheeses.

TABLE 25. Dairy Fat Comparison by Percentage of Fat.

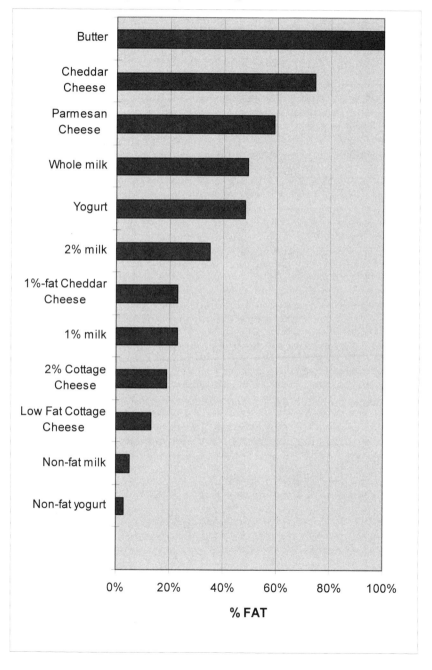

DAIRY FAT CONTENT			
1 Cup Serving	Saturated Fat	Total Fat	% Calories as Fat
Whole Milk	5.1 grams	8.2 grams	49%
2 % Milk	2.9 grams	4.7 grams	35%
1 % Milk	1.6 grams	2.6 grams	23%
Nonfat (Skim) Milk	0.3 grams	0.4 grams	5%

TABLE 26. Grams of Fat in Milk: Note the difference between the claim "2% Milk" and its actual percent of calories from fat!

Lactose Intolerance

Lactose is the primary sugar in milk and dairy products. To digest lactose without difficulty, we need lactase, an enzyme. Lactose intolerance can cause chronic intestinal problems, such as bloating, excess gas, and abdominal cramping. If you have chronic intestinal problems, try omitting dairy products for a month to see if your condition improves.

Most of the world's adult population lacks adequate lactase to digest dairy products regularly. Eighty percent of people in certain parts of the world (Native Americans, Asia, Africa) develop intestinal complaints with regular dairy consumption. People with northern European ancestors tend to have fewer problems from dairy products.

Yogurt and cheese have lower lactose levels and are better tolerated than milk and ice cream.

Milk Allergy

A milk allergy is more serious than lactose intolerance: it can actually make you sick. A milk allergy means you are so allergic to milk protein, you can't even eat yogurt. In addition to intestinal problems, there can be flushing, rashes, and more. Fortunately, this condition is very rare.

THE BENEFITS OF DAIRY PRODUCTS

Calcium Source

Dairy foods are a good source of calcium. Young women who ingest more calcium have stronger, denser bones than young women who have low calcium intake. Forming strong bones early in life (ages 12-25) helps prevent osteoporosis and debilitating fractures later in life.

Other excellent sources of calcium include soy products, green leafy vegetables and whole grains. Dairy products remain the most common dietary source of calcium in the United States. Look to Table 4 on page 19 to estimate your calcium intake.

Vitamin B-12 Source

Vitamin B-12 is an essential vitamin and dairy products are a convenient source. It is vital to your nervous system and blood cells. If you don't eat or drink any animal products, take a Vitamin B-12 supplement, or check your Vitamin B-12 blood level annually.

Vitamin D Source

Vitamin D plays a critical role in forming strong bones. It is added to dairy products, just as it is added to One-A-Day Vitamins and many breakfast cereals, like "Total" and "Product 19." Sunshine exposure on the skin also stimulates Vitamin D production. In fact, 15 minutes of sunshine on your hands and face during three separate exposures each week is adequate to form all the Vitamin D you need.

YOGURT AND LACTOBACILLI

Of all the dairy products, yogurt is the healthiest. Yogurt is loaded with lactobacilli. These friendly bacteria consume the lactose sugar in milk, and convert milk to yogurt. As the lactobacilli increase, the lactose sugars disappear. The Hindus in Asia have used yogurt both as food source and medicinally for thousands of years.

Lactobacillus bacteria live within our intestines whether we eat yogurt or not, protecting us from harmful bacteria. Medical treatments with antibiotics often decrease the amount of lactobacillus bacteria in our intestines and cause intestinal problems. In some cases, non-pasteurized (live) yogurt can be used to treat intestinal problems as the microscopic-sized living lactobacillus bacteria restore the normal intestinal tract environment.

Acidophilus, a type of lactobacillus, is commonly added to milk and other dairy products. Acidophilus kills bad bacteria and helps prevent intestinal infections. Several studies indicate that it may also enhance our immune systems by stimulating white blood cell activity.

Lactobacillus bacteria also convert chemical compounds (ligans) from fiber sources into active compounds that fight cancer. Eventually, we may develop lactobacillus strains that can actually remove cholesterol from our intestines.

Lactobacillus is also the predominant bacteria in the vagina. When they decrease in number, vaginal discharge and irritation may follow. Some medical practitioners use lactobacillus vaginal suppositories to help restore the normal bacteria and decrease vaginal irritation, especially during courses of antibiotics. You can find these live lactobacillus treatments in health food stores and even in some pharmacies.

As a food choice, I'll take yogurt over any other dairy product. Non-fat yogurt is great for dips and sauces. I love to mix it with lemon juice, herbs, mustard, or soy sauce to form a variety of veggie dips.

If you have a whim for ice cream at times, use non-fat frozen yogurt instead. You can add yogurt to dishes at the last moment, like curries, to provide a creamy sauce and blend the spices. In place of sour cream in soup, drop in a spoonful of non-fat yogurt; it lends a touch of tartness that you'll enjoy. However, be careful not to cook yogurt even for a few seconds, as it will curdle with heat.

EGG WHITES

Egg whites versus egg yolks

What's in egg yolks and why are they getting such bad reputations? Egg yolks contain fat and cholesterol, two additions we *don't need* in our diets. Lately, the poultry industry has improved eggs by feeding chickens seaweed and flax oil. These expensive egg yolks are not quite as bad for us. Someday, they may come up with a non-fat egg, but they haven't yet.

What's in an egg white? Good things! Egg whites are an excellent source of low-fat protein. For the average American eating a high protein diet, the true benefit of egg whites is not their nutritional content, but their versatility in baking. Beaten egg whites change a food's appearance and make it light and fluffy.

Whip egg whites into an artistic meal. Soufflés and Meringue pies are elegant, easy to make, and delicious, even without the fat. Pancakes rise better with whipped egg whites.

So what do I do with the yolk? The same thing you do with the egg shells–throw them out, or cook them for your dog or cat. (Many animals can physiologically handle cholesterol better than humans.)

ALCOHOL

Why is alcohol listed on my food pyramid? You may be surprised to learn that a moderate intake of alcohol appears to be compatible with better health. We know that alcohol increases healthy HDL cholesterol levels and decreases our risk of cardio-vascular disease.

But on the dark side, we also know that it increases our risk of high blood pressure and breast cancer. Consuming alcohol also decreases our folic acid blood levels; if you drink alcohol, make sure you eat foods rich in folic acid (beans, green leafy vegetables, citrus fruits). Alcohol can cause severe fetal defects if used during pregnancy.

Alcohol comprises a significant portion of daily calories in diets worldwide. One serving of wine per day equals 4% of all our calories, and 2 drinks per day leaps to 8% of our caloric intake. It has also been reported to slow down our metabolism and the fat-burning process. Thus, not only does alcohol add calories, but it causes weight gain.

Another negative is that some people develop headaches when they drink red wine. Red wine (like chocolate, aged cheeses, and bananas) contains tyramine, a known blood vessel dilator. If you develop migraine headaches, try avoiding these products to see if you are tyramine sensitive.

When you drink alcohol, your liver converts it to an intermediate, more toxic compound, and then converts it again to enhance its excretion. However, if you drink in excess, your liver continues to make the alcohol more toxic, but fails to keep up with the conversion. You will then unintentionally produce excess toxic, free radicals that you can't excrete. As you continue to drink, the free radicals run amuck, injuring liver and brain tissue. No wonder you have a headache and nausea the day after drinking too much alcohol!

As this book notes repeatedly, drinking more than two alcoholic beverages per day for men, or more than one for women, is harmful; drink less or don't drink. Pregnant women should not drink at all.

Overall, there appears to be a small benefit to 1-2 servings of alcohol per day. But first, lets look at a benefit / harm balance. Then, you decide.

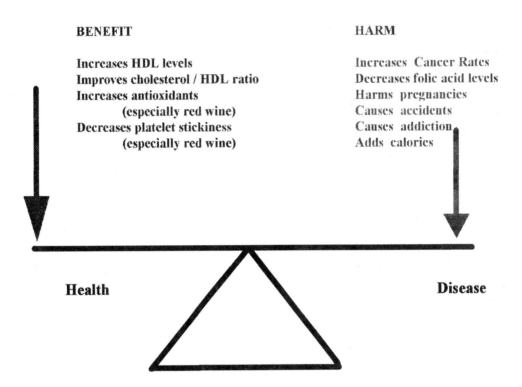

Alcohol–Pros and Cons

BENEFIT

Increases HDL levels
Improves cholesterol / HDL ratio
Increases antioxidants
(especially red wine)
Decreases platelet stickiness
(especially red wine)

HARM

Increases Cancer Rates
Decreases folic acid levels
Harms pregnancies
Causes accidents
Causes addiction
Adds calories

Health

Disease

To limit our alcohol intake at home, when I open a bottle of wine (usually red), I immediately pour half the bottle into a clean, empty half-bottle. I fill it nearly to the rim and cork it and put it back in the cupboard. Now, we have a newly opened half bottle of wine for a dinner for two, which provides about 1 to 1 1/2 glasses of wine per person. The newly full half-bottle of wine in the cupboard stores better and retains its body better than a regular bottle that's half full. That's because the half bottle of air remaining in the regular bottle contains extra oxygen which oxidizes the wine.

The recipe section of this book occasionally uses wine or other alcohol. If you wish to avoid alcohol in uncooked recipes, simply substitute non-alcoholic wine. You'll still get the flavor and some of the antioxidants, minus the alcohol. When a recipe calls for a liqueur, consider using a non-alcoholic rum or orange-flavored extract instead.

Remember, when food is cooked, you rapidly lose all the alcohol.

DESSERTS

For many of us, dessert is the climax of the meal. Yet, many desserts cause harm to our health, thanks to the overemphasis on fat and sugar. How can we eat a delicious dessert without the harm? We must learn to create desserts that are just as tasty, but at least harmless–and preferably, healthful. If we can make desserts healthful and tasty, we'll eat them more often. It's another WIN/WIN situation.

Fruit comes immediately to mind. It comes in all colors, textures, and shapes. Bake it, sauté it, blend it, or freeze it and create pies, crumbles, smoothies, sorbets, and frozen yogurts. Fruit adds natural, healthy sweetness and makes a dessert creamy when blended. Splurge and buy quality fruit for desserts!

Egg whites make desserts light and fluffy, and hold flour together. Think of meringues, angel food cake, crepes (French pancakes), and dessert soufflés.

If you use fat in a recipe, choose canola oil. You can substitute one teaspoon of canola oil for either one egg yolk or two teaspoons of butter.

CHOCOLATE

Here's a pleasant surprise: **chocolate**, in limited quantities, has a place on your dessert table!

Chocolate is soft, dark, and creamy. It tastes fantastic, yet there is more to it than great taste. Chocolate can actually make people feel better. It seems to contain several mysterious nutrients that scientists have just started to understand. For a woman, this emotional influence often gets stronger near the time of her menstrual cycle.

Yet, despite all these wonderful qualities, 50% of the calories in chocolate are from fat. Our goal when eating chocolate is to put it in balance with the rest of our diet.

Chocolate is a rich source of magnesium and provides a limited source of antioxidants. Hence chocolate provides some known benefits.

It was first used by the Mayans in Central America 500-1,000 years ago, almost exclusively by the royal class and priests. Chocolate beans were considered so valuable, they were used as currency.

Chocolate arrived in Europe in the 16th century. Initially, it was used as a drink only by royalty and the extremely wealthy. By the 1800's, improved production methods brought chocolate to the masses. And today, I doubt that anyone could remove chocolate from our lives.

Chocolate comes from the cocoa bean which grows in a pod on the cocoa tree in tropical countries. Chocolate producers process cocoa beans into different grades of chocolate. About 50% of the calories in a cocoa bean come from fat, as cocoa butter. Next they add sugar to sweeten the chocolate and vanilla to flavor it. Milk chocolate has regular milk added and all the saturated fat that comes with it.

TABLE 27. Types of Dessert Fat: Each fat portion represents nearly 60 calories. Compare total fat, saturated fat, and monounsaturated fat.

TYPE OF DESSERT FAT	Calories	Total Fat	Saturated Fat (less stearic acid)	MUFA
Canola oil (1 tsp)	60	6.8 grams	0.5 grams	4.0 grams
SemiSweet Chocolate (2 1/2 tsp)	59	3.7 grams	1.1 grams	1.2 grams
Egg Yolk (1)	59	5.1 grams	1.6 grams	2.0 grams
Butter (1 3/4 tsp)	59	6.6 grams	3.3 grams	1.9 grams
Cream (2 Tbs)	64	6.5 grams	4.1 grams	1.9 grams
Whole milk (3/8 cup)	64	3.1 grams	1.9 grams	0.9 grams

Producers of cheap chocolate sell off the cocoa butter to the cosmetic and pharmaceutical industries and replace it with inexpensive, saturated fats that raise your cholesterol levels. Next, they add extra sugar to cut the chocolate content and put in artificial vanilla instead of real vanilla. *Taste the difference* between cheap and high quality chocolate.

Most Americans eat a mass-produced form of chocolate, with the cocoa butter removed. But we can do better. To distinguish between mass-produced chocolate and fine chocolate, read the label. The first ingredient should be cocoa, which should be at least 50% plain chocolate. If sugar is listed first, watch out; it is the major ingredient in place of chocolate. Next, make sure it's made with real cocoa butter; see if they mention cocoa butter substitutes (CBSs) like vegetable oils, or animal fats. If so, look for another brand. Lastly, check whether they list pure vanilla (vanille bourbon) or artificial vanilla (vanillin). At least the artificial vanilla does not worsen your health, it only detracts from the taste. Lecithin may be added and this is fine, as it is high in Vitamin E and does not lessen the flavor.

Many studies show cocoa butter to have a neutral impact on cholesterol levels. This is an important difference from other fats. While cocoa butter is 63% saturated fat and 37% monounsaturated fat, it contains a lot *"stearic acid."* In chocolate, stearic acid represents half of the saturated fat and nearly one third of the total fat. This unusual saturated fat does not increase your bad LDL cholesterol levels the way butter, poultry or beef fat do. Stearic acid acts like a monounsaturated fat.

My program allows up to 3% of calories as saturated fat. There is room for fine chocolate in limited amounts. If I have a choice between a little, bitter-sweet chocolate on my dessert, a slice of butter with my bread, or 2% milk on my cereal I'll go for the chocolate every time.

However, just because chocolate is less harmful than butter doesn't mean you should go out and eat it by the handful. Chocolate is high in fat, and fattening.

How to use chocolate

Cooking with chocolate is fun. Melt it slowly in a double boiler. A pan placed in simmering water works great. Drop the chocolate into the pan and watch it slowly melt. Be careful not to let water mix in with the chocolate when melting, and don't burn it. Try dipping fruit into the melted chocolate; raspberries are my favorite, but bananas, strawberries, or pineapple are delicious coated with it. Or you can pour it over non-fat frozen yogurt or non-fat ice milk. It's also delicious dribbled over banana bread or carrot cake. As you'll see in the recipes, you can stir in sweetened coffee with melted chocolate to make mocca frosting, too.

When eating quality chocolate, really taste it. Let the chocolate melt in your mouth, and *savor the flavor as it lingers on your taste buds.*

FRUIT

Fruit offers a wide range of delightful, delicious desserts. Fruit can be sautéed, baked, and blended into drinks. Fruit smoothies with non-fat yogurt or with fruit juices are delightful. Slice fruit and serve it on a plate to finish a meal, or pour berries, cherries, or sliced fruit on other desserts.

To me, fresh fruit sorbet (or non-fat frozen yogurt with fresh fruit) rivals the best of ice creams. Don't expect non-fat yogurt to taste like ice cream, it doesn't. The texture without the fat is quite different and clearly not as "creamy." Yet, you can taste the fruit better in a sorbet, and the tartness of frozen yogurt can be very enjoyable.

Try to add fruit to the end of every meal. You can also add diced fruit, dried fruit, or juice as a substitute for sugar in recipes. Natural fruit sweeteners are better for you than sugar, which has problems with its use. First, sugar does not satisfy your appetite, so you keep eating. Second, eating sugar increases insulin production, making you hungry and converting those sugar calories into body fat.

This does not mean that you can't use sugar. Rather, limit your use of sugar in desserts and substitute fruit when possible. You can also substitute artificial sweeteners for sugar, although I haven't emphasized that in the recipes.

TABLE 28. Compare dessert sweetener options. Each serving has nearly 100 calories. Choose natural fruit sweeteners over sugar.

Type of Sweetener	Quantity	Calories
Sugar	2 Tbs (6 tsp)	97
Apple	1 Medium	81
Banana	1 Medium	105
Strawberries	2 1/2 Cups	105
Apricots	1 1/2 Cups	110
Raspberries	1 3/4 Cups	105
Orange	1 Medium	92
Orange Juice (from frozen concentrate	1 Cup	113

FISH AND SEAFOOD

You probably noted that I listed seafood as optional on my antioxidant food pyramid. There are benefits and harmful effects to eating seafood. It provides a source of fat-soluble antioxidants, without the harmful impact of saturated fat. Seafood is also high in omega-3 fats, reported to have a variety of health benefits including: decreased death rates in people with known coronary artery disease, and stabilizing of mood, depression and anxiety. Shellfish provides a rich source of antioxidant-dependent minerals like zinc. Unfortunately, many fish products are contaminated with heavy metals like mercury and PCB's, especially those caught near industrial harbors. Whether you eat seafood is a choice you need to make. If you choose to eat seafood, limit yourself to two servings per week.

Why Don't You List Lean Meats And Poultry In Your Food Pyramid?

I did not list lean meat and poultry products on the food pyramid because I fail to see significant health benefits from eating them. There is ample scientific evidence that they are actually harmful. Yes, meat and poultry are a source of protein, iron and B vitamins. However, anyone following this program will receive plenty of protein, iron and B vitamins. Further, iron (especially heme iron found in meat and poultry) acts like an oxidant and can cause more harm than good.

The meat and poultry industries are working to decrease the fat content of their products. In many cases they have succeeded, as a variety of lean sandwich meats (less than 20% of calories from fat) and products are now available. Skinless chicken and turkey and some fat-trimmed red meats contain less than 20% of their calories as fat. Unfortunately, the fat in these products is still high in saturated fat.

Another worry is that these lean meat and poultry products also contain industrial hormones. Most store-bought poultry in the U.S. has been fed high levels of these and they do affect people. Men, women, and children all appear to have increasing health concerns related to expanding hormone intake. These problems include prostate problems, PMS complaints, and increased cancer rates. Did you know that young girls who eat meat and poultry regularly reach puberty years earlier, increasing their lifetime risk of cancer? This is a big concern! If you choose to eat skinless poultry and lean meats, I suggest you look for organic products that weren't raised on hormones.

One of the worst things you can do to meat is barbecue it. Yes, the American outdoor dinning ritual makes meat more dangerous. The problem with the barbecue is that it covers the meat with soot (activated free radicals). You are better off to wrap barbecue foods in foil or skip the barbecue completely.

You can follow my Antioxidant Diet Program and eat small portions (3 ounces per serving or less) of lean meats and poultry 2-3 servings per week. I will continue to encourage the delicious and nutritious foods listed on my antioxidant diet food pyramid. As always, the choice is yours.

BEVERAGES

Our bodies are 80% water–obviously, we need fluid to survive. But many of us fail to drink enough liquids. We should aim to drink eight cups of fluid (two liters/quarts) per day.

Beware of liquids such as coffee, black tea, caffeinated colas, and alcohol. They increase our urine production and fail to hydrate our tissues.

Many of my patients drink coffee for breakfast, colas for lunch, and a beer or a glass of wine with dinner. In essence, they do not drink anything hydrating all day! No wonder they feel tired and constipated all the time–they are low on fluid. Next time that happens to you, try drinking water instead of coffee for a pick-me-up. It works.

Water is the ultimate hydrator, and it's available to us all. If you don't have good quality drinking water, go to the store and buy some. It's cheaper than colas and sodas, and better for you. Juices and herbal teas are valuable as sources of vitamins, antioxidants, and minerals. Look at the weekly recipe section in Chapter Nine for ideas on how to drink more healthy liquids.

For people not sensitive to sodium intake, miso is a hot beverage that we should use more often. Miso contains calcium, decreases cholesterol levels, helps control blood sugar peaks and lowers a meal's glycemic index. It also helps women with changing levels of estrogen. Women should drink a cup of miso every day, particularly the low-sodium version.

You can find miso in the produce section of most grocery stores near the tofu and soy products. Some stores may keep it in the exotic or Oriental foods section.

TEA

Tea is a wonderful beverage, whether hot or cold. In fact, tea is the most popular beverage in the world. People in southern Asia often drink tea with milk. In the Orient, green tea is the most popular beverage–and for good reason.

Chinese green tea is a good source of antioxidants; it is loaded with flavonoids (antioxidants). Producers make green tea by chopping, rolling, and quickly heating tea leaves. The heating process traps the chemicals and antioxidants in the tea leaves. The high antioxidant content remains intact.

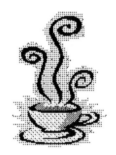

Black tea contains about 20% of the flavonoids of green tea. To make black tea, the leaves are chopped, rolled, and exposed to air (oxygen) for 6-8 hours. In the drying process, the flavonoids become oxidized (by oxygen) which decreases the antioxidant content of black tea compared to green tea. Oolong tea is an intermediate between black tea and green tea. It is exposed to air for only a couple of hours before it is heated.

I feel that flavonoids have not received the attention they deserve as potent antioxidants. You can expect to hear more about these beneficial compounds in tea and red wine in the near future. While tea contains abundant antioxidants, studies to date have not provided compelling evidence that drinking black tea alone prevents common forms of cancer. Regular green tea consumption appears more promising and is associated with reduced cancer rates.

Both green tea and black tea are caffeinated, black tea more than green. The oxidation (or fermentation) of the tea leaves somehow increases its caffeine content. When my wife and I worked in China, local friends often asked if we wanted stimulating tea (black tea) or relaxing tea (green tea). But both teas are caffeinated, so if you wish to avoid caffeine, look for decaffeinated brands.

Green tea has a pleasant, although slightly bitter, flavor that I have learned to enjoy. Make a weak cup at first to appreciate the subtle flavor. If it still seems bitter, you can add 1/4-1/2 teaspoon of honey. To make a traditional flavored green tea, brew it strongly and serve without sweetening.

Never drink scalding beverages, including tea. Recent studies suggest that this may increase your risk of esophageal cancer. Let your tea cool slightly before you start to drink.

Since we're touching on sources of antioxidants, I want to bring up an important point. No single antioxidant, or single source of antioxidants has shown itself to produce strong clinical benefits in large, well-controlled studies. However, in contrast, diets containing multiple antioxidants do show multiple benefits.

Take green tea as an example. Tea may be an important player within a large group of other antioxidants, just as a solo flutist is an important player within a large orchestra performing a symphony. We don't expect a solo flutist to perform a symphony alone; nor should we expect a single source of antioxidants to keep us healthy.

Herbal Teas (herbal infusions)

"Tea" technically refers to a drink made from a plant that produces tea leaves, like black tea or green tea. Many people call herbal infusions "herbal teas." While the correct term for a drink made from herbs and spices is an "herbal infusion," herbal tea has become the more popular term in the United States.

People have brewed herbal teas medicinally for thousands of years. In particular ginger, chamomile, and mint teas are easy to find and are great any time of day, especially before bedtime.

Herbal teas, or infusions, can be powerful healers. Some health care providers recommend garlic or echinacea teas to reduce the duration and severity of a cold. Just chop up a teaspoon of each and add two cups of boiling water. Let cool, and add honey and/or lemon. For nausea, stomach or intestinal problems, ginger is commonly served in a tea. Chop up a teaspoon of fresh ginger root twice a day and brew it in near-boiling water. Add a dash of mint and fennel to balance the flavor.

Green tea (if you are not highly caffeine sensitive) or herbal teas are a nice way to end the day. Just sit back quietly and sip a cup. You will soon find yourself looking forward to your "moment of peace" with a cup of tea in hand.

COFFEE

Most health books discourage coffee use. In reality, there is no clinical evidence that drinking under four cups of coffee per day has any serious health effects for most people. Nor does it appear to affect cholesterol levels, blood sugar levels, or cancer rates.

However, coffee is related to increased heartburn and aggravates bouts of insomnia and anxiety. If these symptoms bother you, skip that cup of coffee. Coffee also increases your urination, so drink extra fluid if you drink coffee.

Coffee likely contains trace amounts of antioxidants, but the quantity is insufficient to add significant benefits. While caffeinated coffee intake can increase alertness, there are many other beverages you can choose that actually benefit your health.

Interestingly, people drink coffee most often first thing in the morning–exactly when we are in need of hydration. If you choose to drink coffee in the morning, be sure to drink another beverage, too.

JUICES

Fruit juices provide us with a generous supply of vitamins and antioxidants. In particular, citrus juices, carrot juice, guava juice, and tomato juice are loaded with nutrients and antioxidants. That's why it's a good idea to drink a glass of juice in the morning, and another in the afternoon with a snack. Because diabetics will note a rise in blood sugar levels after drinking juice, they should limit their intake to 1/2 cup once or twice per day and should drink their juice with a meal.

Frozen juices also provide plenty of nutrients. Best of all is to make your own juice with the vast array of juicing machines available. To me, home made carrot juice tastes wonderful. Because apple and pear juice provide fewer nutrients than other juices, you should limit their use.

CHAPTER 6   *ENHANCING*
YOUR NEW
LIFESTYLE
PYRAMID

If my *28-Day Antioxidant Diet Program* dealt only with food, something important would be missing. The point of this book is to promote overall health and vitality. As such, exercise has a strong influence on our antioxidant-oxidant balance. Furthermore, stress affects our ability to make important food and exercise choices. Lastly, you can add all the right foods and exercise, but if you poison yourself with environmental toxins, your health still suffers. The cornerstones of my program include proper nutrition, regular exercise, mental well-being, and a clean environment. Combined, they will help you lay the foundation for a healthy life.

"Health" means more than being free from disease. It means being in a state of physical, mental, and social well-being. As our health improves, we gain "vitality."

Your life is a continuous experiment, highly modified by the dietary and activity choices you make. I believe your level of vitality is the best indicator that your lifestyle choices are correct for you. My goal is to maximize your sense of vitality in all you do.

EXERCISE: THE FAST TRACK TO SUCCESS

Our bodies were not designed to sit in an office 40 hours per week, and certainly not 60-70 hours per week. <u>Our bodies were built for movement.</u> A 30-minute walk or its equivalent is <u>vital</u> at least 3 times per week, and preferably every day. Unfortunately, many of us fail to attain 30 minutes of exercise, even once or twice per week. Not surprisingly, fitness levels in America are declining while obesity rate are climbing.

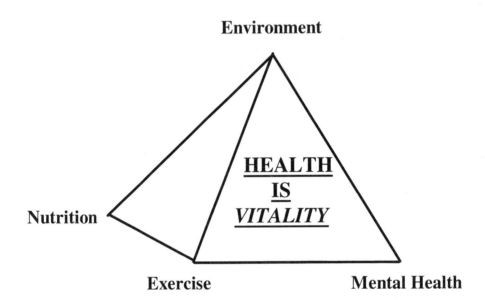

Exercise and Weight Control

Some of my patients say, "I watch what I eat and I exercise 30 minutes a day..........but, I just can't lose weight. What am I doing wrong?"

While some of us can get by with 30 minutes of exercise per day and reach our lean body weight, most of us can't. To really be <u>lean</u>, most people would need an hour or more of daily aerobic activity. It's a matter of genetics–we each live with our unique genes.

In ancient times, people who could exercise all day without losing weight had an advantage during times of famine. Today, a year-round guaranteed food supply has turned that genetic payoff into a disadvantage and a tendency to gain weight.

Like it or not, many people who eat "normally" might need to exercise 30-60 minutes every day to reach within 20 pounds of their lean body weight.

Again, I would emphasize fitness over body shape. Many clinical studies, including the MR FIT study, show that the best predictor of long-term weight control and weight loss is a continuing commitment to regular exercise.

While living at your lean body weight is associated with reaching your maximal lifespan, your health does not usually suffer if you weigh within 20 pounds of your lean body weight. A simple, *approximate* method to calculate lean body weight is to start at 106 pounds for a five foot male; then add six pounds for every inch greater than five foot height. For a female, start at 100 pounds for a five foot height, and add five pounds for every inch over five foot.[1] (Charts allow less weight for women because they have a smaller bone frame than men.)

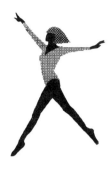

> *For example, to calculate my approximate lean body weight: I am 5 foot 9 inches tall: 106 pounds + 45 pounds = 151 pounds. So, I should weigh no more than 171 pounds to be within 20 pounds of my lean body weight. Fortunately, I'm happy weighing 165 pounds. So I can continue to eat 20% of my calories as fat at my current exercise level. If I wanted to reach my lean body weight, I'd likely need to increase my exercise time of 3-4 hours per week to 6-12 hours per week.*
>
> *To calculate lean body weight for a female who is 5 foot 3 inches: We take 100 pounds + 15 pounds = 115 pounds. If we allow a 20 pound weight margin above lean body weight, a 5 foot 3 inch female should weigh no more than 135 pounds.*

Trying to lose weight without exercise is almost <u>pointless</u>. We eat less, so to save energy, our metabolism slows. We don't lose much weight, and we're often fatigued, as well. When we go back to normal eating, with a reduced metabolism, we gain our weight back in a flash and often gain some extra weight, too.

Thirty minutes of exercise per day increases your metabolism for up to 8 to 12 hours. It helps you lose weight even when you are not exercising. If you want to lose weight, eat well and exercise for 30 minutes twice per day; you'll benefit from an increased metabolism around the clock.

In a well designed study comparing 12 months of interventions with "diet only," "diet plus exercise," and "exercise alone," the "diet only" group initially lost weight during the first year, but after two years had actually gained weight. In contrast, the "exercise only" group lost a smaller amount of weight at one year, but kept it all off at

---

1. This weight estimate works for people with average height and average body frames. Obviously, body builders can weigh 30-40 pounds more than this calculation and be at their lean body weight. People under 5 foot 2 inches in height can also exceed their healthy weight if they are even 15 pounds over their lean body weight, while somebody over 6 foot in height can often carry 30 extra pounds without health problems.

year two. The "diet plus exercise" group lost the most weight at the end of one year, but did no better than the "exercise alone" group at two years. The bottom line is: cutting calories for 3-12 months without exercising doesn't result in long-term weight loss.

Studies show that the exercise equivalent of walking 16-20 miles per week remains the best predictor of long-term weight control. This averages out to a 3 mile walk six days per week. This is also the equivalent of 1,500-2,000 calories burned every week on exercise machines. (It takes me 35-45 minutes to burn 300-400 calories on aerobic exercise machines.)

Here's a success story about one of my patients:

> *Sherrie came to see me six months ago wanting to lose weight. She was working out at the YMCA for 30 minutes, three times per week and she looked fine. She was also eating well, but couldn't lose weight. It didn't seem fair because she tried to do everything right.*
>
> *Surprisingly, moderate workouts for 30 minutes 3 times per week do not seem to result in long-term weight control, although it will improve fitness levels.*
>
> *Sherrie started five one-hour workouts per week on a variety of exercise machines and burned about 400 calories each session. She lost 4-5 pounds every month over the next three months without changing her eating habits one bit. If she keeps up the exercise, she will continue to lose weight and won't gain it back.*

Obesity and Weight Control

Webster's dictionary defines *obesity* as "being very fat or stout." We medical professionals often define obesity as "excessive weight that hurts one's health and ability to function."[1] Obesity often disables people both physically and mentally.

I define being *overweight* as when a person's weight is more than 20 pounds over their ideal weight, without any bearing on functional capacity.

I avoid focusing on body shape, but I am deeply concerned by the emotional and physical harm caused by obesity. In a country where obesity rates are climbing, we need to pay attention to factors that contribute to weight gain. This is not a cosmetic concern about body shape; this is a serious national health problem that threatens our health and independence. To put this national health crisis in perspective, at least two thirds of

---

1. A technical definition of obesity is when a Body Mass Index (BMI) exceeds 30. To calculate your body mass index, take your weight in kilograms and divide by your height in meters squared (BMI = Weight (kg) / height (meters) x height (meters). This definition doesn't work for body builders and athletes.

Americans are overweight. (A Harris poll, February 1996, noted that 74% of Americans were overweight.) Even more alarming, one third of adult Americans are not just overweight, but obese, and 25% of American adolescents are obese. The national cost in sick days and medical care for obesity in America now exceeds $140 billion yearly.

While I am convinced that some people are genetically prone to weight gain, and that these same people may become obese, I personally don't attribute obesity to genetic makeup. My reasoning is simple; most countries don't have obesity. Yes, you can find overweight people in other countries, but you do not find severe obesity in large numbers outside of the United States. This is good news, because if obesity was caused by our genetic makeup, weight control would seem hopeless. Yet, if lifestyle choices play a decisive role in long-term weight management, then there is real hope. I believe inactivity remains a primary factor in the cause of obesity in the United States. And if true, activity becomes the cure.

I know that weight gain is an emotional and sensitive issue for many people. Many people have worked hard to lose weight, trying diet after diet, only to watch their weight go down, then up again. Dieting is frustrating. Yet, working with patients in physical and mental discomfort has shown me that people need fitness to remain functional and active. While genetic factors largely determine body shape, our fitness levels are usually determined by our lifestyle choices.

Many patients ask me if they can't just take a pill to lose weight. In reality "Redox R" and "Phen-Fen" diet pills have taken many by storm. Unfortunately, they are only minimally effective. Yes, you hear the story about the rare person who lost 40-50 pounds on diet pills, but some people taking placebo pills also lost this amount of weight, too. In reality, diet pills work, and at one year most people lose 10% of their body weight. But by three years, studies show the actual weight loss for those still taking the pill to be only 5-7% less than their original body weight.

Consider the cost of taking diet pills, combined with provider visits, the expenses often exceed $700 yearly. If you ever stop the pills, every study has shown that you gain ALL the weight back. Thus over 10 years, it would cost nearly $1,000 for every 1% of weight loss achieved. To me, this high cost negates any benefit from the small weight loss associated with diet pills. And, after realizing the cost of the benefit, consider that these pills come with clear risks. Although short-term risks include death; they are exceedingly rare (only 1 death for every 20,000 people on diet pills). The biggest concern is that we have no idea what the long-term risks of taking diet pills might be.

Long-term successful weight loss does not come from skipping meals, diet pills, or dieting. Success comes from making a long-term commitment to changing your lifestyle. The keys to long-term weight loss and improved function are adequate daily aerobic exercise and major reductions in simple sugar and fat intake.

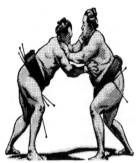

While the public seems to focus on weight and shape, I would rather focus on fitness. Fitness brings health and physical independence. Throughout this book, I will emphasize fitness and vitality. The key to long-term successful weight control is healthful food and daily aerobic activity.

Japanese sumo wrestlers represent fat and fit. They eat extra calories, but don't eat extra fat. They exercise for several hours per day. While they look fat, their liver, heart, and other internal organs are as fat free as the average lean American. In contrast, average obese Americans contain dangerously high quantities of fat in their heart muscle, liver, kidneys and other internal organs. Sumo wrestlers form "healthy fat," meaning while their skin is thick, their arteries and internal organs are clean. Proper nutrition, even to excess, combined with regular exercise is consistent with health.

Exercise and Oxidative Stress

Exercise increases oxygen consumption and increases free radical production. That's not considered good. So why is exercise beneficial?

Researchers recently studied the effects of participating in the Hawaii Ironman World Championship Triathlon. They found that prolonged exercise in world-class trained athletes *improved* the antioxidant-oxidant balance. They particularly noted that the oxidation of bloodstream fats dropped with exercise, without intake of antioxidant supplements. They also found that LDL cholesterol levels decreased while HDL levels increased.

My colleagues and I call those who exercise *frantically* on an occasional basis "weekend warriors." The pain and stiffness following these weekends reflects oxidative stress injuries to musculoskeletal tissues. They hurt! Extreme overuse activities will burn and oxidize your tissues, causing inflammation. While muscles frequently heal quickly, tendons have a limited blood supply; hence, tendonitis injuries can take weeks to months to heal.

Regular fitness activities will promote your antioxidant production and improve your tolerance for oxidative stress injuries. Clearly, regular exercise improves health and vitality and may help to boost immunity.

Imagine 55-year-old Mr. Jones, who after a winter of "activity hibernation," pulls his back mowing the lawn for the first time in the spring. Or 42-year-old Ms. Thompson who tries jogging 2 miles for the first time in 5 years with the new neighbor and tears her hamstring muscle. Both of these people missed over 3 weeks of normal work and Ms.

Thompson had to cancel her vacation to Italy! These episodes represent common, yet preventable injuries.

If you still choose to engage in "weekend warrior activities," load up on antioxidant-rich foods, hydrate yourself well, and avoid oxidants such as alcohol and tobacco that might increase your misery later. You could add antioxidant supplements the day before and after known overexertion, including: 400 IU of Vitamin E, 1000 mg of Vitamin C, and 15 mg of zinc.

Planning an exercise program works. Next year, Mr. Jones will not only be fit enough to mow his lawn, but he will enjoy his summer, thanks to regular, active, outdoor activities. Ms. Thompson rehabilitated her hamstring and started a controlled-speed walking program. By September, she was enjoying a spectacular vacation in Italy, largely because she had tremendous energy and walked happily all day from site to site.

STARTING YOUR PERSONALIZED EXERCISE PROGRAM

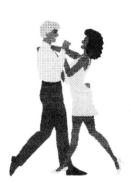

Your current fitness level determines how you start an exercise program. A person who hasn't done any fitness activity in months shouldn't start out the same way as somebody who walks 20 minutes daily.

First, we need to design a program for three levels of activity: "Inactive," "Moderately Active," and "Moderately to Strenuously Active." Then, we need to design activities to promote different forms of fitness using: aerobic activities, strength training, and flexibility.

AEROBIC EXERCISE

Aerobic exercise is a continuous, oxygen-consuming activity that strengthens your heart and lung capacity. Aerobic activities should last at least 20 minutes and preferably reach 30-60 minutes of continuous motion. Brisk walking, swimming, biking, rowing, continuous gardening, dancing, and similar activities are excellent. Many stationary aerobic exercise machines allow all-weather aerobic exercise indoors, including stairclimbers, treadmills, stationary bicycles, and rowing machines.

If you have any medical problems or take medications, always check with your health-care provider prior to starting an exercise program.

Step I: Starting from Inactivity

If you have not been exercising at all, start with 10-minute sessions daily during Week One. You can walk, bicycle or use a variety of cardiovascular exercise equipment. Allow yourself 5 minutes to stretch before and after exercise. Altogether, find 20 minutes each day of the week for exercise–10 minutes to stretch and 10 minutes to exercise.

For Week Two, extend sessions to 15 minutes of exercise per day. For Week Three and Week Four, assuming your legs and feet don't hurt, aim for 20 minutes. For Week Five, try 25 minutes, and aim for 30 minutes of continuous activity by week six. With a newly increased activity level, your muscles will tone and tighten with exercise, making a 5-minute stretch before and after each session extra important.

The first month of a new exercise program can produce injuries. During the first month make an effort to stretch before and after each activity session, and don't overdo the exercise. Give yourself time. It is more important to go slowly for a longer time than to go wild for a few minutes, and suffer later. Particularly during the first month, don't worry about sweating, just concentrate on completing your weekly goal without injury!

If you choose walking as an activity, select comfortable walking shoes and loose clothing. Find a safe walking path with even, flat ground. If the weather is harsh, consider walking laps in a local gymnasium or a shopping mall. If you are exercising too fast to speak, slow down. Monitor your pulse and aim for a pulse rate that is 50-60% of your maximum heart rate.

To calculate your maximum heart rate, take 220 minus your age. This number equals your maximum heart rate.

> *Here's an example: Danielle is 40. Her maximum heart rate = 220 - 40 (her age) = 180. To start an exercise program, her heart rate goal should be 60% of her maximal heart rate: 180 x 60% = 108 beats per minutes.*

> *In time, as her exercise tolerance builds, she will want her heart rate to reach 70% of its maximum. Again, 220 - 40 = 180. 180 x 70% = 126. Therefore, when she exercises, she should aim to keep her heart rate near 126 (say 115-130) beats per minute for at least 30 minutes.*

Your primary goals for a new exercise program are: (1) Not to injure yourself, and (2) To relax and enjoy yourself.

Here is a helpful hint. Look for a walking or exercise partner! Walking partners can boost your morale and success, and help you stay on track without skipped days.

Most of the medical benefits from exercise occur when people move from inactivity to Step 1 activities. For many people, simply continuing Step 1 activities meets their goals of improved health, greater energy, and general well-being. If, however, you want to lose weight, maximize your energy, and improve your cholesterol and blood sugar levels, you should move to Step 2 activities. If you have been previously inactive, you should be ready for Step 2 activities within 1-2 months of regular Step 1 activities.

Step 2: Mild to Moderate Aerobic Activity

If you work out occasionally, or have successfully competed Step 1, you're ready to further boost your aerobic capacity, burn more calories and fat, and increase your stamina. Regular Step 2 level activities bring the maximal benefit from aerobic exercise.

Plan on 40-60 minute workouts daily (at least 5-6 days per week). Increase your activities gradually, as rapid increases can cause injuries and more oxidative stress. Increase your workouts by an extra 5 minutes every 2 weeks. Keep your pulse rate at 60-70% of your maximum heart rate during your workout. Then, allow yourself a 5-minute cool down and stretch at the end of your workout.

Speedwalking, swimming, and cross-country skiing are terrific moderate aerobic activities. Jogging, while popular, increases pounding on your back, feet, and joints. While you don't burn more calories jogging than speedwalking, you do sustain more injuries. Speedwalking with 2-3 pound hand weights also provides a nice upper-body workout over a 30-60 minute time span.

Cross-train and pursue a variety of activities. By alternating your walking, swimming, bicycling, or use of cardiovascular equipment you'll maximize the fitness of a variety of muscle groups.

Personally, I like a 20-minute warm-up on a stationary bike, as I can read a few journal articles while I exercise. Next, I move to 20 minutes on the stairmaster. I alternate my third station between a rowing machine, or weight training with 8-10 stations of weight lifting over 20-30 minutes.

Step 3: Moderate to Strenuous Activities

As your stamina grows, you may start to push your limits. Avoid exercise intensity that pushes your pulse rate over 80% of your maximal heart rate. You won't gain much physically, but you'll greatly increase your production of free radicals. While you can improve your cardiovascular fitness with more strenuous activities, you'll also increase your possibility of injuries.

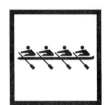

There is still hot controversy as to whether there are long-term benefits to intense exercise. There is strong evidence that strenuous activities increase oxidative stress, generate excess free radicals, and significantly increase soft tissue problems like tendonitis and bursitis. There are also theories that regular strenuous activities may lower the immune response. Therefore, you shouldn't be surprised to discover that many competitive athletes suffer from frequent infections and injuries.

On the other hand, benefits of regular vigorous exercise include rapid calorie burning, improved cardiovascular endurance, and appetite suppression.

TABLE 29. The pros and cons of different exercise equipment.

	Cost	Space	Impact	Other
Treadmill Machines	High	Generous	Smooth	Easy, interactive
Stationary Bike	Low-Mod.	Small	Smooth	Easy, boring but great for reading
Stairmaster	Mod-High	Medium	Knee stress	Smooth, high fat burner
Video or TV Aerobics	Minimal	Variable	Variable Low-impact preferred	Need good shoes and motivation
Rowing Machine	Low-Mod	Generous	Smooth	Need good form to protect your back and knees
Nordic Track	Low-Mod	Generous	Smooth	Great exercise, but requires skill

Strenuous training increases calorie requirements. If you exercise over 8-12 hours per week, extra healthy fats become an essential calorie source. Snack on monounsaturated rich nuts (cashews, filberts, pecans, almonds, and macadamias), eat avocados, and add extra olive oil and canola oil when preparing meals. Seafood offers another option for healthy fat.

Women who overdo endurance activities can suppress more than their appetites; they can stop their normal menstrual cycles. Once the menstrual cycle is suppressed, the bones lose calcium, reducing strength and density just like after menopause. Studies have shown that calcium supplements don't offset this exercise-induced bone weakening. Only by modifying the intensity of workouts until menstrual cycles normalize, will normal bone density be restored.

Strength Training

Increasing muscle mass can improve your health in many important ways. Consider the following benefits of adding muscle to your frame:

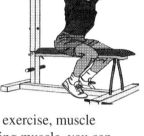

- Increased metabolic rate (According to Dr. Joel Prosner, a physician-researcher in Philadelphia, adding muscle in overweight people increases their metabolism and helps them burn calories.)
- Increased ability to burn calories with exercise (During exercise, muscle burns calories like crazy, while fat sits inactive. By adding muscle, you can exercise and eat extra without gaining weight.)
- Decreased injury rates (Adding muscle helps to prevent tendon and muscle strains. Increasing strength also slows joint damage caused by arthritis.)

Muscle mass manufactures a vital amino acid called "glutamine." Glutamine represents 30% of the protein in human muscle and breast milk. We don't normally consume glutamine in our diet, so we rely upon our muscle tissue to produce it. Our muscles then release it into the blood stream during illnesses and times of physical stress.

Glutamine acts as an important nutrient in many ways. It:
- Promotes intestinal healing
- Stimulates immune system function
- Nourishes your liver and kidney
- Provides the building blocks to make "glutathione," (an essential compound in your antioxidant system)
- Stimulates muscle mass formation

Reduced muscle mass is related to increased rates of intestinal and infectious complications following surgery. There is a growing body of evidence that giving glutamine intravenously before and after surgery can help prevent complications in those with a reduced muscle mass. These benefits have been especially effective in patients with intestinal trauma and burns. The elderly with muscle waisting appear at highest risk of complications during illnesses and appear to benefit from glutamine supplements.

Regular strength training builds muscle mass and your glutamine reserve.

Most people associate strength training with weight-lifting, yet isometric (non-motion) exercises and elastic band workouts work well, too. Two to three strengthening sessions per week, lasting 20-60 minutes each, can markedly improve strength and fitness.

Both free weights and weight-training machines can be used for strength training. Free weights require more skill and produce more functional strength, but have a higher injury rate with their use. Given the choice, I encourage the novice strength trainer to start with weight-training machines because they are simple and safe to use.

Your most important objective with a new strengthening program is not to injure yourself during the first few weeks. Start slowly and build slowly. Find weights (or motions) that you can lift smoothly 12-20 times.

Pick 6-10 work stations that focus on working specific muscle groups. My preferred lifts include: leg press (quad), leg curls (hamstring), abdominal crunches, overhead presses, overhead pull-down, biceps curls, arm extensions (triceps), and bench presses. Avoid knee extension machines, as this activity overloads the knee cap (patella) and commonly causes pain or injuries.

Here are some weight training tips:

- Optimize your strength training with 2-3 workouts per week.
- Choose weights that you can lift a minimum of 12 times, and preferably 12-20 repetitions per session. Try 1-3 sets of repetitions per station.
- Lift the weight and let it return with slow, smooth, non-jerky motions.
- When you comfortably reach 2 sets of 16-20 repetitions, it is time to increase your weight with your next training session.

Flexibility Training

Running, jogging, and weight training often build muscle mass and reduce flexibility. Loss in flexibility produces low back pain, hamstring and calf injuries, and poor athletic performance.

If you jog or run, especially while developing a new exercise program, take a couple of minutes to stretch your back, hamstrings, and calves before and after you run. For strength training, I advocate at least 5 minutes of low back, hamstring, and calf stretches after your workout.

Swimming promotes flexibility. The ideal exercise program combines speed-walking, swimming, weight training, and stretching activities.

HOW TO BEAT THOSE BARRIERS TO EXERCISING

Increase Your Energy

The more you exercise, the more energy you usually have. The goal is to establish a regular pattern of exercise and to change your cycle: you'll exercise more, feel better, have more energy, and exercise more.

Here are some helpful hints to add energy:

- Exercise early in the morning before your energy level drops.
- Skip high-sugar foods that give you a quick energy surge and a long-lasting energy low.
- Go to bed earlier and get your rest. Skip the late night TV shows.
- Remind yourself that the more you exercise regularly, the better you'll feel.
- Walk to work, or park your car and walk the last 20 minutes. You'll find you arrive alert and refreshed.

Increase Your Efficiency

There are 168 hours in a week. People who get daily exercise usually sleep better, are more productive during the day, more alert, and in better health. If you spend five hours per week exercising, you still have 163 hours per week left. If you can become just 10% more efficient at doing tasks during the 16 hours per day that you are awake, you just gained 7.2 *extra hours* per week!

Personally, my efficiency goes up 10-20% when I exercise regularly. I am more alert, and I get more things done in less time. I can't do all that I want unless I exercise at least 3-5 times per week.

Look at these hints that create time for exercising:

- Workout with a friend or significant other. You get to exercise and socialize at the same time.
- Take your children or a pet for a walk. Even infants benefit from walks in the stroller. A walk counts as quality family time spent together.
- Park 20-30 minutes from work and walk. Or use part of your lunch time for a walk.
- Workout on cardiovascular machines so you can read the paper, your journals, or other work related reading material while you exercise. Maximize your time.

- If you watch TV, pick programs you watch regularly and plan to use that time for push-ups, stomach crunches, free weight lifting, stretches, or use of an exercise machine.

Decrease Your Skeletal Pains with Exercise

Spinal arthritis leaves people debilitated. Knee and hip arthritis disable, too. Despite a billion dollar pharmaceutical industry that treats these problems, medications do nothing to slow the arthritic disease process. So, what can slow the disease process? Exercise! Studies show that regular exercise effectively slows arthritis.

Let me share an example from my practice on how exercise can rejuvenate your muscles and joints.

> *Jerry, a 40-year-old accountant, blew out his left knee playing basketball in high school. Over the years, the pain had progressed and he dropped many of his normal activities. By the time he saw me six months ago, he had gained 20 pounds and his fitness level had deteriorated. At his young age, he was __desperate__ because he felt worse every month. He hobbled into my office very depressed. We reviewed his options at length, and I asked him to start a water aerobics program 4 days per week for a couple of months.*
>
> *Over several months, he increased his workouts from 15 minutes to 45 minutes, lost 20 pounds, rebuilt his fitness level, and strengthened his leg muscles. Now he walks without pain. He still has knee arthritis, so I have advised him to stick with water aerobic activities __permanently__. Recently, he started strength training at the gym and continues to do well.*

Water aerobics represent a wonderful activity for people who can't otherwise participate in weight-bearing activities. It feels terrific to work out in a nearly gravity-free environment, especially if spinal, joint, or weight problems limit you.

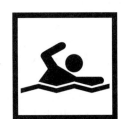

BENEFITS OF REGULAR, MODERATE EXERCISE

- Improves your antioxidant balance
- Decreases stress
- Treats depression and anxiety
- Burns calories

- Suppresses your appetite
- Improves brain chemistry and promotes relaxation
- Increases energy and concentration
- Improves intestinal function
- Improves sexual function
- Increases fitness levels
- Controls blood sugar and insulin levels
- Improves immune response and reduces infections
- Prevents injuries

If you remember Mary, the school teacher, from the discussion on glycemic foods and hunger, you may have wondered if she ever lost weight without adding an exercise program. In reality, she lost about 15 pounds by choosing low glycemic foods. Mary had been doing aerobic tapes at home three days per week for 30 minutes. Not surprisingly, although it helped her fitness level greatly, that wasn't enough for her to lose weight, and she still weighed over 200 pounds.

I asked her to walk 12 times around the track at the school (3 miles) five days per week rain or shine. She could walk before school, at lunch, or after school, but she would do so before heading home. As usual, Mary was ready and willing for a change. At first, the walk took her one hour. Within a couple of months, she had cut her time to 40-45 minutes. It took one year, but for the first time in 20 years her weight fell to under 140 pounds. This wasn't a quick weight-loss program, and I expect that if she gives up her new lifestyle she may regain some of her weight. Fortunately, Mary feels fabulous. I believe she will stick with this new lifestyle that, like her new wardrobe, fits her so well.

EXERCISE SUMMARY

- Exercise a minimum of 3-5 hours per week
- Make each session last at least 30 minutes
- Aim for a target heart rate of 60-70% of your maximal heart rate
- Start a regular program today! The greatest health benefit occurs when changing from no regular exercise to three, 20-minutes sessions of moderate activity per week. There is an additional health benefit when changing from this regular moderate activity to more prolonged, regular activity.

- Increase your endurance gradually to control your weight. For most people, weight control doesn't occur until you reach longer, moderate workouts for 40-60 minutes, 5-6 days per week.
- Don't exercise intensely and infrequently; it's harmful.

REDUCING STRESS

MENTAL HEALTH AND OXIDATIVE STRESS

On a long-term basis, stress-induced oxidation can wear us down, age us, and make us prone to chronic disease and frequent illnesses. When we become stressed, physically or mentally, we increase our production of adrenaline. Adrenaline makes our pulse rush, strengthens our heartbeat, and shunts blood to our vital organs. These are valuable physiological changes in the face of an emergency.

But the response mechanism also has a biochemical dark side. In increasing our adrenaline production, we use more oxygen, which generates greater quantities of free radicals.

Thus, if we want to protect our own tissues from aging and illness, we need to better manage our stress.

Stress is the most common problem I see among my patients. Day in and day out, people appear in my office with stress-induced problems. The list seems endless: stomach ulcers, asthma, back and neck pain, headaches, rashes, intestinal cramps, menstrual cramps, irregular menstrual cycles, recurrent infections and colds, dizziness, heart palpitations, increased urinary frequency, diarrhea, and more.

Diet may influence our ability to handle stress. Many of the electrical connections in our brains require a delicate balance between chemicals and fats. In particular, omega-3 fat deficiencies are related to depression and to poor stress management.

If you find yourself yelling at the car in front of you because it made you miss the light, you're under *stress*. Slow down. Negative thoughts cause negative things to happen, so start turning negative thoughts into positive ones.

Establish a Relationship with Nature

One of the most relaxing, de-stressing things we can do is get back to nature. Many of us live and work under artificial lighting. We breathe air in large buildings that lack fresh air. We eat canned, frozen, and packaged foods that have no connection with our current seasons. We have truly become separated from our natural world.

I personally believe that our mental well-being depends partly on connecting with our natural environment and the seasons. Plant foods contain more than vitamins and nutrients. They also provide plant hormones that are intrinsically in tune with the seasons and might improve our internal ability to adapt to seasonal changes.

Choose locally grown, organic produce year round. Look for fresh greens in the spring, fruit and vegetables throughout the summer. Enjoy squash, nuts, apples, and pears in the fall. Continue to eat rich nuts, winter squash, hearty grains, root vegetables, and citrus fruit in the winter. This is one way to keep hormonally in contact with the seasons.

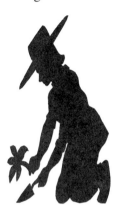

Go outside daily, for at least a half hour. Breathe the fresh air and feel nature around you. Walking outdoors is a uniquely beneficial activity. It is a good source of exercise, exposes us to natural light, and is a source of fresh air. Go for it!

Share Affection

Many of us rush through our days, and hardly take the time to share a hug or an affectionate greeting. I believe optimal mental health depends on warmth and affection. Give hugs daily and feel the warmth that passes between two beings.

Build a Social Network

Because Americans change homes and jobs so often, many of us have lost contact with a close social structure. Yet, social contact benefits our health greatly. Pet owners enjoy better health than people who live alone. People with illnesses who join support groups tend to live longer. In contrast, isolation increases death rates.

Start to grow social roots. Use the recipes in this book and invite friends over for dinner once a week, or arrange regular potlucks. Volunteer at your local food bank, school, health clinic, YMCA, or religious place of worship. Call or visit with a family member weekly. Social networks are good for your social life and your health!

Tips to De-Stress Your Life

- Take a stress management class.
- Listen to a relaxation tape.
- Spend 10-30 minutes per day meditating, praying, or just appreciating beauty in a quiet, relaxed state.
- Get at least 30 minutes of aerobic exercise per day.

- Eat well. A diet full of green leafy and yellow vegetables, fruits, legumes and whole grains gives us clean energy and appears to improve brain chemistry. Omega-3 fat sources (like green, leafy veggies and nuts such as pecans, almonds, cashews, and hazelnuts) may prevent depression and stress. Moods can also improve by increasing your carbohydrate intake.
- Retreat to a hot bathtub with a cup of herbal tea for 15-30 minutes per day and relax. If necessary, lock the door.
- Share at least 5 hugs per day! Hugs should not be limited to romantic partners. Hugs are an essential part of the energy exchange between living beings. Hug your significant other, hug a friend, and hug your pet. If you have a child, hug her/him several times per day.
- If none of these ideas help, talk to a mental health professional or your own medical provider.

There are two books that deal with pain and stress management that I found enlightening. Both offer help for stress management and chronic pain relief.

- *Who Dies?* by Stephen Levine (Written for people with cancer and their families)
- *Full Catastrophe Living, Using the Wisdom of Your Body and Mind to Face Stress, Pain, and Illness,* by Jon Kabat-Zinn Ph.D. (Written for people with chronic pain and stress)

PURIFYING YOUR LIVING ENVIRONMENT

You can eat well, exercise daily, and manage your stress, but if you poison yourself your health suffers. The purity of the air we breath and the food and water we drink greatly affects us.

I have discussed how to improve your positive antioxidant balance throughout this book. Now, I want to highlight a few everyday "pro-oxidants" to watch out for that accelerate aging and threaten your health.

STOP SMOKING NOW!

A book about antioxidants wouldn't be complete without a brief reference to tobacco use. Tobacco is one of the most powerful oxidants in our environment. Tobacco products cause extensive tissue aging and damage through oxidative stress.

As a medical provider, there are three things that I can do to help people <u>markedly</u> improve their health. First, I teach them to eat healthy foods. Second, I encourage them to get moderate exercise regularly. Third, I help smokers quit smoking. Everything else I do pales in comparison to these top three objectives.

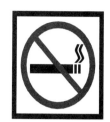

The harm caused by tobacco use is profound, and is <u>not</u> limited to lung cancer. I see some of the following problems aggravated by tobacco use, nearly every day:

TABLE 30. Problems Related to Tobacco Use

Insomnia	Heart attacks & strokes	Kidney and bladder cancer
Stomach ulcers	Irritable bowel pains	Cervical cancer
Lung infections	High blood pressure	Male impotence
Sinus infections	Foul breath	Bone weakening (osteoporosis)

Yes, our bodies develop bladder cancer while trying to urinate the toxic oxidants out of our bodies. If you smoke, I strongly advise you to quit; it is likely to be the best thing you will ever do for your health.

First Steps To Quitting Smoking

- Make a quit date, and tell your friends, family, and co-workers about it.
- Identify when and why you smoke. How else could you satisfy your needs at those times?
- Enroll in a "quit smoking" class. Many classes now offer nicotine replacement with patches or lozenges. Nicotine replacement is much more effective when <u>combined</u> with personal instruction.
- If at first you don't succeed, try, try again. Learning to quit smoking can be like learning to ride a bicycle. You need to get back on and go for it. Many people need to quit 4-5 times before they finally succeed.

AVOID PESTICIDES

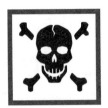

Pesticides are potent oxidants that can accelerate aging, cause cancer, and destroy health. The large quantity of agricultural pesticides used in the United States remains a serious problem.

The American public ingests large quantities of pesticides. Many pesticides are fat-soluble; therefore, they are commonly found in high-fat foods. Fortunately, by choosing low-fat food products, you decrease your intake of pesticides. In the American diet, 55% of pesticide residues are supplied by meat, 35% are supplied by dairy products, 6% by vegetables, 4% by fruits, and 1% by grains.

You will cut your pesticide intake drastically by picking foods from my antioxidant food pyramid!

Try these tips to avoid pesticides

- Buy organic! Organic products do not use pesticides. The price of organic foods is somewhat higher now, but as more and more people buy organic, the prices will drop. Buying organic also means buying crops that aren't raised on fertilizers. Organic grains and produce usually have a higher nutrient and mineral content.
- Increase your intake of vegetables, fruits, grains, and legumes to decrease your intake of pesticides. And always wash your produce at home before you eat it, preferably before you put it in the refrigerator or in a serving bowl. See "Pesticide removal:" on page 174.
- Eat more vegetarian meals. Breast-feeding mothers who eat meat products and vegetable products have a 35-times higher concentration of pesticide contamination in their breast milk than vegetarian mothers.
- Buy hormone-free animal products. If you choose to eat dairy products, poultry, or meat, buy organically raised products. Many meat, poultry, and dairy products contain lots of pesticides. They are also commonly loaded with hormones. Eating these hormone-filled animal foods likely increases cancer rates in men and women and worsens female hormonal problems. For an extra three cents per egg, you can buy free-range chicken eggs, free from antibiotics, hormones, and pesticides. Likewise, for a few extra cents you can buy non-fat, organic dairy products without added hormones. Ask for these improved products in your own grocery stores.

OLESTRA: A Fat You Can't Absorb

What about *"Olestra R,"* the amazing new snack fat with no calories? Olestra is not a pesticide, nor is it a toxin. So why did I place it with tobacco use and pesticides? Olestra is already in America's food chain, and soon, many Olestra-like products may be available in pill form, too.

Olestra is a fat compound so big that the body can't absorb it from the intestines. But is this really good news? Let's consider how it works, because there is more to this than meets the eye.

Olestra tastes and "feels" like fat but theoretically it doesn't make you fat; such a deal! But there are some serious drawbacks to eating Olestra products that outweigh the "no-cal, no-fat" hype it's receiving.

The primary concern is that Olestra does not just pass through your intestinal tract alone–it drags other critical fat-soluble vitamins and nutrients with it. In particular, Olestra prevents our intestines from absorbing carotenoids and other fat soluble antioxidants, those valuable components in fruits and vegetables associated with lower rates of heart attacks, strokes, cancer, and blindness. Olestra isn't a free radical or a pro-oxidant itself; but it acts like one by blocking the absorption of normal antioxidants.

In response to concerns about losing valuable nutrients from Olestra intake, Procter and Gamble has offered to supplement their Olestra-containing chips and crackers with Vitamins A, D, E, and K. Unfortunately, they are not replacing the carotenoids and flavonoids. In fairness to Procter and Gamble, it would be hard to replace carotenoids and phytochemicals when we don't know yet which carotenoids and phytochemicals do what. We haven't even identified all the essential carotenoids, flavonoids, and phytochemicals in vegetables and fruits, so we can't expect them to replace what we don't fully understand.

Procter and Gamble's own studies prove that these reductions in carotenoid levels are significant. Lutein blood levels drop 20% after eating one cup of Olestra-containing chips per day. (Lutein is the carotenoid that is associated with preventing blindness.) Worse, lycopene blood levels dropped 60% with this small serving of Olestra snacks per day. (Lycopene is associated with decreasing prostate cancer, heart attacks, and strokes.)

At a recent medical conference, I spoke with representatives from Procter and Gamble about the long-term impact of decreasing the absorption of carotenoids, flavonoids, and other fat soluble phytochemicals. They told me that Procter and Gamble continues to study the long-term impact of Olestra intake.

Antioxidants impact our health over decades, not just weeks to months. Therefore, studies to assess the long-term impact of Olestra on health would also take decades.

Meanwhile, millions of people might eat Olestra products for 10-20 years, and later find that their risk of death and disease has increased tremendously.

One of the unpleasant results of eating Olestra is that it can cause loose stools and digestive problems. Since you can't absorb it, it goes right on through your intestinal tract, causing bloating, cramping, and diarrhea.

Some people may find the intestinal complaints mild, while others will find them severe. When you stop eating the Olestra products, the intestinal problems go away. Hopefully, most people will be bothered by the abdominal complaints and shy away from Olestra.

While Procter and Gamble initially contended that eating low-calorie, fatty snacks could help Americans lose weight, there is no evidence that eating Olestra containing chips will help with weight loss. In fact, controlled studies with Olestra and a placebo showed that people who ate Olestra snacks did not reduce their caloric intake.

Once again the choice is yours. You can find Olestra in chips and crackers now. Next, it will be in salad dressings, French fries, and hamburgers.

The FDA will require a label on all products that contain Olestra. What this product needs is a label that accurately portrays the risk of eating Olestra products regularly. I would suggest a label more like this.

TABLE 31. Olestra Warning

> This product contains Olestra. Olestra inhibits the absorption of critical vitamins and nutrients. Eating Olestra may increase your risk of cancer, heart attacks, strokes, and blindness. Vitamins A, D, E, and K have been added, but there is no evidence that these additions will prevent you from increasing your risk of these serious diseases. Olestra may also cause abdominal cramping and loose stools.

The food industry will not wait for a food product to be proven safe. It wants to sell you Olestra products NOW. I would suggest waiting until more is know about Olestra and its long-term health risks.

CHAPTER 7 *SUCCEED IN CHANGING YOUR DIET*

*T*here are three fronts on which you must stage your attack on old eating habits: the home, the supermarket, and the restaurant. This section outlines how to make these life-style changes easier. The first step is all important–it's making that "*Commitment.*"

There are two possible approaches. First, I designed this book to help you change the way you eat. The next two chapters deal with changing both your eating and shopping patterns.

Second, you could seek professional help at the beginning by consulting dietitians, nutritionists, and other health care professionals who can help you learn new food skills. They can guide you with meal planning and improve your understanding of food choices. They can also teach you how to keep food records.

If you decide on seeking professional assistance, try to find someone who advocates a low-fat eating program emphasizing vegetables, fruits, grains, and legumes. Seek programs like my *28-Day Antioxidant Diet Program*, the *Ornish Program*, or the *McDougall Program*.

Cookbooks can also be a big help in learning new recipes. There are many low-fat cookbooks that use ample grains, fruits, legumes, and vegetables. The New Vegetarian Cuisine by Linda Rosensweig is full of delicious recipes, and is one of my favorites.

You can also keep current with lifestyle magazines for regular, up-to-date information on recipes, food preparation, shopping, and kitchen equipment. In particular, try the *Health Letter* (published by the Center for Science in the Public Interest.) and *The Vegetarian Times*.

EMPHASIZE SIMPLE FOOD CHANGES

Complex diets can be hard to follow. Counting calories and fat grams is difficult, and often discouraging. To succeed in eating well and feeling better, try making these simple changes:

1. Eat more colorful vegetables and fruits at each meal.

2. Eat more whole grains.

3. Eat at least one to two servings of beans or soy products per day.

4. Eat less fat, and avoid margarine and saturated fat.

5. If you use dairy, choose non-fat dairy products.

6. Choose simple non-fat snacks.

7. Emphasize feeling better when you make food choices.

MONITORING YOUR FOODS

Monthly food monitoring is a powerful tool for improving eating habits. Food records can be simple and do not require extensive food knowledge or math skills. Food records, filled out five days per month, teach us about the foods we eat, and can help us become experts on the fat and vitamin content of commonly eaten foods. If you choose to see a dietitian or nutritionist, bring food records to your appointment. It is a big help to your health care provider.

A simplified version of a food record only counts fat, servings of whole grains (like bread, cereals, rice), and servings of vegetables and fruits. You can copy the food monitoring chart on the next page. Your goal is to write down what you eat on three weekdays and two weekend days per month. By writing down what you chose to eat, it forces you to evaluate your food choices. Studies show that monthly monitoring over six months helps improve one's food choices, improves cholesterol levels, and aids in weight loss.

Many people will cut their fat content by 10% just by keeping a record of their food intake. For example, use a measuring spoon. You may use substantially more oil than you thought. If you eat meat, see how far you can stretch 3 ounces per person. You may surprise yourself by quantifying how much you really eat. Try it!

Try these monitoring charts 5 days monthly. You'll have 100 possible points each month. Do it monthly for 6 months. You'll see your scores climbing as you eat and feel better.

TABLE 32. Food Monitoring Chart: 14 points are possible on this chart from "Foods Items to Add" and 6 points are possible on the chart from "Fat Items to Cut." 20 points total are possible. Many readers have found that copying these monitoring charts and placing them on the refrigerator door helped them make better food choices. Go for it!

Food Items to Add	Possible points (14)	Actual points	Notes
3 Fruits per day (minimum)	1 point for each fruit item		100% citrus juice or vegetable juice can count as 1 point. No other juices count. 1/2 cup equals 1 serving
4 Vegetable Servings per Day (minimum)	1 point for each vegetable		1/2 cup equals one serving. Try to have at least one serving per day of a green leafy vegetable
5 Servings of Cereals and Grains per day (minimum)	1 point for each serving		Whole grain breads, pasta, rice, whole grain cereals. Do not count white bread, or refined grain products
1 Serving of Legumes or Soy products per day (minimum)	2 points		1/4 to 1/2 cup equals 1 serving

TABLE 33. Food Monitoring Chart.

Fat Items to cut			Substitutions
No high fat spreads like mayonnaise, butter, or margarine	1 point if avoided		Try using non-fat spreads, fruit preserves, or non-fat refried bean spreads instead
No fatty meats like hamburgers, sausage, sandwich meats, bacon, or hot dogs	1 point if avoided		Read the labels, find products that are less than 30% calories from fat. Try soy products such as tofu hot dogs, or soy-veggie burgers
No fatty chips, donuts, or fatty snacks.	1 point if avoided		Find non-fat chips or fruit snacks. Check the label and find snacks that have less than 30% of calories from fat.
Limit meat, poultry, and egg yolks to 1-3 servings per week	1 point if limited		If you eat meat or poultry, limit them to 3-4 ounce servings
Limit dairy products to non-fat or 1% fat only.	1 point if used		Use non-fat milk & non-fat yogurt. OK to have 1-2 ounces of cheese per day.
Limit cooking oils to 1-2 teaspoons per person per meal. Only use canola oil or olive oil.	1 point if followed		No deep fried food, i.e., French fries.
Six points possible per day Total:			

Fat Reduction

Most diet programs today focus on cutting down on fat intake. We know that we feel better, are healthier, and lose weight if we eat less fat.

Average Americans eat 38-40% of calories from fat, and that means over 1/3 of their energy intake often comes from artery-clogging grease. This sort of diet causes weight gain, increases the risks of heart attacks, diabetes, cancers, and strokes, and causes many digestive problems. After adding all the delicious and healthy foods we need, my goal is to help people cut their fat intake to less than 20% of total calories. People with coronary artery disease should consider a goal of less than 10% of their calories from fat.

Most people trying a diet try to cut back a little, and that's what they achieve–*little*. When their fat consumption drops from 38% to 34%, they don't feel any better. Then, 2-3 months later, they go back to their same old habits. So, how can people do better?

Rather than changing from regular mayonnaise to half the fat mayo, stop using mayonnaise altogether. Try non-fat refried beans as a spread instead. Rather than a change from whole milk to 2%, only use "non-fat" dairy products. Don't try to eat just one fried potato chip; stop buying them. Or find baked chips that have no fat. Do not buy hot dogs and burgers that are 70% fat. Buy the children veggie-soy burgers and soy dogs; they taste good, they are better for us, and kids will eat them. So can you.

Of course not everything you eat needs to have less than 20% of its calories from fat. You want the total calories to average less than 20% fat. And, if you are willing to exercise for more than 45-60 minutes in a day, you can eat more healthy fats that day, too. (See "MEET FATS THAT ARE GOOD FOR YOU" on page 55.)

There are advantages to knowing how to screen your food purchases. First, by reading food labels you can immediately eliminate many unhealthy foods that exceed a 20% fat limit. Second, when you choose to buy healthy foods that are higher in fat (like sliced almonds, tofu, or olive oil) you know instantly to limit their use.

If you want to reduce your fat intake below the 20% found in my recipes, follow two simple steps. First, use half the oil or nuts called for in my recipes. Second, whenever a recipe calls for grated parmesan cheese, use non-fat grated cheese instead.

Counting Fat Grams

No, I am not going to ask you to learn to count your daily fat gram intake. But some of you already have gone to the painstaking trouble of learning how to do this.

If you know how to count fat grams, great. To limit your fat intake to under 20% of your total calories, allow yourself 44 grams of fat per day. If you have a history of heart disease, consider a 22 gram daily fat limit. Many people who count fat grams only count high fat food sources, like chicken, oils, spreads, etc. They don't actually count the fat in their low fat food choices, like vegetables, grains, fruits, and beans. The result is that they drastically underestimate their actual fat intake. If you choose to count fat grams, make sure you count all the fat.

An advantage of following a Dr. Ornish diet is that you don't have to do any counting or figuring. But you do have to avoid all foods that contain fat. Essentially an Ornish diet means no nuts, no dairy unless non-fat, no oils, no fats, no avocados, etc. It also means no breads, pastas, or sauces that contain these fatty products. The Ornish Program is not only simple, it works if you're willing to accept all its restrictions.

In contrast, with my *28-Day Antioxidant Diet Program* you can still eat chocolate and nuts and cook with olive oil in limited quantities. The advantage of setting a 20% limit on caloric fat intake is that it allows you to use many delicious food products that are loaded with antioxidants and may, in spite of their fat content, be good for you. Just remember to use them in moderation. Find what works for you!

LEARNING THE TRUTH ABOUT FOOD LABELS

Sorting through the maze of information on a food label can be challenging, even for the sophisticated label reader. Not only does label reading require some math calculations, but the information in some of them can be downright misleading. Think of this section as a class in **"Food Label Reading 101."**

For example, foods labeled "low fat" or "reduced fat" may actually have a high fat content. (It's all relative to "reduced from what" or "lower than what"). Products said to contain "no cholesterol" may still contain large amounts of fat.

A perfect example of deceptive advertising is "2%" milk. Many of us have blindly believed that 2% means 2% fat. It doesn't. In fact, 2% milk actually contains 35% fat!

If our goal is to eat meals with fewer than 20% of calories from fat, we'll need to know how to calculate the fat content from a label. Here's how to quickly assess the percent of calories from fat:

- Find the calories from fat.
- Find the total calories per serving.
- Divide the fat calories by the total calories. You will get a number behind a decimal point. Move the decimal point to the right two places and this is your percentage. If you get more than 20% of calories as fat, put the product back and look for a lower fat alternate.[1]

Label Reading Practice

Are you ready to practice some "label analysis?" Look at the examples below. Begin with a typical *Fancy Spreadable Cheese* on the market. The front label often announces that the cheese is "50% less fat."

---

1. Occasionally, you'll come across a food label that does not list the calories from fat. To calculate them, simply multiply the number of grams of fat by 9 to find the calories from fat. (Each gram of fat has 9 calories.)

```
┌─────────────────────────────┐
│  ┌───────────────────────┐  │
│  │      BUY  OUR  NEW     │  │
│  │                        │  │
│  │       FANCY            │  │
│  │                        │  │
│  │     SPREADABLE         │  │
│  │                        │  │
│  │       CHEESE           │  │
│  │                        │  │
│  │    50 % LESS FAT!      │  │
│  │                        │  │
│  └───────────────────────┘  │
└─────────────────────────────┘
```

Before you toss this into your shopping cart, look at the "Nutrition Facts" section on the back label.

- Step 1: Fat Cal = 35.
- Step 2: Total calories = 50.
- Step 3:   35 (fat calories) divided by 50 (total calories) = .7, which is 70% calories from FAT.

Wait a minute. How did 50% less fat become 70% fat?   Unfortunately, putting this on a cracker is NOT going to create the low-fat snack you were hoping for.

Notice that the Total Fat of 4 grams is listed as 6% of the Daily Value (DV%). This sounds deceptively better than the 70% fat it actually contains. The bottom line is, if you eat much of this product, you'll get fat, too!

NUTRITION FACTS

Serving Size: 2 Tbsp.

	Amount/Serving	DV%
Calories 50	Total Fat 4 gm	6%
Fat Cal 35	Sat. Fat 3 gm	15%
	Chol. 20 mg	7%

```
╭─────────────────────────────╮
│                             │
│      WHOLE WHEAT            │
│                             │
│    FLOUR TORTILLAS         │
│                             │
│    Home Style Freshness!   │
│                             │
╰─────────────────────────────╯
```

Look at another product. How about trying WHOLE WHEAT FLOUR TORTILLAS. There's no reference on the front label to fat content.

Now, look to the next page for the back label with the Nutrition Facts section.

NUTRITION FACTS
Serving Size: One Tortilla

Cal   120
Fat Cal   20

Amount Serving		DV%
Tot Fat	2 gm	3%
Sat Fat	0 gm	0%
Chol	0 gm	0%

- Step 1: Fat calories listed as 20.
- Step 2: Total calories = 120.
- Step 3: 20 (fat cal) divided by 120 (total cal) = .166, or 17% fat.

17% fat sounds great to me.

What about good, healthy *tofu*? According to the front label, it's a "cholesterol free" and "lactose" free food. Does that mean it's also fat free?

- Step 1: Fat calories listed as 70
- Step 2: Total calories = 120
- Step 3   70 (fat cal) divided by 120 (total fat) = 58% fat.

Tofu contains 58% of its calories from fat! However, since tofu has multiple health benefits, you might want to find a way to use it despite its high fat content. If you add a little tofu to a lot of low-fat food (like veggies, beans, pasta, and rice) you'll get a whole meal with under 20% fat. (Check out my recipes with tofu. All are under 20% fat.)

MOUNTAIN FRESH

TOFU

Cholesterol Free, Lactose Free

NUTRITION FACTS
Serving Size: 3 Ounces

Cal   120
Fat Cal   70

Amount Serving		DV%
Total Fat	7 gm	11%
Sat Fat	1 gm	5%
Chol	0 gm	0%

Next, try a *Whole Grain Cereal*. The front label says, "made from whole grains."
Now look at the Nutrition Facts section on the back label.

FRONT   *BACK*

THE BEST

WHOLE GRAIN

CEREAL

Made From Whole Grains

Low in Fat!

NUTRITION FACTS
Serving Size: 1 cup

Cal   110
Fat Cal 18

Amount	Serving	DV%
Total Fat	2 gm	3%
Sat Fat	0 gm	0%

- Step 1: Fat calories = 18.
- Step 2: Total calories = 110.
- Step 3: 18 (fat cal) divided by 110 (total cal) = .16, or 16% fat.

Add non-fat milk and you have a meal that's a deal!

Don't even think of putting whole milk on this or your calculation will change drastically (see below).

	Cereal	+	1/2 Cup Whole milk		Total
Total calories	110	+	75	=	185
Fat calories	18	+	37	=	55

- Step 1: Fat calories 55
- Step 2: Total calories 185
- Step 3: 55 divided by 185 = 30% calories from fat.

30% fat doesn't seem too bad, but remember that it's mostly saturated fat. Therefore, it's worse than you thought. Stick to non-fat milk**!**

Imagine another typically vague label to decipher. The product is *Light Sour Cream.* The front label says "1/3 fewer calories" and "2/3 less fat." Having read the label, you might well ask, " Fewer than what?" and "Less than what?"

- Step 1: Calories from fat = 15
- Step 2: Total calories per serving = 35
- Step 3: 15 (fat cal) divided by 35 (total cal) = 43% fat.

This might be better than regular sour cream, which is pure fat. Yet, this is a dairy product, so again, most of the fat is saturated fat.

A 43% fat rating is slightly lower than tofu, but in contrast, there is nothing healthful or redeeming about sour cream. What if you add 2 tablespoons to 1 cup of veggies?

	1 Cup Steamed Broccoli	2 Tbs Light Sour Cream		Total
Total Calories	45	+ 35	=	80
Fat Calories	4.5	+ 15	=	19.5

- Step 1: 19.5 calories from fat
- Step 2: 80 total calories
- Step 3: 19.5 divided by 80 = 24% calories as fat.

Even this small amount of "Light" sour cream is slightly too much fat, particularly saturated fat. So now, you have some choices to consider:

- Eat it and absorb the saturated fat.
- Avoid these high fat products altogether.
- Use even a smaller amount per serving, like one tablespoon of "Light" sour cream (one half serving) per one cup of steamed vegetables (two servings). Don't even think of using regular sour cream.
- Buy nonfat sour cream instead. (This is what I do.)

Practice these calculations in the grocery store when you buy products. Don't worry about exact math, but aim to buy products with fewer than 20% fat calories.

If you find a food item that's clearly over 30-50% fat, consider whether or not it has some redeeming nutritional value, despite its high fat content (like almonds, cashews, tofu, avocados, olive oil, or high quality chocolate that will be used sparingly). If not, put it back on the shelf and congratulate yourself for using your label-reading skills to avoid another fatty pitfall!

DON'T BE FOOLED BY THE FRONT LABEL; READ THE NUTRITION FACTS TABLE ON THE BACK.

INVOLVING YOUR SIGNIFICANT OTHERS

Family involvement can make or break dietary goals, particularly if a significant other does the shopping or the cooking. Invite your spouse or companion to a nutrition class or to a health professional visit. A two-for-one visit is one way of getting a bargain and treating two for the price of one. When we get our families involved, we no longer have to cook separate meals.

Eating together as a family does more than just ease the transition. Meals bring us together. Food is a unifying experience. Poor eating habits overtake us when we nibble all day without a proper meal. During a family dinner, focus on interacting with your loved ones and tasting your food. Turn off the TV, put the newspaper and magazines away, and enjoy the experience of sharing food with family.

Involving your significant others in your dietary changes does not necessarily mean that they will adopt your new eating preferences. The first step in involving family is to explain why you want to make this change. (You're seeking better health, weight loss, lower cholesterol levels, or to feel better and more energetic.) The second step is getting them to agree to help you change the way you eat. Ask if they are willing to read this book to help "you" make needed changes. A distant third step could involve seeing if they are interested in changing how they eat, too.

A reluctant significant other presents a bigger challenge. You can't force somebody to eat what you cook. Try choosing food items that they like and build from there. If your housemate wants her/his own food, lectures about disease will likely alienate them and make them more firm in their resolve not to change. Actions speak louder than words, so be consistent and set a healthy example.

If you live with a *"gotta-have-my-meat-everyday"* person, here are some tricks. Try cooking stir-fries, rice dishes, or casseroles that you can eat and enjoy, and let your significant others (S.O.'s) add meat to their meals. If you don't want to cook their meat, let them cook it. That way, you only need to cook one meal, and your S.O. can use your main dish as a side dish. Hopefully, this will ensure that your S.O. receives the important antioxidants, veggies, and whole grains they need. Pasta dishes are also easy to divide into two parts; you can even keep different sauces on hand in the refrigerator. Mexican food, like burritos and tacos are equally easy to prepare; add beans to one dish, and let your S.O. add meat to their dish.

Involving children in diet changes is tricky. You need to ensure that your changes provide their special nutritional needs. Let's briefly address how a family with children can improve their food choices. Then I'll address how my program works for women during pregnancy. If you don't have children to feed in your home, and you don't plan on pregnancies, feel free to jump to the next chapter.

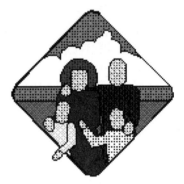

INVOLVING CHILDREN IN DIETARY CHANGES

Children have unique nutritional needs that vary at different ages.

1 year to 4 years

During these years, children learn food habits that will last a long time. Encourage them to eat a variety of grains, vegetables, and fruits at these ages, and food battles will be fewer in the future. Beans and legumes provide a great source of zinc and iron that children need.

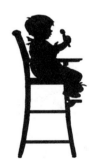

Until age 2, children can drink whole milk, as they need the extra calories. You'll have two types of milk in the refrigerator, non-fat for you and whole milk for them. Most children need at least 30% of their total calories from fat. Don't place adult fat-restrictions on this age group unless you and your medical provider discuss it first.

4 years to 12 years

Now that the children eat regular table food, food choices represent food preferences, not their understanding of proper nutrition. You may never get your children to like and eat vegetables, fruits, and whole grains if you don't do so now. This is the time to enforce long-term eating habits.

Avoid food battles at home by having only healthy foods and snacks available. Keep sugar-coated cereals, cookies, white bread, and candy out of the house during these formative years. Don't let unhealthy high-fat foods like regular hot dogs, extra-cheese pizza, and sandwich meats in the house. This way you won't be tempted by "junk food," either!

The key to developing lifelong healthy taste preferences occurs at this age. It is essential in a child's development to learn to enjoy fruits, vegetables, legumes, and whole grains. Don't give in; rather, keep trying new ways of serving healthy foods.

Some parents actually over-restrict fat intake for their children, misunderstanding recommendations intended for adults. If your child is on the slim to skinny side, extra calories and fats may be necessary, but you need to choose healthy fats. At this age, rather than letting them eat just any type of fat, some types should be avoided, like whole milk, 2% milk, high fat cheese, regular high-fat hot dogs, and high-fat chips. These food sources contain the "wrong types" of fat.

Instead, let them eat nuts (like almonds, cashews, hazelnuts, and pecans) and avocados. Add extra canola or olive oil to foods you cook especially for them. Children at these ages can excel by eating the recipes in my program.

Children love to cook at this age. Involve them in baking wholesome cookies and making pancakes. Let them rinse vegetables and fruits before you put them in the refrigerator after grocery shopping. Ask them to plan dinner, and assist them in cooking as they get older.

Some parents complain that their children won't eat vegetables. Since vegetables are the most important food group that children eat, this is a serious concern. By 5-6 years of age, I explain to children in my office that eating vegetables is not a choice, but something they must do to become athletic and healthy. I offer the following suggestions to encourage children to eat produce:

- Serve veggies as snacks during the day. You can serve them raw with non-fat or truly low-fat dips. You can lightly blanch veggies by boiling them for 1-3 minutes, then plunging them into cold water to stop the cooking process. Children often prefer slightly cooked veggies, cooked al dente, for snacks. Eliminate high fat chips and other junk food snacks.
- Give your children a choice as to which vegetables they want. Don't ask if they want veggies, ask them if they want them raw, steamed, blanched, or sautéed. Offer to squeeze on lemon juice, soy sauce, or vinegar. Offer non-fat bean or yogurt dips so that children can have fun dipping veggies.

- Serve children vegetables first. After the children are seated, put some veggies on their plates. Later add the rice, pasta, or other things you know they will eat.
- If all else fails, tell them not to eat their vegetables. It is a similar technique to telling screaming children in the back of a car "not to smile." Be firm in telling them, "no smiling and no laughing," and the screaming usually stops immediately. Telling children not to eat their broccoli creates a similar WIN/WIN situation. It is a game that many children enjoy playing over and over. Personally, I am quite tired of this game in my house as my boys want me to forbid them from eating dinner all the time, but it works.

12 years to 18 years

Teens have already established many patterns by this age. The best you can do is buy healthy foods so your teenagers have only healthy choices before them. Encourage cooking during these years. It is an important skill, and can be a big help to a busy family. Teenagers establish eating patterns now that will determine how they eat throughout their adult years.

As they strive for independence, encourage them to pick recipes, to shop for groceries, and to cook. You can establish nutritional boundaries, like low-fat pizza.

Encourage teens to read food labels and educate them on how to decide if a food is a healthy choice. Many teens enjoy deciding if a food really is "low-fat" as marked on the label, so they can avoid being manipulated by the food industry.

Rapidly growing teenagers need extra calories. Encourage them to choose healthy fats during these "growth spurts."

Teens Girls

Teenage girls have special nutritional needs. As noted in the bone health section, women have a once-in-a-lifetime opportunity to build bone mass between the ages of 13-25. Encourage calcium intake during this critical time. Green leafy vegetables, whole grains, non-fat dairy, and soy products provide good calcium sources. As noted in the health benefits section, cutting down on salt, meat, and cola intake will also produce stronger bones.

I asked Dr. Connie Weaver, professor at Purdue University and Chair of a National Nutrition Board evaluating calcium intake, about the high variability in calcium needs in teenage girls. We agreed that an inactive teenage girl with a high salt and animal protein intake needs at least 1500 mg of calcium per day. On the other hand, an actively exercising vegan female with a low salt intake may need only 700 mg per day to reach peak bone density. (See Table 4 on page 19 for calcium sources.)

Unfortunately, most teenage girls fail to obtain an adequate calcium intake to form strong bones. While added salt intake remains a problem in increasing calcium losses, the solution is simple. You can either cut salt intake, or add an extra 1/4-1/2 cup of non-fat milk (soy milk or cow's milk) per day to make up for the difference between a low salt and high salt diet.

Folic acid intake is especially important in teenage girls who often fail to eat high folic acid containing foods (green leafy veggies, beans, orange juice) and are therefore, commonly folic acid deficient.

Because teen pregnancies are on the rise, it is vital that young women have adequate folic acid stores. Folic acid deficiency at conception increases the risk of newborn spinal defects (spina bifida). This condition produces devastating problems and can largely be prevented by eating enough folic acid before getting pregnant; taking folic acid after getting pregnant is too late. I see the simplest solution to preventing spinal bifida in newborns is to have young women during their reproductive years take a One-A-Day Vitamin or eat a fortified cereal like "Total" or "Product 19" daily.

PREGNANCY

If you are thinking about getting pregnant, consider three things:

1. Eat folic acid to prevent birth defects. Food sources rich in folic acid include green leafy veggies, beans, orange juice, and whole grains. See Table 36 on page 271 for Folic Acid Food Content to be sure your intake is adequate. To repeat myself, if in any doubt, take a supplement! (This is an unusual case where supplements might be better than food sources, since folic acid supplements increase folic acid blood levels more effectively than do folic acid rich foods.)

2. Before getting pregnant, confirm that your blood count is normal. Meat and poultry provide iron, but these foods are not good for you. Beans, seafood (limited to two servings per week), whole grains, and green leafy vegetables are other healthy sources of iron. If in doubt, especially if you are a woman with heavy menses (heavy menstrual flows cause excess blood and iron loss), have your health care provider check your blood count; a simple hematocrit will do as a screening test.

3. Make sure you are immunized for German measles (rubella) before you get pregnant. Once you're pregnant, it's too late to get immunized without harming the baby.

What if I'm Pregnant?

If you think you're pregnant, it's the perfect time to start eating healthier foods! Pregnancy requires a balanced healthy diet, both for your health and comfort, and the health of your baby. My diet program provides all the essential nutrients for your pregnancy.

Having provided maternity care for 10 years, I believe this book represents a wonderful diet for a pregnant woman. It offers recipes and a program highlighting foods with extra fiber, vitamins, and nutrients. Proper nutrition means more than just taking prenatal vitamin supplements–it encompasses everything we eat.

A normal weight gain during pregnancy is 25-30 pounds. Most women can easily lose those pounds later with nursing, normal exercise, and sensible eating.

Women need more dietary iron when pregnant. Green leafy vegetables, legumes, and whole grains are a great source of iron. Cooking with cast iron pots and pans can increase your iron intake, too.

Foods rich in Vitamin C help increase iron absorption, too. A *pregnant vegan* woman will be challenged to obtain adequate dietary iron for a growing baby unless she eats iron-rich foods at each meal.

Despite the best diet, many women will need iron supplements (in addition to prenatal vitamins) when pregnant. Take them only if your blood count is low, as excessive iron supplements can decrease zinc absorption.

Avoid processed sugary foods (candy bars, candies, sugar frosted cereals, etc.) anytime, but especially when you are pregnant. These sugary foods can cause you to gain excessive weight and increase your risk of sugar intolerance and gestational diabetes, a form of diabetes that occurs during pregnancy.

And at this time, you should avoid all alcohol until after the birth.

Do indulge in green leafy vegetables which provide essential supplies of zinc, iron, Vitamin C, omega-3 fats, folic acid, carotenoids, calcium, and other important vitamins and minerals during your pregnancy. Eat at least two servings of green leafy veggies per day: kale, greens, leafy lettuce, broccoli, and beet greens are top choices.

Vegans have special needs during pregnancy. In particular, confirm that your zinc and Vitamin B 12 intake are adequate, or take a supplement.

Protein intake is important during pregnancy. You do not need to start eating poultry and meat during your pregnancy, but you do need other daily protein sources such as beans, soy products, non-fat dairy products, and ample grains and vegetables. Seafood can provide a good source of protein, iron, and omega-3 fats, but be cautious with sources that may be high in mercury, such as tuna.

CHAPTER 8   *SHARPENING*
YOUR SHOPPING
AND DINING
SKILLS

SHOPPING: DO'S AND DON'T'S

*T*HE BIGGEST CHANGE I AM ASKING OF YOU, IS TO CHANGE HOW YOU SHOP FOR FOOD. Your trip down the food aisles with a grocery cart can make the difference between health and vitality, and weight gain and disease.

We have to shop well to eat well. We can only cook foods that are in the house. To shop well, we need to know what to buy. Shopping is the first step to better health and more energy.

Most of us have a pattern as to how we shop. We know how often we need to make our ritual collection. We know the store we want to use. We even know which aisle has which ingredients. We usually buy the same bread, the same pasta, and the same veggies. We are creatures of habit, so let's build better food-buying styles.

Check your food supplies

Before you make your list and head to the local grocery store, see what you have in the refrigerator and in the cupboards. If you have never followed an antioxidant-rich, low-fat diet, you will likely find butter, margarine, potato chips, hot dogs, candy, and other forms of health-harming fats and sweets.

If you plan to slowly ease into this diet program, you can finish the products you find on your shelves. However, if you are ready to make a radical lifestyle change and want to feel much better, I encourage you to think of other options for these unhealthy foods.

- Donate the food to the local food bank.
- Throw the food away.
- Give it to a friend.

Choose Colorful Produce–for better taste, appearance, and health

Adding color to a meal doesn't just make it more attractive, it improves its taste and usually adds a wallop of antioxidants to any meal. When you are preparing a shopping list or shopping, think of:

- Reds: red bell peppers and tomatoes
- Greens: broccoli, kale, spinach, and herbs like parsley and cilantro
- Yellows: corn, carrots, yams and sweet potato
- Purple: kale and cabbage

Many of these colors fade quickly if overcooked, so only add them during the last 3-5 minutes of food preparation.

The mistake I make too often is to add these veggies, then turn off the heat because of some delay. When I reheat them, they end up overcooked and I lose some of their color and flavor.

THE SHOPPING LIST

You don't normally need a list to go shopping, although it helps. When you are trying to change your shopping habits, take along a list. Go through your cupboards, drawers, refrigerator, and freezer and establish what you have and what you need. In this section, I will help create a shopping list by food groups, although as you go through your kitchen supplies, you will likely search through one cupboard at a time. Verify what you have, think of what you need, and write down what you will buy at the store.

The appendix has four weekly shopping lists, which can help you to follow my *28-Day Antioxidant Diet Program's* meal plan.

Grains and cereals

Start with the basics: grains, breads, pasta, etc. Go through your cupboards and establish your supplies of pasta, rice, and grains like bulgur wheat or other unusual grains like couscous, quinoa, or amaranth. Do you need whole wheat tortillas? Do you ever cook with polenta (Italian corn meal)?

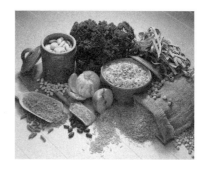

Next, look at breakfast cereals, such as whole grain oatmeal or grapenuts or a fortified cereal that has 100% of the RDA for zinc, folic acid, Vitamin C and Vitamin D. "Total" or "Product 19" are two of my favorites. Choose whole grain breads, or at least whole meal grain breads. Avoid sugar-coated cereals.

For baking, I like whole wheat pastry flour, plus we have whole grain rye flour and soy flour for making bread. I use white flour for dusting pans and equipment.

Legumes and soy products

How are your bean supplies, either canned or dried? Think of soy products, such as tofu, miso, and soy sausage. Soy burgers and tofu hot-dogs work well as snacks and on sandwiches. My favorite treat is sesame tofu. Dry lentils cook quickly, 10-25 minutes, but for super fast meals try canned lentils or other canned beans; they come in handy for soups and many dishes.

Oils and Condiments

Choose canola oil and/or olive oil. When you buy oils, stick to smaller containers (1 liter or less) as old oils can go rancid. Since you will limit the amount of oil you use, go ahead and get good quality.

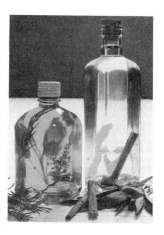

Plan to buy virgin olive oil and canola oil sprays to minimize the oil you use. I also use a squirt bottle that squirts precisely 1/2 teaspoon of oil with each shot; it works perfectly!

How about salsa, non-fat refried beans, tomato sauces, mustard, marmalade, and vinegars (balsamic vinegar in particular)? Look for new flavorings in the condiment and spice section in place of fat, such as sliced almonds, capers, curry spices, cayenne, and others.

Dairy products

If you eat dairy, choose non-fat milk, non-fat cottage cheese, and non-fat yogurt. Think about a non-fat cheese like mozzarella or another cheese that is at most listed as 1% low fat (less than 23% of calories from fat). If you want grated cheese, consider some hard parmesan, or plan to grate non-fat cheese. If you cook with egg whites, add eggs to your list, or consider the non-cholesterol egg beater products.

Planning for produce: Fruits and Vegetables.

Plan on a serving of juice per day per person (4 people equals 25-30 servings per week of juice). Pick highly rated juices (See Table 16 on page 80.) such as orange juice, pink grapefruit, or carrot juice. Also look for low-sodium tomato and vegetable juices. You need at least 1-2 pieces of fruit per day per person for the week. Without planning we seem to run out of fruit by the end of the week in our home. Four people will require at least 30 servings of fruit: melons, apples, oranges, kiwis, pears, berries, etc.

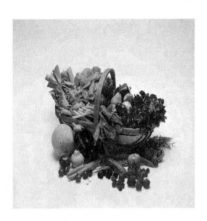

Calculate your veggies, too. Each person should eat 1-2 cups of vegetables per day, primarily green leafy, red, and yellow vegetables. Consider bell peppers, broccoli, sweet potato, carrots, spinach, kale, peas, and beans. If you have two people at home, you'll need the equivalent of 20 cups of vegetables for the week, for four people you'll need 40 cups for the week.

Check your freezer for frozen peas, broccoli, stir-fry mixes, etc. Frozen veggies come in handy for quick meals. Some of the frozen stir-fry combinations are excellent: broccoli, carrots, snow pea pods, cauliflower, and red pepper come in an easy packet that needs only steaming, microwaving, or sautéing. Although fresh is better, the nutritional quality of frozen vegetables remains excellent.

Canned beans are excellent food sources. They help make meal preparation quick and easy. Plan to rinse the beans well before adding to dishes. Canned vegetables are better than none, but they do lose vitamin content and are often loaded with salt and sugar.

This seems like a lot of vegetables and fruits if you aren't used to buying produce. Here is what Janet, a journalist and parent from Olympia, WA, found following this shopping plan.

> *"When I read the chapter on shopping tips I was surprised at the amounts of fruits and vegetables Dr. Masley recommended each time we shopped. But as I thought about it, those were the first things to disappear from the cupboard before our next shopping trip or were slighted from our diet a day or two each week. The next time I shopped at the produce sections I felt I had the "OK" to indulge in a wide variety of vegetables and fruits. Now I purchase a lot more fresh produce and we tend to eat it all. It makes for more interesting meals and more fun on shopping days.*

Do you have supplies of garlic, onion, and leeks? Calculate for one serving from this group per person per day. Include other spices like ginger root, parsley, cilantro, and dried spices too. The most common spice combination I use is Italian Herbs, a mix of thyme, oregano, basil, rosemary, and sage (similar to Fine Herbs and Herbes de Provence).

Beverages

Again, look at your supplies, calculate what you need to buy, and add those items to your shopping list. Consider green tea, herbal teas, tea, seltzers, or other beverages–even red wine. If you buy wine, it may be cheaper to buy a case every 1-2 months than to buy a few bottles at a time.

Add miso to your list if you like to drink broth, and so you can flavor grains or soups. Try soy or rice milk; some are flavored with almond or vanilla and are delicious.

Snacks

Watch out here! Many snacks are loaded with fat. Others are highly refined and send your blood sugar level surging. If you struggle to control your weight, try the habit of drinking tea instead of eating a food snack.

If you usually buy chips, plan to look for non-fat baked chips and serve them with bean dips. Don't eat non-fat chips alone or your sugar level can skyrocket.

Don't plan on nuts as snacks because of their high fat content, unless you can eat only 1-2 tablespoons at one time. Nuts are better used chopped or sliced and sprinkled over a main dish.

Children who are slim or at their normal weight often need more calories and snacks can supply them. Nuts represent a good choice of snack food for these children. Hazelnuts, almonds, pecans, macadamias and cashews provide the healthiest choices because most of their fat is monounsaturated. They also provide a good dietary source of Vitamin E and omega-3 fats.

If you buy crackers, plan to check the fat content before you put them in your cart. Avoid buying them if they have more than 20% of their calories as fat. Rye crisp is a great low fat cracker, and whole grain rye crisp is loaded with antioxidants.

However, if you have weight control problems, I recommend you avoid chips and crackers because they make your blood sugar level rise. You are better off eating fresh fruit, or choosing vegetables with non-fat dips.

Non-fat yogurt with lemon and dill weed makes a lovely dip for vegetables. Look to my *Hors d'oeurves and Dips* recipes for ideas. Salsa and non-fat refried beans make a great dip too.

What about cookies and candies? *I try to avoid them!* First, they should contain less than 20% of their calories from fat. Second, watch out for the sugar content and total calories. An apple provides roughly 85 calories; if your standard snack has more than 100 calories, maybe you need another food type.

Desserts

Lastly, plan for dessert. Fruit always works. You can slice fruit and put it on a plate to make it more attractive. Squeeze on lemon or lime juice or add non-fat yogurt, or have non-fat frozen yogurt by itself.

Consider adding 100% frozen fruit bars to your list, but skip those that are only 10-20% juice.

If you are a cookie person, consider whole wheat fig bars that have less than 20% of their calories as fat. When it comes to sugar and sweets, you should consider a 100-150 calorie limit. Personally, I dislike even thinking about calories, but I don't eat candies, cakes, and cookies except once or twice per month.

If you plan to buy chocolate, buy a small quantity of *high quality chocolate* and make something special.

Frozen dinners

Believe it or not, frozen dinners are often healthier than canned meals. You can check the labels for fat content, if they're less than 20% and have appeal, buy them and add fresh veggies to them.

If you buy frozen pizzas, try buying only the crust and add the topping at home. After heating the crust briefly, add tomato sauce, peppers, tomatoes, mushrooms, pineapple (if you like), onions, garlic, and herbs like basil, thyme, and oregano. Sprinkle on grated, non-fat cheese lightly, or skip it altogether. Add a few teaspoons of chopped cashews and pop the pizza in the oven. Serve with a glass of red wine or a glass of water with a lemon slice. Make a green salad on the side or steam some veggies as a side dish as the pizza bakes in the oven.

GOING TO THE STORE:

Now your list is ready. Give yourself extra time to go shopping this first trip; you'll need it. Not only will you need to read labels, you'll be looking for new ingredients which may take time to find. The next time you go shopping it will be easier, and by the fourth time, "you'll be a pro." If your math skills are weak take a calculator with you. You should be able to do ballpark math, i.e., 35 divided by 120 equals more than 1/5th (>20%) and nearly 1/3rd (<33%); if you're not confident with your ballpark math skills, a calculator comes in handy.

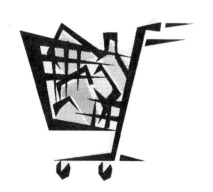

Shopping rule #1:

Don't go to the grocery store hungry. Your willpower will be low, and you'll tend to spend more money than you planned. Eat a piece of fruit or eat a meal before going shopping.

Shopping rule #2:

Take a list the first few times.

Shopping rule #3:

Read the back food value section and calculate the fat content. Don't be fooled by labels like "low-fat," "light," or "50% less fat."

Grocery store design

Grocery stores plan their attack on your wallet carefully; they set up their aisles so that you will buy products. Having a grocery list helps you establish a pattern of action so you can be efficient and quick. Once you're familiar with the design of your grocery store, you can plan your list accordingly.

Consider yourself lucky to shop in the United States. We have a huge choice during four seasons, especially in the produce department. During the winter, we have fruits and vegetables from Hawaii, Mexico, Florida, and California. Most other temperate countries offer a very limited selection in their produce section during the winter.

STORING YOUR GROCERIES

Pesticide removal:

If you are not used to buying and rinsing fresh fruits and vegetables, here are some tips:

1. Buy organic whenever you can. Yes, it is a little more expensive, but the more often we buy organic produce, the cheaper it will get. In particular, I look for organic produce when shopping for items that are covered with wax in the non-organic section (like cucumbers and apples) and those items that have a large surface area (like broccoli and lettuce). If they have a thick waxy coating, and you can't find organic products, consider peeling off the skin.

When shopping, *I head straight to the organic part of the produce section.* I find what looks good and then I look for non-organic produce items. Most days I can find appealing carrots, broccoli, leafy lettuce, apples and oranges.

2. Rinse all produce well. I put in a squirt of dishwashing soap and soak the veggies and fruits, and then I rinse the whole batch again.

3. Remove the outer leaves on lettuce or cabbage where pesticides are concentrated.

4. Scrub potatoes, carrots, and other root vegetables with a sponge or scrub brush; it's better to scrub them than peel them as many of their nutrients are in the skin.

5. High-fat foods contain more pesticides. Take heart that eating low-fat can help reduce your pesticide intake, too.

6. Rinse and clean all produce BEFORE you put it into the refrigerator. You don't want pesticide residues in there.

Tofu

Rinse tofu before putting it away. Review the section on Tofu, page 98, for tips on marinating it before you put it in the refrigerator.

The Cupboards

Some air-tight, see-through containers work well for pasta, beans, grains, flour, etc. Our shelves look like a shoe department at times with all those boxes but it is very practical and quick for food preparation.

Keep oils, vinegars, wines, etc. in a cool, dark place. Oils in particular will go rancid more quickly if exposed to light; if you buy them in bulk, consider storing the extra oil in the refrigerator.

The Refrigerator

Airtight, see-through plastic containers work great in the refrigerator. Leftovers, herbs, marinating tofu, cheeses, and sauces do well packed inside. Herbs such as parsley, cilantro, and basil do much better in a sealed container with a little water than by dropping them into the produce bin. Carrots, celery, and asparagus remain fresher if you stand them upright in an inch of water in a tall container; it makes the difference between limp carrots or crisp carrots after a few days.

Keep a container of juice on hand. The better rated juices make an easy snack.

The Freezer

We seldom cook just enough for one meal. We usually make extra portions, pop them into a sealable container, and put them in the freezer. Frozen food containers make quick, easy lunches on the average hectic morning. Non-fat and low-fat foods freeze very well. It is always nice to have a supply of frozen veggies, like an Asian stir-fry mix, peas, corn, or broccoli for quick additions to meals.

ORGANIZING YOUR 20-MINUTE MEALS AT HOME

How do I become organized?

Most of us no longer have the luxury of spending 1-2 hours cooking dinner every day. Those days are gone. Most of the dinners I cook at home take 15 to 30 minutes to prepare. Lunches take far less time, because we plan to use leftovers.

1. Pasta meals are quick and healthy. Put water on to boil and start chopping and slicing veggies. Plan a sauce (see recipes for ideas), throw in pasta when water boils (usually takes 10 minutes), and start warming or preparing your sauce. Begin steaming or sautéing veggies when pasta has 5-7 minutes to go. Set the table and eat.

2. Cook grains in bulk. When you cook rice, especially wild rice, cook enough for a second or third meal. It takes almost no extra work, just planning. You can sauté garlic and spices, and throw in rice (or other grains like couscous) with veggies, nuts, marinated tofu, or grated cheese for quick meals.

3. Keep extra sauces in the freezer or refrigerator. Why make tomato sauce for only one dinner? For nearly the same amount of work, you can make 4-8 dinners with the same sauce preparation. Freeze the sauce in muffin pans, Ziplock bags, or Tupperware. Try to keep sauces on hand for quick meals.

4. Keep a variety of grains, legumes, veggies, and condiments on hand so you have some variety in your kitchen. You can quickly add canned beans to a meal; just open and rinse. Nothing slows down cooking like having to run to the store. Try to get in a pattern of shopping once or twice per week and keep the basics on hand.

5. Consider how you organized your kitchen. Can you easily reach your grains, legumes, veggies, spices, sauces and condiments, or do you spend much time searching for things you think you have? I have a whole drawer full of spices which are kept in alphabetical order to save time and frustration.

6. Be cautious buying meals-in-a-box or frozen meals as these are often jammed with sodium (salt) and fat. Read the labels. Many of the low-salt, truly low fat versions are great; they just lack vegetables. So throw in some fresh sliced veggies or pull some from the freezer and add them to their prepared meal. Squeeze on lemon or lime juice, pour on some balsamic vinegar, add some marinated tofu or a few tablespoons of beans and you have greatly improved the nutritional value and the taste of a packaged meal. If you use packaged meals as the foundation for your dinners, remember to add antioxidant-rich condiments and vegetables.

DINING OUT

My wife and I eat out with our children about twice per month and are careful how we choose food out of the home. Many people eat at least half of their meals outside the home. Those who eat out frequently need a plan to survive all the "fat" floating out there.

Many restaurants and fast food places serve food with more than 70% of calories from fat. This type of eating leads rapidly to weight gain and poor health.

Let's look at some strategies to eat better when out of the home.

FAST FOOD

Fast food restaurants are notorious for serving food that is very high in fat. A few requests can help greatly. Ask them to skip the mayonnaise, and ask if they have any heart-healthy meals on the menu. When dining out, *"heart-healthy"* should mean that the meal has 30% or fewer of calories from fat, which is much better than items like French fries, where 80-90% of the calories come from fat.[1]

Taco Time and Taco Bell have many types of veggie tacos and low-fat poultry meals that have less than 30% of calories from fat. Be sure to skip the sour cream, and don't get the fries. Rather, order an extra burrito or taco.

Look for salad bars. Load up on veggies and choose fat-free salad dressings.

Many of the "burger joints" are starting to offer veggie burgers. Choose them, and skip the mayo or butter on the bun for a nutritious meal. If you are hungry, instead of ordering a side of fries, ask for two veggie burgers or get a salad on the side. You will feel more satisfied, get a more nutritious meal, and end up eating fewer calories.

RESTAURANTS

It is a pleasure to eat out in a restaurant. There's nothing to cook, no table to set, no dishes to clean; just sit back and be served. Meeting friends or family in a favorite restaurant can be a pleasant social event. The good news is that most restaurants are flexible and will serve you food the way you want it prepared, even with a smile.

My goal when eating in a nice restaurant is to order a delicious, healthy meal, and to feel great when I'm finished. See Table 34 for tips on ordering.

If you eat out rarely, I wouldn't worry about the fat quantity in a restaurant meal. Instead, aim to *add* plenty of healthy foods and *pick the best types of fat* for your meal–olive oil, canola oil, nuts, tofu, or seafood.

However, if you have medical problems, you struggle with weight control, or you eat out frequently, aim for a *"top score"* when ordering. The *type and quantity of fat* are both important to you. For better success when ordering, tell your server your specific preferences with a smile. You can request "low-fat," "no butter please," or "no added oil." You can also ask for "extra veggies" with your meal.

---

1. I wish that heart-healthy indicated that the food was less than 30% fat, and that they used healthy fats. For example, I'd rather eat a meal with 30-40% fat from olive oil or nuts than something with 20-25% fat from margarine or butter. For now, expect a heart-health insignia to refer to a 30% fat limit. If you want to know more, just ask your server.

Score on Your Dining Experience

Start your meal with a colorful salad with leafy greens or other colorful veggies. (Don't bother eating a salad with iceburg lettuce because of its low-nutrient content.) Choose a fat-free dressing and skip the cheese. Or, order an olive oil vinaigrette on the side and *lightly* (1-2 teaspoons) drizzle it over your salad. Alternatively, start with a hearty bean and veggie soup, but skip cream based soups.

TABLE 34. Dr. Masley's Dining Score: A ten equals a perfect score.

Possible Points	Items	Your Score
2 pts	If you have at least two or more servings of veggies (1/2 cup equals one serving). Don't count french fries or mashed potatoes. A small colorful salad counts as one serving.	
1 pt	If your meal was flavored richly with condiments, such as garlic, ginger, spices, herbs, or curry.	
1 pt	If your meal featured whole grains, such as brown rice, whole grain pasta, or dense whole grain bread. Don't count white bread, refined pasta or white rice.	
1 pt	If your meal had beans or soy products.	
1 pt	If you had one serving of fruit with dessert or with your meal (1/2 cup of fruit equals one serving).	
1 pt	If your meal was heart-healthy, either non-fat or with fewer than 30% of calories from fat.	
1 pt	If your meal was fat free, or made with olive oil or canola oil. No score if it contained fatty meats, fatty dairy, or cream sauces.	
1 pt	If you exercised for at least 30 minutes today. Or, you can go for a walk after your meal.	
1 pt	If your restaurant uses organic products and they wash non-organic produce.	
10 pts	Total	

Choose entrées that feature exciting combinations of vegetables, nuts, and whole grains. If you want something with fish or lean poultry, that's OK, but pick a dish that entices you with healthful foods. Choose whole grain side dishes with brown rice, fresh whole grain pasta, amaranth, or bulgur wheat. Skip the white fluffy bread.

Drink water with a slice of lemon or mint. If you like wine, order "*one glass of red wine with your entrée.*"

Do order a dessert featuring fruit. Sorbets taste fabulous and fruit crumbles and fruit tarts are delicious. If you want *high quality chocolate*, go for it and have it with fruit, Make sure your dessert isn't loaded with butter or cream such as ice cream. Don't cheat yourself with poor quality chocolate sauces or candy bars.

Having eaten a fantastic meal, enjoy a walk. Walking is a great way to enhance your digestion and brings *quality time* to any relationship.

Types of Restaurants

Restaurants vary greatly, but many have a healthy-heart insignia next to items that are less than 30% fat. If not, ask the server and they are usually delighted to help.

Japanese and Thai restaurants often start off with a wonderful soup. They usually have delicious, low-fat, items on the menu. Rice, noodles, and vegetables are important staples. Beware of sodium and MSG hidden in the food. Ask the server to recommend items for your meal with *your preferences* in mind.

Pizzas can be low in fat if you skip the sausage and pepperoni, and ask for 1/3 the usual cheese. Salad bars in pizza restaurants often offer a variety of options.

Italian restaurants usually have several tomato flavored items on the menu; look for those made with marinara sauce. Have a whole wheat roll in place of butter covered garlic bread, and dip your bread into tomato and garlic sauces. Do ask that your food be served with extra garlic (if you tolerate garlic well). Order a green salad with non-fat dressing. Lastly, save room for dessert, as Italian restaurants often serve excellent sorbets.

Chinese restaurants should serve low-fat food, but often don't. Insist on low-fat preparations; they can do it, and frankly I like them better than a stir-fry dish swimming in oil. Ask for colorful veggie, tofu, and mushroom dishes served with steamed brown rice. Again, beware of hidden sodium and MSG.

Mexican restaurants are the biggest challenge; frequently everything is dripping with fat. First, *skip the very high-fat tortilla chips.* Second, avoid the sour cream. Third, ask them what menu items might be rich in veggies and low in fat. While often high in fat, enjoy the healthy guacamole. Other best bets are tostadas, chile rellenos, burritos, and tacos with a side of rice and beans. I always ask if the refried beans are made with lard; upon request they'll often offer cooked whole beans without lard and mixed with a wonderful salsa.

Breakfast in a Restaurant

Breakfast should be an easy meal to eat at a restaurant. Yet too often, pancakes, waffles, hash-browns, and omelets lack produce, are dripping in fat, and covered with butter.

Remember to order pancakes and waffles without that scoop of butter on top; I ask for extra fruit instead! Toast and marmalade, fruit plates, and cereals make great healthy meals. Skip saturated fat-packed bacon and sausage at all cost. Many restaurants now serve soy sausage that is low-fat, healthy, and delicious. Spicy Mexican or Greek omelets, made with no-cholesterol egg-substitutes, also tastes great.

EATING AT FRIENDS' HOMES

When friends ask you to their home, state your food preferences up front. It is unfair to let them work hours cooking dinner and then learn that you can't eat it.

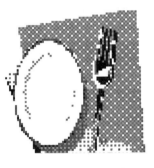

After nearly two decades of dealing with this, I have learned that speaking out at the time of the invitation is the easiest and fairest thing for my host-to-be. If Ms. X asks you over for dinner on Saturday night, thank her for the invitation and state that you have switched to a very low-fat diet. If you are now vegetarian, tell her that, too. If you hear silence, or uncertainty about what to make, suggest a potluck and offer to bring a dish. Most of the time, they will turn your offer down, but be prepared to make or suggest a delicious low-fat entrée if need be. Look for an occasion to ask Ms. X over for a meal at your place for a delicious low-fat, antioxidant rich meal.

Let me share my initial experiences when I drastically changed my diet in 1979.

I had been working and traveling in Asia for six months and quit eating meat. At times after coming home, I felt harassed by some of my friends and family because of my change in diet and lifestyle. People seemed to ask the same questions over and over: Did I think tomatoes suffered when I ate them? At first I ignored them, but later I would usually retort that their slice of beef sure suffered–and give details! I went through an unfortunate militant, vegetarian stage. Rather than being able to share in the joy of my new diet, all I did was alienate people.

Fortunately, that experience was short-lived and I have since learned to avoid discussing controversial nutrition topics with people while eating.

There is a fine line between answering someone's questions on nutrition and getting stuck in a debate with someone who wants to argue about food. I now attempt to answer questions openly, without placing a judgment on people's choices.

To maintain proper social etiquette, try not to discuss your new eating habits over a meal. Deflect the conversation until after dinner or get it out of the way before you sit down at the table. Having stated your preferences, if you are served a dish "floating in fat," or something you don't want to eat, you can either gracefully decline or just take a courtesy taste without offending your host.

BUSINESS MEALS

The trendy term for business meals has changed to *"power lunch,"* or power meals. I like the term as it emphasizes the need to be alert. Drinking alcohol decreases our thinking power, but so does eating fat. High-fat food makes us tired by sending our blood supply to digest all that food. When your stomach feels "stuffed," your thinking power suffers.

Look for heart-friendly signs on the side of the menu. Again, order salads with non-fat dressings or ask for the dressing on the side. (Restaurants often drench their salads with dressing fat.) Try pasta dishes without a heavy white sauce. Avoid fried food, like French fries or fish and chips. By ordering low-fat power meals, your mind <u>performs</u> better, plus you benefit your health.

If you order alcohol during a business meeting, don't drink until the food arrives. Cocktails on an empty stomach greatly decrease your thinking power. Order "one" glass of wine, and ask them to bring it with your meal. Drink water, or order a glass of tonic water with a slice of lemon, or a seltzer until the food arrives.

If you are vegetarian, one option is to call in advance to review your food preferences, perhaps while making a reservation. This can prevent your playing "20 questions" with the server in front of your business associates. Personally, I find restaurants very *"veggie-friendly"* these days; the key is to smile and be friendly. Even if they fail to have a vegetarian dish on the menu, usually they will happily whip up a tantalizing pasta dish for you on the spot.

AIRPLANE FOOD

The variety of food on airplanes has improved greatly in the last 10 years, if your flight has a meal service. Vegetarian and low-fat meals are available upon request. Remember to ask for these when you make your reservation. Request special meals at least 24 hours in advance. With luck, I've received veggie meals with just a couple of hours' notice, but don't count on it. When traveling with children, we invariably carry snacks that they enjoy; it makes the flight more enjoyable for everyone.

CHAPTER 9   *HOW TO START*
THE 28-DAY
ANTIOXIDANT
DIET PROGRAM

*D*uring my ten years of clinical work as a family physician, I have urged my patients to try my Antioxidant Diet Program. Thousands–yes, thousands–of times, I've suggested that health will improve and energy will rebound within 2-4 weeks if people will give healthy lifestyle changes a chance. And in fact, most people report feeling more ener-getic and more "alive" very quickly. Others who are struggling with chronic aches and pains may need 3-4 weeks on the program before they feel its rejuvenating effects. I've found that a month is a good trial period for people to try out my nutrition plan, hence *THE 28-DAY ANTIOXIDANT DIET PROGRAM.*

The program is not limited to 28 days, however. It may well be the beginning of a lifetime of weight control, better health, and vitality.

Most diet or weight loss programs restrict calories and produce short-term weight loss, but with a sacrifice. Denial is part of the price one pays for the loss of a few pounds, which are usually gained back when the diet ends. These "No-No" diets almost always result in "Yo-Yo" weight gain later.

High protein diets cause rapid weight loss because they favor the loss of water, electrolytes, and muscle while you lose fat. If you lose more than one pound per week, you are losing healthy lean body mass, too. Rapid weight loss diets also increase oxidative stress, as your body cannibalizes itself.

My own "writer's nightmare" was that I would be tempted into writing a quick weight-loss diet program. But I have held firm, realizing that the consistent overall health improvements that come with this diet program speak for themselves. Try this program; really follow it for one month. You should feel terrific, and so will your clothes!

PLUNGERS AND WADERS

Each of us is a unique individual, with our own special blend of likes and dislikes. Therefore, no one program or diet plan will work for everyone. My goal is to help you find a program that will work with your distinct needs and preferences.

Often, I watch people about to go for a swim. I've noticed that there are those who courageously take a running plunge, and those who thoughtfully and carefully wade into the water. I've designed *THE 28-DAY ANTIOXIDANT DIET PROGRAM* to meet the needs of both plungers and waders. Here are two patients–one a Plunger, the other a Wader–who found the diet easy to access and to fit into their lifestyles.

Plunging in

Jeff is a 31-year-old self-employed carpenter who works outdoors year-round. He likes being in charge of his life, and is very conscientious about the work he performs. He moved out of his girlfriend's apartment last year and began to eat donuts with coffee instead of the cereal he had been accustomed to eating with his girlfriend. He also switched from eating dinner leftovers for lunch, to eating at fast-food joints.

Jeff drank beer with dinners that varied from pizza, to burgers, to fried chicken. Although he worked hard, he had lost his jogging partner and his aerobic exercise and began to put on weight.

In the 12 months that followed his breakup, he gained 35 pounds. He had no energy, despite the fact that he slept like a log. He also had terrible stomach cramps and gas. Now, even Jeff's blood pressure had increased from his previous healthy 130/85 to a concerning 150/102.

When I spoke with Jeff, I realized that he didn't need a major medical workup. Instead, I gave him a month to try out my program. I outlined it in detail, and he plunged in with zeal. To my amazement, the very next day he gave all the junk food in his house to a local shelter. He began eating 7 servings of fruits and veggies, 5 servings of whole grains, and a serving of beans every day. He also walked 2 1/2 miles per day, every day as prescribed. I had asked him not to jog for at least the first month, since he hadn't worked out in almost a year.

Within a week, Jeff's stomach had settled down. By three weeks, he had lost 3 pounds and felt terrific, with extra energy at the end of the day. By a month, he had lost 5 pounds, his blood pressure had dropped 15 points, and he decided to stay with the program.

Jeff is the determined type, a guy who makes things happen when he sets his mind to it. By the time he had come to see me, he was ready to do anything to feel better. Using my 28-Day Antioxidant Diet Plan, he went after his goal, and achieved it.

Wading In

Martha is a 30-year-old woman I've known since I helped deliver her baby girl seven years ago. She's a delightful woman, a kind, shy, helpful and caring mother. In contrast, her husband, Jake, is a friendly weekend-warrior sort of guy.

Martha had spent most of her energy caring for her family and working as a secretary for the state. Gradually, she had less and less energy for her job. She had gained 35 pounds over the last two years. Her overall health had deteriorated over the last year with weekly headaches, frequent colds, and monthly "PMS" complaints.

Jake had pushed her into running with him, reciting "No pain, no gain." But following a strained back and a case of hip bursitis, she stopped walking or running altogether.

Martha's checkup was normal, and I offered her the essentials of my program. She had several reservations about changing her lifestyle. Jake wanted those "meat and potato dinners" every night and her daughter "hated vegetables." She was worried about anemia and diabetes, and about her thyroid.

We checked her thyroid, blood count, and a fasting blood sugar reading. All were normal.

One month later, Martha was encouraged by reading some handouts I had given her on feeling better. She agreed to walk 15-20 minutes a day for a month, and to eat 3-5 servings of produce daily.

At two months, she had more energy but weighed the same and was still plagued by headaches and PMS complaints. She then agreed to walk 30 minutes per day, added 1-2 servings of soy products daily for her PMS complaints, and added five servings of vegetables and fruits per day. But still cooked meat and potatoes for Jake and her daughter.

Two months later, Martha had lost 8 pounds and her headaches and PMS complaints were gone.

At 6 months, I saw her daughter for stomach aches related to constipation. I recommended that her daughter get on my program, and Martha finally decided it was time for the whole family to take the plunge.

I didn't see them for 8 months until her daughter came for a well-child checkup. Both mother and daughter were doing well. Martha had no more PMS symptoms, nor headaches; she didn't have an appointment, but wanted to tell me how thrilled she was that she had lost another 12 pounds. Her daughter's stomach aches were gone.

Martha's gradual approach to trying this program worked for her over time. As often happens, it took a child's symptoms to transform the lifestyle and health of other members of the family. Even Jake, who still has his lean meat or poultry serving 2-3 nights per week, learned to enjoy more antioxidant-rich foods at every meal.

TAKING THE PLUNGE

The plunge works well for many people. Get ready, get set, GO! Start by picking a calendar date. Tell friends, family, and significant others about why you want to make this change and when you plan to make it. Often the first day of the month or the first day of the week works well as a start date. Put a note with your start date on the refrigerator and/or the bathroom mirror.

To take this plunge towards more energy and better health look through the shopping guide from Week 1 at the end of this chapter, and Weeks 2-4 in the appendix. You can even buy your food from the shopping lists provided in the appendix. If you are committed to feeling better right away, clean out the cupboards and give away all the white bread, candy, butter, and frozen hamburger meat, to your local shelter.

I don't expect everyone to follow the diet plan exactly. If you really like a meal in Week One, you can substitute and make it again in Week Two or Week Three. You can also choose to add 1-2 seafood meals to your week.

Plan for a regular exercise program. Design activities that work for you and lay out times when you can do them. Don't overdo your exercise plan and injure yourself. Far too often, one of my patients starts a new exercise program, pushes too hard at the start, and within the first month needs 2-4 weeks of rest to recover from an injury. The exercise guide in Chapter Six will help you benefit from your exercise without overdoing it. (See "EXERCISE: THE FAST TRACK TO SUCCESS" on page 129.)

The plunge approach works well for those already committed to changing to feel better. Skip the urge to hesitate and go for it. You'll feel better right away and overall you have fewer choices to make. After a month, you may find that feeling fantastic makes sticking with the program worth it.

WADING IN

For those contemplating a slower rate of change, ease into this program and see how it feels. You can sample recipes as you read through this book and see how this information might impact your lifestyle. Mix in new habits with old ones, but give yourself a time line to adjust your food choices and activity levels.

Try some of my favorite and easy to make recipes for 3-4 meals per week. Plan to eat 7 or more servings of colorful vegetables and fruits daily.

Slowly add more recipes during the week. Focus on breakfast first, the most important meal of the day. Look to the weekly menus for wholesome breakfast ideas. Drink fluid in the morning to start your day, such as citrus or vegetable juice and water.

Aim to reach at least 30 minutes of activity per day within 6-8 weeks. At some point, you'll need to shift from contemplation to action. It takes longer to feel better this way, but for some people, a slower process provides better long-term success.

With either approach, you will learn to make changes that improve your lifelong energy level and slow the aging process. Nobody will live forever, but we can live happier and healthier.

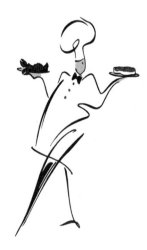

HIGHLIGHTS OF THE 28-DAY ANTIOXIDANT DIET PROGRAM

Here are ten simple steps–in my personal order of importance–to achieving anti-aging benefits, increased vitality, and enhanced health with my *28-Day Antioxidant Diet Program*. Remember, one of the advantages of this program is the focus on ADDING delicious, healthy foods to your diet daily.

1. Eat 7-10 servings of fruits and vegetables daily. Choose 1-2 servings of green leafy vegetables per day and enjoy other colorful produce. Splurge and buy great produce.

2. Eat 1-2 servings of legumes and soy products per day. Emphasize soy products daily.

3. Exercise, giving yourself time to build your activity level. Within 4-8 weeks you should reach at least 30-60 minutes of continuous, moderate activity every day.

4. Limit your fat intake and pick the best fats. Choose fats from canola oil, olive oil, avocados, cashews, almonds, hazelnuts, pecans, or soy products.

5. Drink at least 2-3 quarts (liters) of hydrating fluid per day.

6. Eat 5 servings of whole grains per day. Choose grain products that control blood sugar levels and suppress hunger.

7. Take 10-15 minutes every day to relax. Quietly calm your thoughts during this time. Share warmth and kindness with people around you throughout the day.

8. Avoid exposure to toxins and pollutants, which will increase oxidation in your cells. Limit alcohol intake to 1-2 drinks per day or don't drink at all. Avoid even "passive" tobacco smoke.

9. When you can, buy organic foods that are pesticide and hormone free.

10. Improve your muscular strength, so that you can avoid injuries and increase your ability to handle physical stress and illness.

ENJOY THE RECIPES. GOOD HEALTH AND BON APPÉTIT!

THE 28-DAY ANTIOXIDANT MEAL PLAN

WEEK ONE

Look at a one-week meal plan, then give it a try. Continue on with weeks two, three, and four.

If the Plunger or Wader approaches don't fit your lifestyle, form your own plan. Write out a plan on paper and go for it. Feel free to substitute one day for another. You can also swap a lunch with a dinner. If you like a particular meal from Week One, feel free to repeat it in Weeks Two and Three. Pick meals that work for you. If you want to eat seafood or lean meats during the week, be sure to add antioxidant rich herbs, vegetables, legumes, and grains to the meal you make.

You can compare this meal plan with the RDA recommendations for vitamins, fat, and mineral content. For help with grocery lists, see the shopping lists in the Appendix.

Breakfast

Today, most breakfasts in American homes are rushed, and bear little resemblance to the sit-down breakfast meals of years past. Breakfasts have become quicker to make and eat. Given the choice, choose whole grain bagels or toast and spread marmalade, jams, or nut spreads on them. Or, have a bowl of whole grain, fortified cereal with non-fat milk.

Avoid sugar-frosted cereals, sweet rolls, or toast without a substantial spread. Otherwise your sugar level will skyrocket, only to bottom out later in the morning. Remember to drink hydrating fluid in the morning.

You can substitute non-fat yogurt with fruit any morning you like. If you want eggs, try the egg substitute products. Sauté garlic, onions, fennel, herbs, and/or mushrooms. Stir in egg substitutes (no yolks) and enjoy scrambled eggs with these flavorful veggies.

Lunch

The lunches listed are wholesome and designed to take less than five minutes to prepare. Not many of us have time in the morning to make lunch before dashing off to work. Often, I'll use leftovers from a previous dinner for a lunch. I wrote many of the recipes in this book for six people, assuming that only four people will eat them; this provides you with two ready-made lunches. If you cook for six people, try cooking for eight to get a few lunches out of your preparation time. Be sure to drink a hydrating beverage at noon. You need the fluid, or your day will drag.

AVERAGE DAILY VITAMIN AND MINERAL CONTENT:

If we add Week One's nutrient content and divide by seven we can see our daily average intake of essential vitamins and nutrients.   Nutrient and Vitamin Content of Week One Meal Plan

	DAILY INTAKE	US RDA
Calories	2019 / day	2000 / day
Vit C	498 mg	60 mg
Vit A	35,218 (IU)	5,015 (IU)
Fiber	38 grams	Not specified
Folic acid	917 mcg	400 mcg
B 12	2.6 mcg	2.0 mcg
Calcium	976 mg	800 mg (varies with age) 1,200 mg (by NIH)
Iron	26 mg	15 mg
Total fat	37 grams (16.5% of calories)	60 grams (30% of calories)
Saturated fat	5.6 grams (2.5% of calories)	(not specified)
Monounsaturated fat plus Omega-3 fats	23 grams (10.5% of calories)	(not specified)
Polyunsaturated fat	7.4 grams (3.3% cal)	(not specified)
Protein	67 grams (13% of cal)	(70 grams for 154 lb adult)
Zinc	14 mg	12 mg
Alcohol	10 grams	(not specified)
Calcium/Protein ratio	14.7	14
Sodium	2300 mg	2400 mg (FDA recommendation)

Snack

Do you have time for a snack in the afternoon? If you make healthy food choices, and you have the time, you should have a midafternoon snack. A piece of fruit, veggie sticks, or non-fat fruit yogurt can provide energy for the end of the day. Avoid candies that provide a quick sugar fix, insulin surge, and subsequent sugar low. High-fat foods (like chips) will suck your energy away for digestion at the end of the day when you need energy the most. If you don't have time to eat a snack, at least have a beverage like a glass of selzter, water, juice, or tea.

Dinner

The weekly menus assume that you have 15-30 minutes to cook dinner most weeknight evenings and more time at least once per week. Learn to cook in quantity. For a family of four, cook a lasagna for eight; freeze half and serve it for dinner next week. When cooking pasta sauce for four, cook for 12, and freeze two dinners for a later date. You can cook better in less time.

I include dessert every night. Fruit is a perfect dessert. Look for a non-fat yogurt flavor you enjoy. Bake a pineapple-carrot cake or banana-pecan cake per week, and have a slice with frozen non-fat yogurt or fruit sorbet each night.

WEEKS TWO, THREE, AND FOUR

For these weeks, read "Week Two Sample Recipes" on page 283. Following these tables, you will find the shopping lists for each week. The shopping lists will let you shop <u>once</u> per week over the weekend and enjoy wonderful meals all week.

The appendix also contains a section on "Antioxidant Supplements" and a "Further Reading List."

TABLE 35. Week One Sample Meal Plan

DAY	Breakfast	Lunch	Snack	Dinner	Dessert
♦Sun			Bake Pine-apple Carrot Cake	Spaghetti with Roasted Tomato Sauce. Green Salad. Whole Grain Bread. (Make & freeze extra sauce)	Sorbet with fresh fruit
Mon	Coffee or tea, Whole grain toast with orange marmalade & 1 tsp almond. Orange juice	Veggie Burger, microwaved on whole wheat with tomato and non-fat bean spread. Carrot sticks	Green tea	Pasta Stuffed with roasted peppers, parsley & cheese, and Steamed Broccoli 1 glass wine or water	Sliced Apple &/or Pear. Pineapple-Carrot cake (from weekend)
Tues	Coffee or tea. Bowl of Total cereal with non-fat milk and berries. Grapefruit juice	TACO TIME: Natural soft veggie taco (no sour cream). Apple. Water	1 Glass of Carrot Juice or Tea	Miso soup. Stir-fry with black bean sauce. Rice. 1 Glass wine, sake or water	Slice of cantaloupe. with Pineapple-Carrot Cake
Wed	Coffee or tea. Bowl of oatmeal with fruit. Orange juice	(Leftovers) Pasta with tomatoes, garlic, broccoli. Orange Water	1 Pear and water	Peperonata with Pasta. Whole wheat bread. (Cook extra for a lunch or dinner next week) Green Salad with mustard vinaigrette dressing 1 Glass wine or water	Cantaloupe with Sorbet

Thur	Coffee or tea. Whole wheat toast with marmalade & 1 tsp Almond spread. Orange juice.	(Leftovers) Peperonata with Pasta. 1 Apple Water	Tea	Tabboulleh (bulgur wheat with parsley, tomatoes, sliced almonds and lemon juice). Steamed green beans. 1 Glass wine or other drink. (Cook extra if you need lunch tomorrow)	Frozen non-fat Yogurt blended with fresh or frozen black-berries
Fri	Coffee or tea. Bowl of Total cereal with non-fat milk, & fruit. Tomato Juice	(Restaurant Lunch) Spinach salad (no bacon, non-fat drsg on the side) Whole wheat roll. Iced tea; (or, bring leftover Taboulleh Salad)	1 Apple and tea	Sweet & Sour Stir Fry (with cashews, mushrooms, broccoli, tofu, and pineapple). Rice. (Cook extra for a lunch or dinner next week.) Green Tea or Wine	Sorbet with slices of fruit Enjoy 1/2 ounce of fine chocolate
Sat	Coffee or tea. Apricot & Tofu Pancakes. Banana-Cantaloupe Smoothie. Water	Hiking Lunch: Whole wheat bread sandwiches with tomatoes, cucumber, mustard, & non-fat cheese. Dried Fruit & Water	Trail Mix	Adults: Leek Soufflé. Steamed broccoli. Whole wheat bread. Wine or water Children: Pasta with frozen peas, corn, and sliced tofu hot dogs	Crepes Suzette
Sun	Coffee or tea. Whole rye toast with marmalade & 1 tsp almond spread. Orange Juice	Pizza: with Roasted red bell peppers, leeks, and mushrooms. Steamed Broccoli Water		Borscht Soup. Whole wheat bread. Green Salad. Water with a slice of lemon. (Cook enough to serve with dinner later in the week)	Home made frozen yogurt with blue-berries and port

CHAPTER 10   *FABULOUS ANTIOXIDANT-RICH RECIPES*

INTRODUCTION

The recipe section is organized like a traditional cookbook with sections created by food groups. The main course section is divided into ethnic regions. The sections flow in the following order:

Breakfasts

Starters

- Hors d'oeuvres (Appetizers) and Dips
- Sauces
- Soups
- Salads

Main Courses

- Pasta
- European Cuisine
- Oriental Cuisine
- Asian and Middle Eastern Cuisine
- Southwestern American Cuisine

Finales

- Desserts
- Beverages

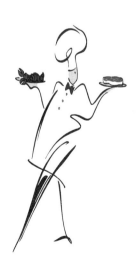

INGREDIENTS

I have tried to limit myself to ingredients that I can find at regular grocery stores in my area. If I have chosen something more unusual, I will make that clear and try to give you an alternative ingredient.

I use alcoholic beverages in some of these recipes. When we cook or sauté with alcohol, the alcohol evaporates and all that remains is the flavor. To avoid alcohol entirely, you can either use non-alcoholic wine in place of wine, or orange extract in place of orange liqueurs, changing very little in the recipe.

The only exception to this rule is adding alcohol to frozen yogurt or ice milk. In this case, the alcohol itself plays an important role in the texture and consistency produced by preventing the frozen dessert from freezing rock hard. If you want to avoid alcohol entirely, skip it but be sure to eat the frozen dessert within a couple of hours before it freezes hard in the freezer or ice cream maker.

Whole wheat pastry flour may be hard to find in some stores. If you can't find whole wheat pastry flour, just mix half whole wheat flour with half all-purpose flour. I list recipes with whole wheat pastry flour, and with half whole wheat flour and half all-purpose in this book.

You can use canned, cooked beans or cook your beans from scratch. Always rinse canned beans well. Don't overcook canned, cooked beans in your dishes or they turn mushy.

I encourage you to try interchanging fruits, berries, beans, nuts, grains, and vegetables in these recipes. You can modify these recipes to fit your tastes, or to take advantage of your crop in the garden, or you can check your local grocery store for fresh seasonal produce.

When sautéing, I use a small amount of oil. If the food starts to dry out in the pan, or starts to stick, don't add more oil. Rather, add a splash of vegetable stock or wine as it will provide moisture, flavor, and accelerate cooking times.

Chile spice varies greatly in "hotness" (enchiloso). One teaspoon of chile paste or sauce may be hotter than one tablespoon of another brand. Add chile spice to these recipes cautiously, depending on your taste preferences.

PIE CHARTS

The pie charts that accompany each recipe represent the energy portion, or calories for each meal. The ingredients listed determine the portion of energy in the pie charts. If I suggest a salad in the introduction, and it is not listed under the ingredients, that portion of energy will not be included in the pie chart.

I developed the pie charts by entering all ingredients on a software program called *Key Gourmet for Windows*. The program calculated the percentages of energy by calories, and I transferred that information to an Excel pie chart format.

The pie charts divide the percent of energy from a meal into: *"Carbohydrates (Carbo's), Protein, and Fat."*

If you skipped the nutrition part of this book, let me very briefly explain why I listed fat as *"MUFA fat"* and *"other fat."* MUFA is an abbreviation for monounsaturated fatty acids. This type of fat (found in canola oil, olive oil, many nuts, and avocados) in limited amounts decreases cholesterol levels, helps prevent blood clots from blocking our blood supply, and slows tissue damage caused by oxidation. In short, monounsaturated fats in limited quantities may be good for us. Omega-3 fats appear beneficial to our health too, and are included under the MUFA part of the pie chart.

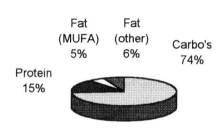

Other fats include saturated fats (from many animal meats and fatty dairy products) and polyunsaturated fats (from grain oils like corn, peanut oil and animal meats). Saturated fats are clearly harmful to our health and should be avoided. Polyunsaturated fats should be limited.

KITCHEN EQUIPMENT

You do not need a gourmet, high-cost kitchen to cook delicious meals. All of the recipes in this book were created with a regular oven and ordinary pots, pans, and utensils. Yet, there are several items that I find essential and timesaving.

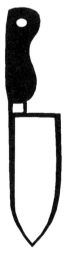

More than any kitchen tool, you'll need a high-quality, sharp *knife*. This tool can last a lifetime, so you can splurge at the kitchen equipment store. I prefer a chopping blade at least 8-9 inches long and 1 1/2 inches wide at the base. You'll also need a tool to keep your blade sharp.

A large, solid *cutting board* complements a knife well. I always run out of cutting space on smaller cutting boards. If you use a sliding cutting board, pull it out and place it solidly on the kitchen counter. You'll cut more adeptly and safely when the cutting board doesn't wiggle.

A metal collapsible *steamer* works wonders with veggies. One steamer seems to fit all my pots and pans. Oriental bamboo steamers are also handy, as they stack on top of each other.

A *blender* can make fruit smoothies, blend soups, form sauces, and mix fruit and yogurt for frozen yogurt. A step up is a *food processor* that can blend the above, and also cut and slice veggies, grate cheese, beat egg whites, and knead dough.

Non-stick skillets are essential. They help us sauté foods without using excess fats and oils. On occasion, I need a second skillet to prepare one full meal. A large *stainless steel pot* is great for soups, sauces, or boiling water for pasta. To make pasta for six people, I add at least six quarts of water and need additional space for the pasta.

I personally avoid aluminum pots and pans. While the press often condemns aluminum, there is insufficient scientific evidence to say that cooking with aluminum is harmful. However, stainless steel or fancier metals make better pans that last longer, and in the long run saving you money. If scientists ever prove that aluminum pans are harmful, you'll be glad you switched to quality cooking pans a long time ago.

Extra *measuring spoons, cups, and bottles* make cooking easy. Keep spares on hand. Measuring oils is easy with all the new tools. Squirt bottles squirt precisely 1/2 teaspoon of liquid. Many spray bottles spray about 1/6 of a teaspoon per second; just count one thousand one, one thousand two out loud and stop. You use far less oil by spraying a thin film than by pouring it out of the bottle.

See-through *sealable containers* help store food. Use tall skinny ones for carrots, asparagus, and broccoli; add an inch of water to the bottom and place them in the fridge to keep veggies fresh and crisp. Use short, flat ones for herbs with a splash of water to keep the herbs from spoiling. Fill medium sized ones with lunches. It helps to have only three sizes that use the same lids, and you can stack the same size containers in a drawer or cupboard. Store left-overs or extra rice in them, and stack them with food in the fridge to save space. Make sure that they are microwave safe if you reheat food in them.

INGREDIENTS FOR SPECIAL MEDICAL CONDITIONS

The majority of these recipes will help you to improve your health if you have medical problems. However, you may need to modify a few of the ingredients in this book if you have medical conditions such as coronary artery disease, diabetes, or hypertension.

People with coronary artery disease will want to go further than reducing saturated fat intake; they'll want to eliminate it. While the saturated fat in my recipes is very low, occasionally I have chosen recipes that include grated parmesan cheese, which contains small amounts of saturated fat. If you have coronary artery disease or diabetes, I recommend that you use non-fat cheese and non-fat dairy products. Simply substitute two tablespoons of non-fat parmesan or another non-fat cheese for two tablespoons of regular parmesan cheese. You can also substitute 1-2 tablespoons of nuts for each tablespoon of regular parmesan cheese.

If you have hypertension, you may need to limit your salt intake. Ask your health care provider if you are salt sensitive. Your medical provider may suggest a sodium-free salt substitute. One cup of sodium-free vegetable stock is a good substitute for one cup of water with one tablespoon of miso.

Diabetics need to avoid sugar. In recipes that use sugar, either skip the sugar, use a sweetener substitute, or avoid that recipe altogether. If you have diabetes, try to add more beans than I called for in these recipes and choose pasta dishes more often.

If you avoid dairy products for medical or other reasons, choose soy milk or calcium fortified rice milk in recipes that use milk. Many recipes use grated cheese as a garnish. Simply avoid the cheese in these recipes and substitute either tofu or chopped nuts instead.

COOKING TIMES

I included cooking times with the recipes to help you plan your time. These times assume you can slice and dice vegetables quickly, and that you have all the ingredients and equipment within easy reach.

If this style of cooking is new to you, when planning meals, give yourself an extra 5-10 minutes per recipe. Soon you'll reach the cooking times set; eventually you might even beat them!

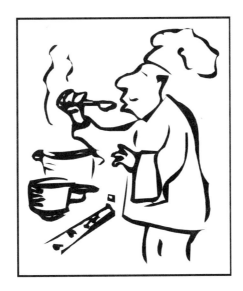

BREAKFASTS

Breakfasts and brunches are enjoyable when we give them the time they deserve. A brunch can be light or filling. Fresh squeezed citrus juice or carrot juice complements a brunch well.

FRENCH TOAST

This is a delicious, low-fat version of the usual high cholesterol French toast. The Apricot, Ginger, and Pear Sauce goes well with this breakfast.

Preparation Time: 15 Minutes
Serves: Four

1	*cup*	*Egg substitute, (or four egg whites lightly beaten)*
1	*cup*	*Milk, non-fat*
2	*Tbs*	*Brown sugar*
1	*medium*	*Orange, grate the rind*
1/8	*tsp*	*Salt*
1/2	*tsp*	*Cinnamon*
1/8	*tsp*	*Ground nutmeg*
1	*Tbs*	*Grand Marnier*
1-2	*tsp*	*Canola oil*
8	*Slices*	*Whole wheat bread*
1/3	*cup*	*Maple syrup, (or use*

"APRICOT, GINGER, AND PEAR SAUCE" on page 210, optional)

2	*cups*	*Peaches, sliced (canned or fresh)*

Mix the egg substitute and milk in a bowl. Stir in the brown sugar, orange rind, salt, cinnamon, nutmeg, Grand Marnier, and 1 teaspoon of oil.

Spray skillet with canola oil and heat. Dip bread slices into the egg mixture, and cook each side until golden. Continue until all the toast is prepared.

Meanwhile, heat topping sauce. To serve, place golden bread slices on the plate and pour topping over each serving with fruit slices.

Per Serving;		
Calories:		323
Saturated Fat:		0.8 grams
Total Fat:		5.9 grams
Fiber:		7.3 grams
Vitamin A:		69% RDA

Fat (MUFA) 6%

Fat (other) 5%

Carbo's 74%

Protein 14%

APRICOT & TOFU PANCAKES

Surprise! Tofu adds a wonderful, fluffy texture to pancakes. This is an easy recipe that both children and adults enjoy. You can substitute any fruit in the pancake batter; try bananas, strawberries, or blueberries.

Preparation Time: 20 Minutes
Serves: Four (makes 16-20 Pancakes)

2	cups	**Whole wheat pastry flour**
1	cup	**All-purpose flour**
4	tsp	**Baking powder**
1/2	tsp	**Salt**
1/4	cup	**Sugar**
2 1/2	cups	**Non-fat milk**
2	large	**Egg whites (optional)**
1/2	pound	**Tofu, soft**
1	cup	**Apricots, chopped (frozen or fresh)**
2	tsp	**Canola oil, for the pan**

Topping:

2/3	cup	**Maple syrup**
1/2	cup	**Apricots, chopped (canned or fresh)**

Mix flours, baking powder, salt, and sugar together in a bowl.

Lightly whip milk and egg whites, stir into dry ingredients. Don't over-mix (a few small lumps are OK).

Cut tofu and pat dry with a paper or cloth towel. Mash tofu, and gently fold into batter with apricots.

Cook on a non-stick frypan or griddle on medium heat. Makes 16-20 four inch pancakes.

If you use oil for the pan, brush on gradually or use canola spray.

Instead of plain syrup, try pouring a mixture of syrup, marmalade, and apricots over your pancakes. Warm syrup in microwave for 30 seconds, if desired. Or try Apricot-Ginger-Pear-Sauce Recipe.

Per serving: Calories: 724
             Saturated Fat: 1.4 grams
             Total Fat: 9.6 grams
             Fiber: 8.3 grams

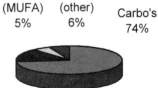

Fat (MUFA) 5%
Fat (other) 6%
Carbo's 74%
Protein 15%

WAFFLES WITH BERRIES

Waffles are a favorite weekend breakfast in our home. You can use your choice of berries and fruit.

Preparation Time: 15 minutes for the first, and 20-30 minutes to finish the batch.
Serves: Four

1/2	tsp	*Canola oil*
2	cups	*Pastry whole wheat flour (or 1/2 all purpose & 1/2 all wheat flour)*
2	tsp	*Baking powder*
1/4	tsp	*Salt*
1	Tbs	*Sugar*
1	medium	*Banana, mashed*
1/2	tsp	*Vanilla extract*
1 1/2	cups	*Non-fat milk*
1	Tbs	*Canola oil*
3	large	*Egg whites, whipped until stiff*
2/3	cup	*Maple syrup*
2	cups	*Blueberries, frozen or fresh*

Preheat waffle iron and brush or spray on oil.

Combine dry ingredients in a large bowl, set aside.

Mix mashed banana, vanilla, milk, and oil together. Then, mix with dry ingredients.

Beat egg whites until peaks form. Fold in with batter.

Warm syrup and berries in microwave or in pan over burner.

Pour batter onto waffle iron until about 2/3 full. Cook until golden and waffle comes free when lid is lifted. Serve with warmed berry syrup.

Per Serving:
Calories:	512
Saturated Fat:	0.6 grams
Total Fat:	5.8 grams
Fiber:	6.5 grams
Zinc:	3.8 mg

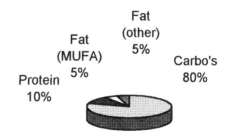

Fat (other) 5%
Fat (MUFA) 5%
Protein 10%
Carbo's 80%

WHEAT BRAN MUFFINS
WITH DRIED APRICOTS

These bran muffins are high in fiber and low in fat. They make a great snack, or can be eaten as a simple breakfast. A couple of muffins per day will greatly increase your fiber intake.

Preparation Time: 10 Minutes
Baking Time: 25-30 Minutes
Makes: 12 Muffins

1 1/2	*cups*	*Whole wheat pastry flour*
1	*cup*	*Wheat bran*
1/2	*tsp*	*Salt*
2	*tsp*	*Baking powder*
2	*large*	*Egg whites, beaten*
1	*cup*	*Non-fat milk*
1/4	*cup*	*Molasses*
4	*tsp*	*Canola oil*
1	*cup*	*Dried apricots, chopped*
1	*medium*	*Yam, cooked & mashed*
1/3	*cup*	*Pecans*

Preheat oven to 375° F.

Mix dry ingredients in a bowl. Combine wet ingredients with apricots in a separate bowl. Combine both and stir in mashed yam.

Spray a non-stick muffin pan lightly with canola oil, pour muffin batter into each depression.

Bake for 25-30 minutes. Muffins are done when a toothpick inserted comes out dry. Let cool prior to serving.

Per Serving: (1 Muffin)		
Calories:	165	
Saturated Fat:	0.4 grams	
Total Fat:	4.2 grams	
Fiber:	4.6 grams	
Vitamin A:	69% RDA	

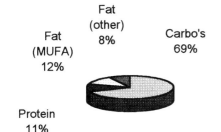

Fat (other) 8%
Fat (MUFA) 12%
Carbo's 69%
Protein 11%

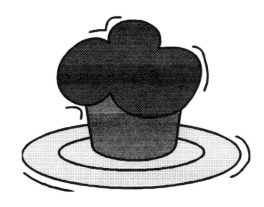

HORS D'OEUVRES AND DIPS

Hors d'oeuvres (appetizers) warm up the palate for a main course. Or, on occasion, a potluck with different hors d'oeuvres provides an assortment of tastes and delights.

Dips can accompany hors d'oeuvres. These can be healthy, low-fat, and flavorful. Choose healthy dippers too, such as jicama slices, veggies, or non-fat chips.

LEMON-YOGURT DIP

This dip goes well with vegetables, stuffed grape leaves, and steamed artichoke leaves. It's also great in sandwiches and veggie burgers.

Preparation Time: 5 minutes
Serves: Eight

1	*cup*	*Yogurt, non-fat plain*
4	*medium*	*Lemons, juiced*
1/4	*tsp*	*Dill weed*
1/2	*tsp*	*Honey or sugar*
1	*pinch*	*Salt*

Garnish with: *Fresh dill, mint or parsley sprigs and a dash of paprika*

Pour off clear liquid floating on top of the yogurt. Mix remaining yogurt, lemon juice, dill weed, honey, and salt in a bowl. Chill and serve. Garnish with a dash of paprika and sprigs of fresh herbs.

Per Serving:	Calories:	37
	Saturated Fat:	0.1 grams
	Total Fat:	0.2 grams
	Vitamin C:	17% RDA

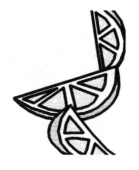

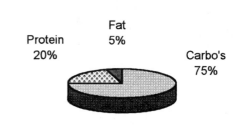

Protein 20% Fat 5% Carbo's 75%

QUESADILLAS

Quesadillas are essentially a cheese and tortilla sandwich. They provide a quick and easy way to make an appetizer or a simple meal. This version adds peppers and refried beans. Serve with your favorite salsa. Use whole wheat or corn tortillas.

Preparation Time: 10-15 Minutes
Serves: Side Dish For Six

12	**medium**	**Whole wheat tortillas**
1	**medium**	**Bell pepper, chopped**
4	**medium**	**Garlic cloves, diced**
1/2	**tsp**	**Virgin olive oil**
1/2	**cup**	**Non-fat refried beans**
2	**Tbs**	**Cilantro, chopped**
1/2	**cup**	**Non-fat cheese (like Monterey Jack), grated**
1/2	**cup**	**Salsa**
Garnish with:		**Fresh cilantro sprigs**

Sauté the pepper and garlic with oil for 2 minutes on moderate heat, stirring occasionally. Add the refried beans and heat until bubbling. Stir in the cilantro and remove from the heat.

Place one tortilla in the heated skillet, pour on 2 tablespoons of beans and spread the beans out over the tortilla. Sprinkle on 2 tablespoons of cheese, and place another tortilla on top. Heat each side about 1 minute. You can use two pans at a time to cook faster.

Cut each tortilla into six triangles and lay out on a plate. Serve with your favorite salsa and garnish with a few sprigs of cilantro.

Per Serving:	Calories:	155
	Saturated Fat:	0.2 grams
	Total Fat:	1.8 grams
	Fiber:	4.2 grams

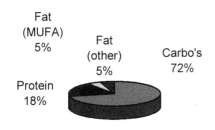

Fat (MUFA) 5%
Fat (other) 5%
Carbo's 72%
Protein 18%

JULIENNED VEGETABLES

*F*lash-cook vegetables to create great snacks and hors d'oeuvres. Toss with a tangy mustard vinaigrette, or skip the dressing and use with dips.

Preparation Time: 15 Minutes
Serves: Four

2	cups	**Broccoli florettes, sliced into thin strips**
2	cups	**Carrots, sliced into 3 inch long thin strips**
1	cup	**Cauliflower florettes, sliced into long thin strips**
1	cup	**Asparagus (if in season), cut in 3 inch lengths**
1	medium	**Red bell pepper, cut into long thin strips**

Dressing:

2	Tbs	**Balsamic vinegar**
2	Tbs	**White wine**
1	medium	**Lemon, juiced**
1	Tbs	**Extra virgin olive oil**
1/2	tsp	**Mustard**
1/2	tsp	**Italian Herbs**
1/2	tsp	**Soy sauce, low sodium**

Garnish with: **Fresh herbs**

Bring several quarts of water to a boil. Have a tub of very cold water with plenty of ice nearby.

Add broccoli, carrots, and cauliflower to boiling water. After 30 seconds, add asparagus and pepper and boil another 30 seconds until tender, but still chewy (*al dente*). Strain veggies and immerse immediately in ice water to stop the cooking process. Mix dressing in a bowl. When veggies are chilled, strain and add to bowl. Toss and garnish with fresh herbs before serving.

Per Serving:	Calories:	30
	Saturated Fat:	0 grams
	Total Fat:	0.1 grams
	Vitamin C:	74% RDA

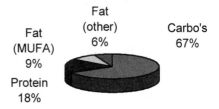

Fat (other) 6%

Carbo's 67%

Fat (MUFA) 9%

Protein 18%

GUACAMOLE

This is a tangy, low-fat version of Guacamole. Serve it as a side dish, or use as a dip.

Preparation time: 15 minutes
Serves: Six

1	large	Avocado
8	ounces	Garbanzo beans (1 cup)
4	medium	Garlic cloves, minced
1/8-1/4	tsp	Cayenne pepper
1/4	tsp	Salt
2	medium	Lemons, juiced
2	medium	Tomatoes, chopped
1/2	cup	Cilantro, fresh
6	Pockets	Pita bread, whole wheat

Peel and mash the avocado. Drain and rinse the can of garbanzo beans well and purée in a food processor (or mash until smooth).

Mince the garlic and sauté for 1 minute in a non-stick skillet sprayed with olive oil. Then add it to garbanzo purée along with cayenne, salt, and avocado. Blend briefly. Stir in lemon juice, chopped tomatoes and cilantro.

Serve with pita bread cut into triangles, or use non-fat tortilla chips, veggie sticks, jicama slices (my favorite), or whole wheat tortillas. You can use extra cayenne pepper or chopped spicy chilies if you like your guacamole hot *(enchiloso).*

If you like your guacamole creamy, mix in 1/2 cup of non-fat plain yogurt.

Per Serving:	Calories:	299
	Saturated Fat:	1.0 grams
	Total Fat:	6.5 grams
	Vitamin C:	95% RDA

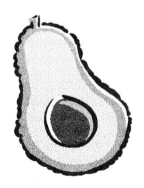

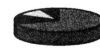

MUFA Fat 11%
Other Fat 7%
Protein 12%
Carbo's 70%

BEAN DIP WITH SALSA

When we eat chips at home, we serve them with a bean dip that is hearty, flavorful, and spicy. Choose or make salsa that provides as much hot, spicy zip as you like. We enjoy this dip warm or cold. Substitute onion, tomatoes, & olive oil for ready-made salsa if preferred.

Preparation Time: 5 Minutes cold, (10 minutes hot)
Serves: Eight with non-fat chips

1/4	*cup*	*Onion, minced*
1	*tsp*	*Extra virgin olive oil*
2	*medium*	*Tomatoes, chopped*
15	*ounces*	*Non-fat refried pinto beans (2 cups)*
1-2	*dashes*	*Cayenne pepper to taste*
1	*medium*	*Lemon, juiced*
1/4	*cup*	*Fresh cilantro, chopped*
1/4	*cup*	*Non-fat sour cream (or cottage cheese)*
1/4	*tsp*	*Cumin powder*
1/4	*tsp*	*Salt*

Garnish with:	*Sprigs of cilantro and a dash of paprika*

To serve cold, mix ingredients into a bowl and serve.

To serve warm, peel and mince onion and sauté with oil for 2 minutes on medium heat. Add tomatoes, beans, and cayenne pepper and heat another 1-2 minutes until bubbling. Remove from heat and add lemon juice, cilantro and sour cream.

Place in a serving bowl and garnish with sprigs of cilantro and a dash of paprika.

Serve with non-fat tortilla chips, veggies, jicama slices, or whole wheat tortillas cut into triangles.

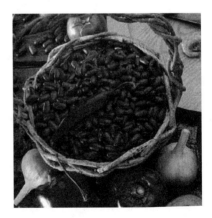

Per Serving:		
	Calories:	80
	Saturated Fat:	0.3 grams
	Total Fat:	1.3 grams
	Fiber:	3.3 grams

MUFA Fat 10% Other Fat 4%

Protein 23%

Carbo's 63%

MEXICAN SALSA

My family loves this version of a traditional Mexican salsa, it goes well with many Latin dishes. Freshly roasted peppers add a rich flavor to this side dish; however, you can use uncooked, canned, or sautéed peppers. For a spicier version, add jalapeño peppers or extra cayenne.

Preparation Time: 15 Minutes (with freshly roasted peppers)
Preparation Time: 5 Minutes (with uncooked peppers)
Serves: Four

1	medium	**Green bell pepper**
1	large	**Garlic clove**
2	Tbs	**Onion, finely diced**
1	medium	**Tomato, coarsely chopped**
3	Tbs	**Cilantro, chopped**
1	medium	**Lime, juiced**
1/2	tsp	**Paprika**
1/8-1/4	tsp	**Cayenne pepper**
1/4	tsp	**Salt**

Roast pepper, See "ROASTING PEPPERS" on page 246. Put garlic in oven with pepper to roast. (If you buy preroasted peppers, you can roast or sauté the garlic, or use raw.)

Dice pepper, mince garlic, and onion and add to tomato and cilantro. Squeeze on juice of 1 lime, add paprika, cayenne pepper, and salt to taste. Stir, chill, and serve.

Per Serving:	Calories:	93
	Saturated Fat:	0.1 grams
	Total Fat:	1.2 grams
	Vitamin C:	237% RDA
	Vitamin A:	40% RDA

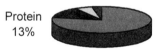

MUFA Fat 6%
Fat (other) 3%
Carb's 78%
Protein 13%

HUMMUS

This recipe provides a more colorful and complex taste than the usual hummus recipe, and with less fat. You can prepare it in advance, or after your guests arrive. Serve with whole wheat pita bread, whole wheat tortillas, or non-fat chips. To form a meal, serve with steamed vegetables, or stuff sprouts and fresh spinach into a pita bread to make a sandwich.

Preparation Time: 15 minutes
Serves: Six

16	ounces	Garbanzo beans, canned
4	medium	Garlic cloves
3/4	cup	Lemon juice
2	Tbs	Sesame tahini
1/8-1/4	tsp	Red pepper flakes
1/4	tsp	Ginger, fresh or ground
1/4	tsp	Salt
2	Tbs	Extra virgin olive oil
3	medium	Tomatoes, chopped
2	cups	Parsley, diced finely
Serve with:		
8	Pockets	Whole wheat pita bread

Rinse garbanzo beans well. Blend in a food processor or mash until smooth.

Sauté garlic for 30-60 seconds on moderate heat until it turns slightly yellow with 1 tsp of the olive oil. Add to garbanzo beans.

Stir in lemon juice along with tahini, red pepper, ginger, salt, and remaining olive oil. Use less lemon juice to taste if you prefer.

Finally, add tomatoes and stir in parsley.

Slice whole wheat pita bread into triangles. If you use whole wheat tortillas, toast lightly on a hot skillet, then cut into triangles. Jicama slices are also great for dipping.

Fat (other) 9%
MUFA Fat 10%
Protein 14%
Carbo's 67%

Per Serving:	Calories:	466
	Saturated Fat:	10.2 grams
	Total Fat:	1.2 grams
	Vitamin C:	145% RDA
	Fiber:	12.1 grams

SAUCES

We use sauces and dips in many meals, from main courses to desserts. They range from tart to spicy to sweet. In these recipes, I use more herbs and spices to take the place of fat.

RASPBERRY SAUCE

Raspberry sauce works well with many desserts. Dribble it on frozen yogurt, use it as the sauce between cake layers, or use it as a dessert dip. You can substitute blackberries for raspberries to make blackberry sauce. Garnish with sprigs of mint leaves and enjoy.

Preparation Time: 10 Minutes
Makes: 1 1/2 to 2 Cups

2	cups	**Raspberries**
1/3	cup	**Sugar**
2	Tbs	**Port wine (or kirsch)**

Thicken with _either_:

2	Tbs	**Non-fat sour cream**
	or,	
1/2	tsp	**Corn starch**

Optionally add:

1-2	tsp	**Freshly squeezed lemon juice**

Heat the raspberries and sugar over medium low heat. Add port and heat until mixture begins to bubble.

Remove from heat and pour through a screen to filter out the seeds.

For cakes or fillers, add either non-fat sour cream or corn starch to thicken.

If you like tartness, add a touch of freshly squeezed lemon juice.

Garnish with fresh mint leaves.

Per Serving:	Fat%:	3%
(Serves 6)	Protein%:	4%
	Carbo's%:	93%
	Calories:	74

APRICOT, GINGER, AND PEAR SAUCE

This is a lovely sauce for pancakes and French toast. You can serve it on frozen yogurt or eat it alone. I enjoy the apricot, pear, and ginger flavor, but you can substitute apples for pears, orange juice for nectar, or peaches for apricots. Canned fruit works, too.

Preparation Time: 10 Minutes
Simmering Time: 10 Minutes
Serves: Six

3	*Tbs*	*Sugar*
2	*tsp*	*Corn starch*
2/3	*cup*	*Apricot nectar*
1/2	*tsp*	*Vanilla extract*
1	*cup*	*Apricots, chopped (fresh or canned)*
1	*medium*	*Bosc pear, sliced*
1-2	*Tbs*	*Candied (crystallized) ginger*
1	*Tbs*	*Grand Marnier liqueur (optional)*

Garnish with: Fresh mint leaves.

Dissolve sugar and corn starch in apricot nectar. Add vanilla and heat until bubbling.

Meanwhile, chop apricots and cut pears into thin slices. Add to heating liquid. Dice candied ginger and add to sauce. (If you can't find crystallized ginger, substitute 1 1/2 tablespoons of fresh ginger root and 1 tablespoon of extra sugar.) Once the sauce bubbles, reduce heat, add Grand Marnier, and simmer for 5-10 minutes. Serve hot, or chill and serve later.

Garnish with mint leaves.

Per Serving:	Calories:	87
	Saturated Fat:	0.1 grams
	Total Fat:	0.4 grams
	Fiber:	2 grams
	Vitamin A:	24% RDA

Protein
4%

Fat
3%

Carbo's
93%

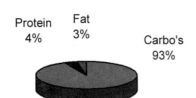

QUICK AND EASY SPAGHETTI SAUCE

This is an Italian-flavored sauce with tofu. It comes in handy for pasta, vegetables, pizza, and casseroles, and it freezes well.

Preparation Time: 15 Minutes
Simmering Time: 30 Minutes to Hours (It gets better with time.)
Serves: Six

4	*medium*	**Garlic cloves, diced**
1	*medium*	**Onion, diced**
2	*medium*	**Celery stalks, finely diced**
1	*Tbs*	**Virgin olive oil**
1	*tsp*	**Italian Herbs**
1	*medium*	**Bay leaf**
32	*ounces*	**Tomato sauce (4 cups)**
12	*ounces*	**Tomato paste (1 1/2 cups)**
1	*pound*	**Tofu, cut into 1/2 inch cubes**
1/2	*cup*	**Red wine**
6	*Tbs*	**Parmesan cheese, grated**

Sauté garlic, onion and celery in olive oil on moderate heat for 2-3 minutes, stirring occasionally. Add the spices and bay leaf, and sauté for another 2 minutes. Pour in the canned tomato sauce, tofu, and tomato paste and let simmer and thicken for 15 minutes.

I often let tofu crumble and disappear in spaghetti sauce; however, you can also roast extra firm tofu cut it into one inch cubes in the oven for 15-20 minutes. It will soak up the sauce flavors and feature tofu balls in your sauce.

Pour in the wine and allow to simmer from 15 minutes to several hours, being careful not to burn the bottom of the sauce.

Serve this sauce over cooked spaghetti noodles and sprinkle with parmesan cheese just before serving.

Serve with:

18	*ounces*	**Pasta**

Per Serving: Calories: 515
Saturated Fat: 1.2 grams
Total Fat: 8.7 grams

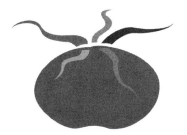

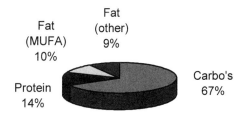

Fat (MUFA) 10%

Fat (other) 9%

Protein 14%

Carbo's 67%

ROASTED TOMATO SAUCE WITH TOFU

You can roast tomatoes and spices in the oven and create a new flavor out of average tomato sauce. Serve this with pasta, put it in sauces, or add it to a casserole. The sauce freezes very well, and saves you precious preparation time later. If you like your tomatoes without the skin, dip them in boiling water for 1-2 minutes and the skin peels away. In August, when beautiful, vine ripe tomatoes are plentiful, pack your freezer with roasted tomato sauce; you'll be glad all winter. You can vary your sauces by adding eggplant or zucchini.

Preparation Time: 15-20 Minutes
Roasting Time: 60-80 Minutes
Serves: Six people at three meals

12	**medium**	**Tomatoes, peeled**
6	**cups**	**Mushrooms, sliced**
3	**Tbs**	**Olive oil**
18	**medium**	**Garlic cloves, diced**
2	**tsp**	**Italian Herbs**
1/2	**tsp**	**Salt**
3	**Tbs**	**Fresh basil, or dried**
3	**medium**	**Onions, chopped**
2	**pounds**	**Tofu, firm**
1/2	**cup**	**Red wine**

Serve 1/3 sauce with:

18	**ounces**	**Pasta**

Set oven on bake at 400° (F).

To skin tomatoes, dip them in boiling water for 1-2 minutes and then peel once cooled.

Sauté mushrooms over medium heat. Once they start to reduce, add oil, garlic, herbs, salt, and onion and cook until onion is yellow to golden.

Slice tomatoes, and place in an oven-proof casserole. Add sautéed mushrooms, spices, onion, and tofu, and let roast in the oven, stirring occasionally. As sauce begins to thicken (about 30 minutes), add red wine, stir, and allow to thicken again (another 20 minutes).

When the sauce is almost thick, turn off heat, leaving in oven for 30 minutes.

Serve part of the sauce. Freeze the rest in separate containers.

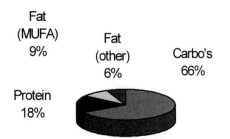

Fat (MUFA) 9%

Fat (other) 6%

Carbo's 66%

Protein 18%

Per Serving:	Calories:	446
	Saturated Fat:	1.2 grams
	Total Fat:	8.4 grams
	Fiber:	4.8 grams

TOMATO SAUCE WITH ROASTED RED PEPPERS & LEEKS OVER PASTA

The leeks and roasted peppers nicely complement the richness of tomato, garlic, and herbs. For people who don't tolerate onions, leeks are a great substitute. This sauce is especially nice in late summer when vine-ripe tomatoes, basil, and red peppers are inexpensive and flavorful. Make a double batch, and freeze some for a winter day.

Preparation Time: 20 Minutes
Simmering Time: 30 Minutes to 2 Hours
Serves: Six

2	*medium*	**Red bell peppers**
6	*medium*	**Tomatoes, peeled & chopped (or 30 ounces of canned tomato sauce)**
4	*medium*	**Leeks**
4	*medium*	**Garlic cloves, diced**
2	*tsp*	**Virgin olive oil**
1/2	*tsp*	**Salt**
1	*tsp*	**Italian Herbs**

Serve with:

18	*ounces*	**Pasta, long**

Per Serving:		
	Calories:	461
	Saturated Fat:	0.6
	Total Fat:	4.1
	Vitamin C:	135% RDA

Start boiling water for tomatoes while roasting peppers, See "ROASTING PEPPERS" on page 246. Add tomatoes to boiling water for 1-2 minutes then strain, cool, and peel.

Wash leeks well and trim tiny roots. Cut leeks 1-inch above where color changes from white to green. Discard tops. Dice and sauté leeks and garlic on medium heat with oil and salt for 2-3 minutes. Add herbs with chopped tomatoes, cover, and allow to simmer.

Chop roasted peppers and add to sauce and continue to simmer slowly for at least another 20 minutes. Leave sauce chunky, or put in the blender to render it smooth. In a large saucepan, bring salted water to a boil, and when boiling briskly, add pasta. Cook until *al dente*, about 10 minutes. Pour sauce over pasta.

Serve with salad or green vegetable.

Fat (MUFA) 4%
Fat (other) 4%
Carbo's 79%
Protein 13%

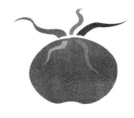

SOUPS

Soups are perhaps the ideal nourishing meal, keeping many of the vitamins and nutrients that are lost in steaming and sautéing. They also offer us valuable fluid, something many of us fail to drink in sufficient quantity. Soups can be warming on a winter day, or refreshing during the summer's heat. Try to prepare and enjoy soup often.

MISO SOUP

This makes an easy starter for any Oriental meal. It has a delicate flavor and awakens one's appetite. To turn this into a simple meal, add a pack of udon noodles (or any pre-cooked pasta) and a green leafy vegetable like spinach, Swiss chard, or kale. Shiitake mushrooms are excellent in this soup, but any mushroom will do.

Preparation Time: 12 Minutes

Serves: Four to Six

Miso Soup:

4	medium	Garlic cloves, diced
1/2	tsp	Ginger root, diced
1	medium	Carrot, diced
1/2	cup	Mushrooms, sliced
1/2	tsp	Canola oil
4	medium	Shallots
3 1/2	cups	Water, warm
3	Tbs	Miso
1/4	pound	Tofu, cubed

Optional ingredients:

6	ounces	Udon or soba noodles, cooked
2	cups	Kale, chopped

In a large saucepan, sauté garlic, ginger, carrot and mushrooms in oil for 2 minutes on medium heat.

Meanwhile, chop shallots and cut tofu into 1/2 inch cubes. Add shallots to the garlic and sauté for another 1-2 minutes on moderate heat. Add 3 cups of water and bring to a boil. Dissolve the miso paste in the remaining 1/2 cup of water. Add tofu and miso broth to the saucepan and let simmer 3-4 minutes. Serve.

Add optional ingredients with the tofu, simmer 3-4 minutes.

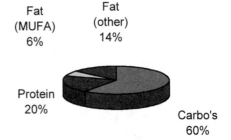

Per serving:	Calories:	106
	Saturated Fat:	0.3 grams
	Total Fat:	2.6 grams
	Vitamin A:	164% RDA

Fat (MUFA) 6%
Fat (other) 14%
Protein 20%
Carbo's 60%

VEGETABLE STOCK

*V*egetable stock is needed in many recipes. When sautéing veggies, add a splash of stock to flavor your sauté, and accelerate the cooking process. You can use ready made powdered varieties, broth cubes, or make your own delicious version. If you use pre-made stock, look for low-sodium brands. Whenever you steam vegetables, save the residue water as liquid for future stock. Don't hesitate to vary the vegetable ingredients listed below. Try adding fennel, beat leaves, spinach, or other root vegetables to create your own favorite flavors.

Preparation Time: 15 Minutes
Simmering Time: 1 Hour
Makes: 6 Cups

1	*Medium*	*Onion, diced*
4	*Medium*	*Garlic cloves, diced*
2	*Medium*	*Celery stalks, diced*
1	*Medium*	*Potato, diced*
2	*Medium*	*Carrots, diced*
1	*Medium*	*Tomato, chopped*
1	*Cup*	*Mushrooms, chopped*
2	*Tsp*	*Virgin olive oil*
1	*Tsp*	*Italian Herbs*
6	*Cups*	*Warm water*
1/2-3	*Tbs*	*Miso*

Peel and dice onion and garlic. Dice celery, potato, carrots, tomato, and mushrooms.

Heat the oil in a soup pot, and add cut vegetables. Stir in spices and sauté for 2-3 minutes, then cover and let simmer for 10 minutes. Add water and bring to a boil. Stir in the miso paste and let simmer for 1 hour.

For a delicate flavored soup, like garlic soup, only add 1/2 to 1 tablespoon of miso paste. For a hearty soup that will have rice or noodles, add 2-3 tablespoons of miso.

After simmering, filter stock from cut vegetables with a screen. Use the stock immediately, or place in the refrigerator in a sealed container.

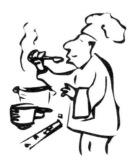

Per Serving:		
	Calories:	58
	Saturated Fat:	0.2 grams
	Total Fat:	1.3 grams
	Fat Calories:	18%
	Carbo Calories:	69%
	Protein Calories:	18%

WON TON SOUP

This soup has a rich, yet delicate flavor. Vary the vegetable ingredients inside the won tons as you like. You can expand this into a complete meal by adding more veggies and tofu.

Preparation Time: 20-30 Minutes
Serves: Four (or Two as a meal)

4	medium	**Garlic cloves, minced**
1	Tbs	**Ginger root, minced**
1	small	**Onion, minced**
1	tsp	**Canola oil**
1	cup	**Broccoli flowerets, finely chopped**
1/4	pound	**Tofu, diced**
20	4 inch	**Won ton wrappers**
1-2	cups	**Shiitake mushrooms, sliced**
1	tsp	**Rice vinegar**
4	cups	**Water**
3	Tbs	**Miso**
1	cup	**Kale, sliced in long strips**
1/4	small	**Lemon, juiced**

Garnish with: **Sprigs of parsley**

Sauté garlic, ginger root, and onion with oil on medium heat for 2 minutes. Add broccoli and tofu and sauté another 3 minutes. Set aside to cool.

Separate won ton wrappers on a dry surface. Place 1 to 1 1/2 teaspoons of sauté mixture into center of each won ton. Brush water along outer edge of won tons. Fold won tons in half, forming a triangle, and press edges firmly together using fingers or a fork. Spray for 1-2 seconds with canola oil and set aside.

Bring water to a boil in a large pot.

Sauté mushrooms for 2 minutes on moderate heat with rice vinegar in a large second pot. Add 4 cups of hot water to this second (soup) pot and heat until the liquid starts to bubble, then turn down to simmer and add kale. Stir in miso until it dissolves. Cover.

Once the first pot boils, reduce the heat to medium and add half the won tons, stirring gently to keep them from sticking. After 3 minutes, remove won tons and add to second soup pot. Repeat this process with remaining won tons.

Just before serving, add lemon juice and garnish with parsley.

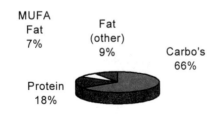

MUFA Fat 7%
Fat (other) 9%
Carbo's 66%
Protein 18%

Per Serving:		
	Calories:	227
	Saturated Fat:	0.6 grams
	Total Fat:	4.2 grams
	Vitamin C:	93% RDA

GAZPACHO

Vine ripened tomatoes and fresh herbs form a delicious, cold summer soup. Serve on a hot summer day with a side green salad and whole grain bread.

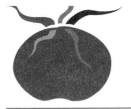

Preparation: 15 Minutes
Chill: 15-30 Minutes
Serves: Six

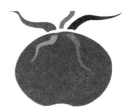

6	*medium*	**Garlic cloves, diced**
1	*large*	**Red bell pepper, chopped**
1/2	*tsp*	**Ground cumin**
1/2	*tsp*	**Paprika**
1/2	*tsp*	**Salt**
1 1/2	*tsp*	**Virgin olive oil**
1 1/2	*pounds*	**Tomatoes (4 med)**
4	*ounces*	**Whole wheat bread, toasted & crumbled (1/2 cup)**
1	*medium*	**Lemon, juiced**
1/4	*cup*	**Parsley**
1/4	*cup*	**Fresh basil**
1/4	*cup*	**Fresh mint leaves**
1	*cup*	**Cold water**
2	*Tbs*	**Balsamic vinegar**
1	*medium*	**Cucumber, peeled and chopped**
Garnish with:		**Fresh herbs**

Sauté garlic with oil on medium heat for 20-30 seconds. Add chopped pepper, cumin, paprika, and salt and heat another 90 seconds. Remove from heat and set aside.

Place tomatoes, bread, lemon juice, herbs, water, and vinegar in a blender and purée. Add the sauté mixture and cucumber and pulse again, leaving some bits of cucumber. Chill for 15-30 minutes.

Pour in bowls and garnish with fresh herb sprigs. Serve tossed green salad and whole wheat bread.

Per Serving:	Calories:	108
	Saturated Fat:	0.4 grams
	Total Fat:	2.5 grams
	Fiber:	2.5 grams
	Vitamin C:	104% RDA

Fat (MUFA) 13%

Fat (PUFA) 4%

Carbo's 70%

Protein 13%

BORSCHT

Here's a low-fat version of the classic Russian winter soup. It's wonderful with a hearty rye bread. The red beet color, with a spoonful of yogurt and a garnish of green parsley pleases the eye. If you don't find beets with greens, you can substitute a cup of Swiss chard or an extra cup of cabbage.

Preparation Time: 20 Minutes
Simmering Time: 20 Minutes
Serves: Six

4	*medium*	*Beets, with chopped greens*
1	*large*	*Onion, diced*
6	*medium*	*Garlic cloves, diced*
1	*Tbs*	*Canola oil*
3	*medium*	*Carrots, cubed*
2	*medium*	*Potatoes, cubed*
1/4	*tsp*	*Caraway seeds, crushed (optional)*
8	*ounces*	*Tomatoes, canned or fresh (1 cup)*
6	*cups*	*Warm water*
1	*cup*	*Cabbage, chopped*

Garnish with:

3/4	*cup*	*Non-fat yogurt*
Sprigs		*Parsley or chives*

Rinse the beets and drop the roots into boiling water for 1 minute to help remove skins. Allow to cool and peel off skins. Set beet greens aside.

In a large saucepan, sauté onion and garlic in oil for 2-3 minutes on moderate heat, until onions appear slightly golden. Meanwhile, scrub and wash carrots and potatoes. Cut the carrots, potatoes, and two of the beets into small cubes. Grate the other two beets. Add all ingredients with crushed caraway seeds to a saucepan and sauté for 1-2 minutes.

Add tomatoes and water, bring to a boil, then simmer for 10 minutes. Add cabbage and beet greens to soup, and simmer for another 10 minutes.

Spoon 2 tablespoons of yogurt onto each serving and garnish with parsley or chives.

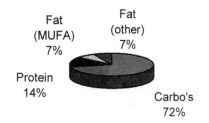

Fat (MUFA) 7%
Fat (other) 7%
Protein 14%
Carbo's 72%

Per Serving:		
	Calories:	297
	Saturated Fat:	0.6 grams
	Total Fat:	4.9 grams
	Vitamin C:	58% RDA
	Vitamin A:	239% RDA
	Fiber:	8.8 grams

SALADS

Salads are very versatile. We serve them either as an introduction to the main course or as a full meal. A tossed green salad cleanses the palate and prepares the way for dessert after a heavy meal. In the nutrition section of this book, I emphasized the importance of greens and vegetables in our diet. Here is a chance to add more greens and veggies to any meal.

RAITA (YOGURT SALAD)

This yogurt dish is served with Indian curries. It is light, refreshing, and cooling if you bite into a hot chile and need relief. It can also be used as a dip.

Preparation Time: 5 Minutes
Serves: Side Dish for Six

1	*cup*	**Yogurt, non-fat plain**
1/2	*medium*	**Cucumber, peeled and diced**
1/4	*cup*	**Cilantro and/or mint leaves, chopped**
1/4	*tsp*	**Paprika**
1/2	*medium*	**Onion, peeled and minced**
1/8	*tsp*	**Anise seeds (optional), or 1/2 small fennel bulb diced**

Combine all the ingredients, saving a sprig of cilantro and a dash of paprika for a garnish. Keep chilled in the refrigerator until ready to serve.

Per Serving:

Calories:	605
Saturated Fat:	2.2 grams
Total Fat:	10 grams

Fat
6%

Protein
32%

Carbo's
62%

TOSSED GREEN SALAD WITH DRESSING

A crisp green salad goes well before the main dish. A salad can also be served after the main course as the French do, to lighten and cleanse the palate before dessert. This dressing is light, tart and has no oil. I prefer colorful lettuce, like bibb, butter, or romaine.

Preparation Time: 5 minutes
Serves: Four

Salad:

6	cups	**Salad greens, washed, dried, and cut**

Mix dressing ingredients in a large salad bowl. Pour the salad on top and set aside. Toss the salad with the vinaigrette dressing (below) just before serving.

Dressing:

Use Vinaigrette dressing below:

Per Serving:	Calories:	19
	Saturated Fat:	0 grams
	Total Fat:	0.2 grams
	Fiber:	2.1 grams
	Vitamin C:	34% RDA

Fat (MUFA) 5%
Fat (other) 5%
Protein 31%
Carbo's 59%

VINAIGRETTE DRESSING

I love this dressing. It's easy to prepare, full of flavor, creamy, tart, and has essentially NO fat. Try it on salad or with steamed vegetables

Serves: Four to Six

2	Tbs	**Balsamic vinegar**
1	Tbs	**White wine**
1	Tbs	**Fresh squeezed lemon juice**
1	tsp	**Soy sauce, low sodium**
1	tsp	**Mustard, dijon**
1/2	tsp	**Italian Herbs**
1	dash	**Ground pepper**

Mix ingredients together in a bowl. Enjoy!

TABBOULEH

This is a wholesome, filling Middle Eastern salad. You can make it in the morning or put it together just before serving. To make a meal, serve steamed green beans or broccoli on the side.

Preparation Time: 20-25 Minutes, (tastes better if it has time to chill)
Serves: Six

2	cups	**Bulgur wheat**
2 1/2	cups	**Water**
1	Tbs	**Miso paste**
1	medium	**Onion**
3	medium	**Garlic cloves**
2	tsp	**Virgin olive oil**
1	tsp	**Italian Herbs**
3	Tbs	**Walnuts, chopped (or hazel nuts)**
2	medium	**Tomatoes, chopped**
1 1/2	cups	**Parsley, diced finely**
1/2	cup	**Mint, diced finely (optional)**
4	medium	**Limes, juiced**
1	Tbs	**Extra virgin olive oil**
1	Tbs	**Balsamic vinegar**
8	ounces	**Garbanzo beans, cooked and drained (1 cup)**

Put 2 cups of bulgur wheat into a large bowl. Bring 2 1/2 cups of water to a boil, then add miso paste and stir until dissolved. Pour hot broth over bulgur wheat, cover, and let sit for 20 minutes. Stir occasionally.

Dice onion and garlic, then sauté in 2 teaspoons olive oil. Add dried herbs and chopped walnuts. Sauté until onion and garlic just turn yellow; don't overcook. Add to bulgur wheat and stir together to absorb flavors.

Meanwhile, combine tomatoes, parsley, mint, and lime juice in a separate bowl. Add 1 tablespoon olive oil, vinegar, and garbanzo beans; if you used canned beans rinse them well.

Once bulgur wheat has soaked for 20 minutes, mix the 2 bowls together in a salad bowl and chill in the refrigerator.

Serve in a large salad bowl, or pour over a bed of lettuce on a large serving plate. Garnish with sprigs of parsley and mint.

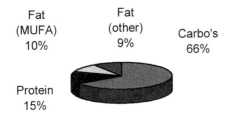

Fat (MUFA) 10%
Fat (other) 9%
Carbo's 66%
Protein 15%

Per Serving:		
	Calories:	550
	Saturated Fat:	1.4 grams
	Total Fat:	13.1 grams
	Fiber:	13 grams
	Vitamin A:	99% RDA
	Vitamin C:	78% RDA

CITRUS & SPINACH SALAD

This is a delicious, light salad with a delicate flavor. Serve prior to a main course, or double the portions and serve as a light meal.

Preparation Time: 10 Minutes
Serves: Four

1	small	**Fennel bulb**
1	Tbs	**Fresh lemon juice**
1	large	**Pink grapefruit**
1	large	**Orange**
1/4	cup	**Fresh mint, chopped**
1	tsp	**Sugar**
4	cups	**Fresh spinach leaves**
1	medium	**Red onion, thinly sliced (optional)**

Bring a pot of water to boil with a dash of salt. Cut fennel into thin slices, and pour lemon juice over the fennel (this helps it's color). Add fennel to boiling water for 2-3 minutes until tender but slightly chewy; don't overcook. Immediately rinse with very cold water until chilled. Place in a bowl.

Cut grapefruit and orange in half, then cut out citrus segments between the membranes and place in a bowl with the fennel. Squeeze remaining juice into the bowl once all the citrus fruit is removed. Add chopped mint and sugar, and stir.

Place thoroughly rinsed and dried spinach in a salad bowl. Pour fennel and citrus contents over spinach, toss lightly, optionally toss with red onion and serve.

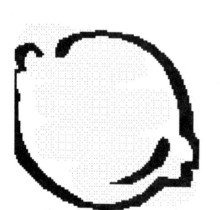

Per Serving:		
	Calories:	75
	Saturated Fat:	0.1 grams
	Total Fat:	0.6 grams
	Vitamin C:	108% RDA
	Fiber:	3.0 grams

PASTA

I adore pasta dishes. While you can make your own pasta or buy it fresh, there are a number of varieties of dry pasta and it's easy to use. Sauces vary and expand the range of delicious pasta meals you can make.

The average recipe book calls for 2 ounces of pasta per person. As these meals are low in fat, and as pasta is healthy, my recipes use 3 ounces of pasta per person. Live it up, and eat pasta more often.

If you are eating pasta to load up on energy the night before an endurance, athletic event, you want at least 4-6 ounces of pasta.

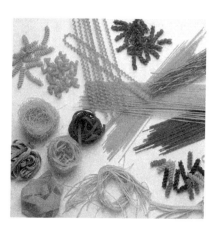

PASTA DOUGH

*M*aking pasta at home is fun. It also produces great pasta. You can vary its color and texture by adding spinach, dried tomatoes, and spices to the dough. Substitute an equal volume of veggie ingredients in place of water; the veggies do not make a significant change in the nutritional value or the taste of the pasta. At home, we use a pasta machine. All you have to do is drop in the dry ingredients & mix, then slowly add the wet ingredients. The machine does the rest. You need only put the pasta in boiling water. Don't substitute regular whole wheat flour for whole wheat pastry flour; it is too coarse. You can substitute semolina or all-purpose flour in place of whole wheat pastry flour.

If you prefer to taste your pasta and sauce distinctly, you don't want the sauce to cling to the pasta. Add 2 teaspoons of olive oil to the boiling water before adding the pasta, and rinse it after draining to remove the starchy film. If you want the pasta flavors to blend with the sauce, don't add oil to the boiling water, don't rinse the pasta after draining, and don't dry it completely with draining; the starchy wet surface on the pasta will join and cling to the sauce.

Preparation Time: 20 Minutes
Serves: Four (Makes about 12 ounces)

Regular Pasta:

1 1/2	cups	**Whole wheat pastry flour**
1 3/4	cups	**Semolina flour**
1/2	tsp	**Salt**
1/2	cup	**Water**
3	large	**Egg whites (lightly whipped)**
2	tsp	**Virgin olive oil**

Spinach Pasta:

Add 1/2 cup chopped, cooked spinach and reduce water to 1/4 cup

Prepare the sauce in advance. You can prepare the pasta dough in advance too; just cover to prevent drying, and cook in boiling water later.

To cook fresh pasta, bring water to a brisk boil, use at least 4 quarts (liters) of water per pound of pasta (12-16 ounces is a serving for four). Add 2 teaspoons of salt per 4 quarts of water; most of the salt goes down the drain with the water after cooking.

Fresh pasta will be cooked in 2-3 minutes, don't overcook the pasta. Drain immediately and serve with your favorite sauce.

Per Serving:	Calories:	462
	Saturated Fat:	1 gram
	Total Fat:	5.1 grams
	Fiber:	8.3 grams)

PASTA WITH BASIL,
TOMATOES, AND ARTICHOKE HEARTS

Summer brings these flavors together with gusto. I like to steam fresh artichokes and serve the leaves as hors d'oeuvres with a yogurt or vinaigrette sauce. You can also use artichoke hearts canned in water. Cherry tomatoes work well, but any flavorful tomato will do.

Preparation: 15 Minutes
Serves: Four

16	*ounces*	*Fresh pasta (2 cups)*
4	*large*	*Garlic cloves, diced*
2	*Tbs*	*Pine nuts (or sliced almonds)*
1	*tsp*	*Italian Herbs*
1/2	*tsp*	*Salt*
1	*Tbs*	*Extra virgin olive oil*
3	*cups*	*Cherry tomatoes, quartered*
2	*cups*	*Artichoke hearts, sliced lengthwise*
1	*cup*	*Fresh basil, chopped, or use 1/2 cup diced parsley*
Garnish with:		*Fresh basil sprigs*

Start heating pasta water and bring to a rolling boil. Separate fresh pasta pieces from each other and set aside.

Prepare and measure all ingredients so you can cook the sauce quickly after adding pasta to the water.

When pasta water boils, add fresh pasta and cook for about 2 1/2 to 3 minutes, until pasta is al dente.

Begin immediately to sauté garlic, pine nuts, herbs, and salt in oil. After 1 minute, add tomatoes and artichoke hearts and heat another 2 minutes. Add basil, cover, and heat 1/2 minute; then remove from heat.

Drain pasta and pour onto a serving plate. Spoon tomato, basil, and artichoke sauce over the pasta. Garnish with sprigs of fresh basil and serve with fresh whole grain bread. This dish goes nicely with a light red wine. Offer with tossed green salad.

Per Serving:	Calories:	472
	Saturated Fat:	1.3 grams
	Total Fat:	9.2 grams
	Fiber:	7.6 grams
	Vitamin C:	65% RDA

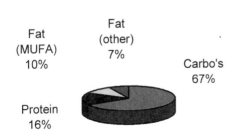

Fat (MUFA) 10%
Fat (other) 7%
Carbo's 67%
Protein 16%

EGGPLANT LASAGNA

This popular eggplant dish can be prepared in many ways. Serve with a tossed green salad or a steamed green vegetable and warm, thick-crusted bread. You can prepare the dish in advance and store it in the refrigerator.

Preparation Time: 40 Minutes (plus time for the sauce to simmer)
Baking Time: 25 Minutes
Serves: Eight

3	cups	Tomato sauce (see recipes)
6	medium	Lasagna noodles
2	medium	Eggplants
4	medium	Garlic cloves, diced
1 1/2	Tbs	Virgin olive oil
1	pound	Mozzarella, non-fat cheese, grated
6	Tbs	Parmesan cheese, grated
1/2	cup	Parsley, chopped
4	cups	Broccoli flowerets
1	medium	Lime, juiced

Preheat oven to 375° F. Prepare sauce. Bring water to a boil, and cook lasagna noodles until *al dente*, about 12 minutes. Then drain, rinse, and set aside to cool.

Meanwhile, slice eggplant widthwise into 1/2 inch slices (making 16 slices). Microwave for 10 minutes (or steam for 5 minutes). Sauté garlic for 30 seconds in oil on moderate heat in a large skillet. Add eggplant and sauté each side until lightly browned on both sides. Set aside to cool.

In a 9x13 inch ovenproof dish, build 8 individual mounds with 3 pasta layers.

Pour 3/4 cup of sauce into dish, then lay 8 slices of eggplant to form 2 rows. Lay 2 strips of pasta over eggplant rows. Sprinkle on 1/3 of the mozzarella cheese, and add another 3/4 cup of sauce. For the second layer, add 8 more eggplant slices, then cut 2 long strips of pasta in half and lay widthwise. Again, add 1/3 of the cheese and 3/4 cup of sauce.

For the top layer, add 2 strips of pasta lengthwise, remaining mozzarella cheese and sauce. Cut lasagna into 8 portions with a sharp knife, creating 8 servings (this makes it visually pleasing, and much easier to serve). Sprinkle parmesan cheese and half the parsley on top. Bake for 20-25 minutes. After baking, sprinkle remaining parsley on top.

Serve with side of steamed broccoli seasoned with lime juice.

Per Serving:	Calories:	602
	Saturated Fat:	2.8 grams
	Total Fat:	13.6 grams
	Fiber:	12 grams
	Vitamin C:	170% RDA
	Fat%:	20%
	Protein%:	23%
	Carbo's%:	57%

PEPPERONATA WITH PASTA

This is a popular Italian pepper stew we enjoy serving on a bed of short pasta noodles. Roasting the peppers creates a wonderful caramel flavor that makes the little extra effort worthwhile. Serve with a hearty, warm, whole grain bread.

Preparation Time: 30 Minutes

Serves: Eight

3	*medium*	*Red bell peppers*
3	*medium*	*Green bell peppers*
2	*medium*	*Yellow bell peppers*
24	*ounces*	*Pasta noodles, short*
1	*large*	*Onion, diced*
8	*medium*	*Garlic cloves, diced*
2	*medium*	*Zucchini*
1 1/2	*tsp*	*Italian Herbs*
1	*tsp*	*Salt*
2	*Tbs*	*Virgin olive oil*
4	*medium*	*Tomatoes*
8	*ounces*	*White beans, cooked and drained*
1/2	*cup*	*Almonds, sliced*
1 1/2	*cups*	*Parsley, chopped*
1	*dash*	*Ground pepper*
1/4	*cup*	*Parmesan cheese, grated*

Roast the peppers. See "ROASTING PEPPERS" on page 246. After removing skin, cut into long, thin strips.

Bring water to a boil for the pasta, adding a dash of salt and oil. When water is boiling vigorously, add pasta and cook until *al dente*.

Meanwhile, sauté onion, garlic, and zucchini with herbs, salt, and olive oil for 2-3 minutes. Slice tomatoes, and add to the sauté, cooking them for another 2-3 minutes. Add roasted peppers and let simmer. Rinse beans well and pour over the stew.

Place nuts in microwave for 60 seconds, or roast in a skillet on medium heat for 1 minute. Mix nuts and 2/3 of the chopped parsley in with pepper stew.

Place cooked pasta on a serving plate and pour pepperonata over it. Sprinkle remaining parsley, a dash of freshly ground pepper, and parmesan cheese over dish. Serve with dense, warmed bread.

Per serving:		
	Calories:	518
	Saturated Fat:	1.7 grams
	Total Fat:	11.3 grams
	Vitamin C:	160% RDA
	Fiber:	10.1 grams

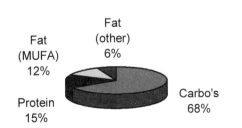

Fat (other) 6%

Fat (MUFA) 12%

Protein 15%

Carbo's 68%

PASTA STUFFED WITH GARLIC, RED PEPPERS, & CHEESE

This is a fun, yet simple meal. You can prepare it in advance and pop in the oven prior to serving.

Preparation Time: 30 Minutes (plus time for the sauce)
Baking Time: 20 Minutes
Serves: Four

1 1/2	cups	Tomato sauce (see recipes)	Prepare sauce and simmer.

1 1/2   cups   **Tomato sauce (see recipes)**

2   large   **Red bell peppers**

12   ounces   **Large Pasta shells (over 1 inch long for stuffing, 1 1/2 cups)**

8   medium   **Garlic cloves, diced**

1   cup   **Celery, diced**

2   cups   **Mushrooms, sliced**

1   Tbs   **Virgin olive oil**

1/8   tsp   **Salt**

1   tsp   **Italian Herbs**

1 1/2   cups   **Non-fat cottage cheese**

1 1/2   cups   **Non-fat mozzarella cheese, grated**

Garnish with: *1/2 cup fresh parsley*

Serve with:

4   cups   **Broccoli flowerets, sliced**

1   medium   **Lemon, juiced**

Prepare sauce and simmer.

Start boiling water for pasta, adding a pinch of salt and a dash of oil.

Roast peppers. (See "ROASTING PEPPERS" on page 246.)

When water reaches a vigorous boil, add pasta shells, stirring occasionally. When the pasta is cooked *al dente*, about 10 minutes, drain and rinse with cold water.

Meanwhile, sauté garlic, celery and mushrooms with oil, salt, and herbs for 3 minutes on medium heat. Chop roasted peppers and add to sauté. Remove from the heat. Allow to cool, and stir in cheeses.

Stuff pasta with veggie and cheese mixture. Lay stuffed shells in an ovenproof baking dish. Pour sauce over stuffed shells. Set aside in the refrigerator for later, or bake in the oven for 20-25 minutes. Garnish with fresh parsley and serve.

Five minutes prior to serving, steam broccoli and season with lemon juice.

Per Serving:		
	Calories:	620
	Saturated Fat:	1.1 grams
	Total Fat:	7.6 grams
	Vitamin C:	392% RDA
	Fiber:	10.6 grams
	Vitamin A:	144% RDA

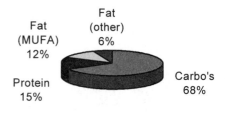

Fat (MUFA) 12%

Fat (other) 6%

Protein 15%

Carbo's 68%

MACARONI & CHEESE
WITH PEAS & CARROTS

My children love this dish. It took them a couple of tries to get used to the veggies, but now it's a big favorite. You may substitute or add other veggies. If you can't find reduced fat cheddar, use half cheddar and half non-fat cheese.

Preparation Time: 15-20 Minutes
Serves: Four

12	ounces	**Macaroni elbows (2 cups)**
1	cup	**Non-fat milk**
2	Tbs	**Corn starch**
1/2	cup	**Non-fat cottage cheese**
1	cup	**Cheddar cheese, reduced fat, grated**
1	tsp	**Mustard**
1	tsp	**Soy sauce, low sodium**
1	cup	**Frozen peas**
1	cup	**Frozen carrots, or cooked diced carrots**
2	Slices	**Whole wheat bread, toasted and broken into crumbs**

Bring water to a boil with a pinch of salt. Cook pasta until *al dente*.

Meanwhile, mix corn starch with milk until dissolved. Add cottage cheese and mix. Then, add grated cheddar cheese, soy sauce, and mustard. Stir. Add peas and carrots to sauce.

When the macaroni is cooked, drain and pour back into the same sauce pan. Stir in sauce, reduce heat to medium low. Stir ingredients until cheese melts and starts to bubble. Pour into a serving bowl and sprinkle bread crumbs over macaroni and cheese. Serve with salad or other green leafy vegetable.

Per Serving:	Calories:	390
	Saturated Fat:	1.6 grams
	Total Fat:	3.6 grams
	Fiber:	5.8 grams
	Vitamin A:	163% RDA

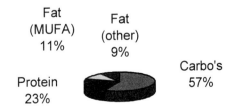

Fat (MUFA) 11% Fat (other) 9% Carbo's 57% Protein 23%

EUROPEAN CUISINE

*E*uropean food is extremely varied. Sauces, garlic, breads, wine, and pasta are important ingredients in European cooking. In particular, my recipes will highlight Mediterranean dishes that reflect some of the healthiest populations in the world.

Mediterranean food is full of color, flavor, and nutrition. Certain flavors dominate the palate, namely, garlic, tomatoes, and Italian Herbs. Italian Herbs is a blend of oregano, basil, thyme, rosemary, and sage. Most grocery stores carry this practical combination. Similar herb blends are "Fine Herbs" and "Herbes de Provence." You are encouraged to buy these herbs individually so that you can vary your recipes.

Red wine is the normal beverage at any Mediterranean meal, and complements flavors that dominate this regional cooking style. If you avoid alcohol, there are now a variety of non-alcoholic red wines available. Water with a slice of lemon goes well with any dish.

Look for whole grain breads that can be warmed in the oven. A firm crust with a soft center that is perfumed by yeast is perfect to dip into soups, or to dunk in a garlic-flavored tomato sauce.

Tossed salads featuring leafy green lettuce and a simple vinaigrette dressing can be served after the main course to cleanse the palate and prepare your taste buds for dessert. Try this lovely French tradition.

WARMING BREAD

Choose pumpernickel, or try dense whole grain breads, such as half whole wheat and half rye. Start the oven 20 minutes before serving and place bread in the oven 10-12 minutes before you serve. Avoid putting butter or margarine on bread. If you must have fat on your bread, sauté garlic and herbs in olive oil for 1 minute and brush it on.

PREPARING LEEKS

Leeks are featured regularly in European cooking. Select leeks with extra whiteness extending up the stalk. Wash well, as they are often gritty. Trim off the tiny roots, and cut off the tops about one inch above where the white turns green. Cut in long, thin strips and then dice. Sauté like an onion, but don't overcook.

I usually save the green tops for making vegetable stock.

LEEK & MUSHROOM SOUFFLÉ

This is a visually spectacular main course. Soufflés are simple to make and this recipe is low in fat, as well. Most of the preparation can be done in advance; just allow 10 minutes to mix the ingredients with the egg whites, then pop into the oven. You can substitute diced broccoli flowerets for leeks to vary the recipe. Serve with a salad, soup, or side of rice for a filling meal.

Preparation Time: 30 Minutes
Baking Time: 30 Minutes
Serves: Six

5	medium	**Garlic cloves, minced**
2	cups	**Leeks, diced**
1	cup	**Wild mushrooms, diced (shiitake, oyster, or other)**
1	Tbs	**Virgin olive oil**
1/8	tsp	**Salt**
1/2	tsp	**Italian Herbs**
1/4	cup	**Whole wheat flour**
1	cup	**Milk, non-fat**
9	medium	**Egg whites**
1/2	cup	**Mozzarella cheese, non-fat, grated**
1	Slice	**Whole wheat bread, toasted and crumbed**
2	Tbs	**Parmesan cheese**

Serve with:

6	cups	**Asparagus spears**
1	medium	**Lemon, juiced**

Per Serving: (for six)	Calories:	196
	Saturated Fat:	0.9 grams
	Total Fat:	4.2 grams
	Vitamin C:	177% RDA
	Fat%:	18%
	Protein%:	39%

Preheat oven to 375° F. Sauté the leeks, mushrooms, and garlic in oil. Add salt and herbs and heat until lightly cooked, 2-3 minutes on medium heat. Add flour, stir gently, and heat another minute. Stir milk into mixture slowly and allow to thicken, 1-2 minutes on low heat. Set aside to cool.

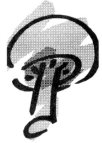

Beat egg whites until stiff but not dry. Gently fold in grated cheese and bread crumbs, followed by sauce. If you over-mix, the egg whites lose air and the soufflé rises poorly. Pour mixture into a soufflé pan, sprayed with olive oil. Sprinkle parmesan cheese on top and place in the oven for 30 minutes.

Five minutes before the soufflé is ready, begin steaming asparagus. When tender but still chewy, place in a serving bowl and season with lemon juice or a vinaigrette sauce.

Remove soufflé from the oven and serve immediately. It will collapse as it cools, or when cut into.

SPINACH SOUFFLÉ

This easy-to-make soufflé dish is colorful and flavorful. It rises less than other soufflés, yet the spinach and basil add flavor and texture. Serve with steamed green beans or another vegetable.

Preparation Time: 30 Minutes
Baking Time: 30 Minutes
Serves: Four

1	medium	Onion, roasted, then diced finely
6	medium	Garlic cloves, diced
2	tsp	Virgin olive oil
1/4	tsp	Salt
1/2	tsp	Italian Herbs
1	Tbs	Whole wheat pastry flour
1/4	cup	Non-fat milk
1/3	cup	Fresh basil leaves
1 1/4	cups	Cooked, drained spinach
1/2	cup	Non-fat mozzarella cheese, grated
1/2	cup	Breadcrumbs, toasted
8	large	Egg whites
2	Tbs	Parmesan cheese, grated

Garnish with: Fresh herbs
Serve with:

4	cups	Green beans with, "VINAIGRETTE DRESSING" on page 220

Set oven at 375° (F), and place onion in the oven to bake, baking 10-30 minutes.

Sauté garlic with oil, salt, and herbs for 2 minutes on medium heat. Add flour and cook another 1-2 minutes, stirring occasionally. Add milk and basil, reduce heat to simmer, and stir until sauce thickens. Add well drained spinach, onion, and simmer another 2 minutes. Remove from heat and set aside.

Beat egg whites until stiff. Gently fold in breadcrumbs and grated cheese, followed by sauce. Spray a soufflé dish lightly with oil and pour in the mixture. Sprinkle parmesan cheese on top. Garnish with fresh herbs. Place in the oven for 30 minutes, until top is golden.

Five minutes before soufflé is done, steam green beans. Toss vinaigrette with cooked beans.

Remove soufflé from the oven and serve immediately. It will collapse as it cools or is cut.

Per Serving:		
	Calories:	167
	Total Fat:	3.6 grams
	Saturated Fat:	0.9 grams
	Fiber:	5.9 grams
	Vitamin C:	82% RDA
	Fat%:	17%

PIZZA DOUGH FOR GREAT PIZZA

*T*o make great pizza, you need great pizza crust. This is a favorite recipe in our family. We have played with many pizza dough recipes and have had repeated success with this variation. If you make pizza often, buy a pizza stone. The stone evens the heat in your oven and benefits most of your baking, not just pizza making. Serve with a side salad.

(I also use this dough to wrap nut loaves and vegetable turnovers.)

Preparation Time: 10 Minutes (Plus Baking Time: 8-10 Minutes)
Dough Rising Time: 5 Minutes with the microwave, about 1 hour otherwise
Makes: (2) 10-inch pizza crusts

1	*cup*	*Warm water*
1	*Tbs*	*Sugar*
1	*Packet*	*Active dry yeast*
1	*cup*	*All-purpose flour*
2	*cups*	*Whole wheat pastry flour*
1	*tsp*	*Salt*
1	*tsp*	*Freshly ground black pepper*
1	*tsp*	*Italian Herbs*
2 1/2	*Tbs*	*Extra virgin olive oil*

Pour warm to hot water, about 110° (F) into a bowl. Stir in sugar, and yeast. Yeast should create foam and bubbles on the surface of water within 3-5 minutes or it is not active.

Mix flours, salt, pepper, and dried herbs into a mixing bowl. When well mixed, form a center depression and slowly pour in the yeast with water and 1 1/2 tablespoons of oil. Mix together.

If using a heavy duty mixer, mix for 5 minutes, preferably with a dough hook. If dough is flaky and dry, add 1 teaspoon of water; if it is overly sticky, add 2 table-spoons of flour and re-mix.

If you knead your dough by hand, knead with floured hands for 10-15 minutes.

To help dough rise, roll it into a ball and spread 1/2 teaspoon of olive oil on the surface with your hands. Put in a bowl in a warm place to rise for 45-75 minutes (doubling time varies with temperature). Cover bowl to prevent drying.

(To accelerate rising, put covered bowl with dough in the microwave on low temp for 5 minutes.)

After dough rises, punch into a smaller ball and divide in half forming two dough balls. On floured surface, spread by hand or rolling pin to form two 10-inch crusts. Leave edges slightly thick. Brush or spray 1/2 tablespoon olive oil on outer rim of crust before baking.

Per Serving:		
	Calories:	300
	Saturated Fat:	1.2 grams
	Total Fat:	8.3 grams
	Fiber:	5.3 grams
	Fat%:	17%

PIZZA-IN-A-HURRY

You can make good pizza at home in a flash, and it is better than the frozen pizzas you buy at the store, or the fat-packed pizzas they sell at restaurants. You'll need to have some ingredients on hand, such as frozen pizza crusts, ready-made sauce, and some veggies. Pick your favorite toppings, such as bell peppers, sautéed mushrooms, garlic, sautéed onion or leeks with herbs, broccoli, corn, cashews, pinenuts, or pineapple. Cheese can be grated in less than one minute. Serve with steamed green vegetables, or a tossed salad for a complete meal.

Preparation Time: 10 Minutes
Baking Time: 8-10 Minutes
Serves: Four

2	*medium*	**Garlic cloves, diced**
1/2	*tsp*	**Italian Herbs**
2	*cups*	**Mushrooms, sliced**
1	*tsp*	**Virgin olive oil**
1	*medium*	**Bell pepper (any color), sliced**
1	*10 inch*	**Frozen pizza crust**
1/2	*cup*	**Pizza or pasta sauce (See recipes)**
3/4	*cup*	**Non-fat mozzarella cheese, grated**
1/2	*cup*	**Pineapple chunks, drained**
1/4	*cup*	**Parmesan cheese, grated**
1	*tsp*	**Chili pepper flakes (optional)**

Preheat oven to 475° F.

Sauté garlic, herbs, and mushrooms in oil for 2-3 minutes on moderate heat, stirring occasionally. Add peppers, heat another 2 minutes.

Meanwhile, place pre-made crust in oven for 1-2 minutes (put frozen crust in oven for 2-3 minutes). Remove from the oven, pour 1/2 cup of tomato sauce, then sprinkle grated mozzarella cheese on pizza.

Arrange sautéed veggies over pizza, add pineapple. Sprinkle grated parmesan cheese. For hot spice on your pizza, add chili pepper flakes. Place pizza in the oven for 8-10 minutes. Remove when crust is golden.

Per Serving:
Calories: 290
Saturated Fat: 1.3 grams
Total Fat: 5.9 grams
Vitamin C: 40% RDA

Fat (MUFA) 12%
Protein 19%
Fat (other) 7%
Carbo's 61%

PIZZA WITH LEEKS, MUSHROOMS AND ROASTED RED PEPPERS

These flavors are wonderful on a pizza. For a great pizza, try the pizza dough recipe in this book. You can use sautéed peppers, but ripe, red peppers are special and fragrant when roasted. Many grocery stores carry roasted peppers in jars, if you want to avoid roasting them. I prefer chanterelle, shiitake, or oyster mushrooms on pizza, but any mushroom will do. Serve pizza with a salad, or steamed green vegetables for a complete meal.

Preparation Time: 15 Minutes (plus time for the crust)
Baking Time: 8-12 Minutes
Serves: 4

1	10 inch	**Pizza crust**
1/2	cup	**Tomato sauce (see recipes)**
2	medium	**Red bell peppers, roasted**
2	cups	**Mushrooms, sliced**
3	medium	**Leeks**
1	tsp	**Extra virgin olive oil**
1/2	cup	**Non-fat mozzarella cheese, grated**
1/2	cup	**Parmesan cheese, grated**

Preheat oven to 500° F.

Prepare pizza crust and sauce according to recipes, or, for ready-made crust or sauce, set them on counter.

Roast peppers, See "ROASTING PEPPERS" on page 246.

Clean leeks well, and cut off tiny roots. Cut leeks in half lengthwise, then slice finely from root outward. Stop after cutting 1-2 inches into the green. Slice mushrooms and sauté with leeks in oil for 2-3 minutes on medium heat.

Pour sauce on pizza, sprinkle on mozzarella cheese, and arrange veggies on pizza. Now, sprinkle on parmesan cheese.

Place pizza on a pizza stone or pizza pan in the. Remove when pizza edges are lightly golden, about 8-10 minutes.

Serve with salad or steamed green vegetables.

Per Serving:		
	Calories:	460
	Saturated Fat:	2.3 grams
	Total Fat:	9.5 grams
	Fiber:	7.4 grams

Fat (other) 6%

Fat (MUFA) 12%

Carb's 62%

Protein 18%

ORIENTAL CUISINE

Food from Thailand to Japan varies greatly, yet many of the same ingredients are used. Presentations are elegant. Vegetables and rice are the dominate energy source in meals, making them tasty and healthy. Seasonings and spices vary greatly from Thailand to Southern China to Northern China to Japan. Tofu provides an important source of protein, fiber, and texture in Oriental cooking.

COOKING RICE

Rice remains the featured grain in most Oriental dishes. Different types of rice require slightly different cooking methods.

To Serve Four: Use 1 1/2 Cups of Rice Cooked with 3 Cups Water

1 1/2	*cup*	*Rice*
3	*cups*	*Water*

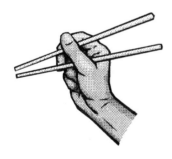

For polished Oriental rice: rinse rice in a pan, stirring until water turns cloudy. Pour out cloudy water, and add new water and stir again. Repeat until water remains fairly clear. I usually rinse, stir, and drain three times. Drain and add measured water. Bring to a boil, then reduce heat to simmer, cover, and cook for about 20 minutes, until rice is tender but still chewy.

For brown rice: put rice and water in a pan, bring to a boil, and immediately reduce to simmer for 30-40 minutes. Cook until rice is tender, but still chewy.

For white rice: cook like brown rice, but for 15-20 minutes.

For wild rice: put 1 part rice with 5 parts water and bring to a boil. Reduce heat and simmer for 50-60 minutes until tender but chewy. Drain, save fluid for soup stock if you like. Add miso broth (1/2 tablespoon per cup of water) or vegetable broth to cooking liquid to flavor the rice.

For basmati (or texmati) rice: sauté rice in oil for 2-3 minutes with onion, garlic, and/or herbs. Then add water and cook like white rice.

SWEET AND SOUR STIR FRY

This version of sweet and sour stir fry is low in fat and delicious. You can serve it with rice or noodles. There are many delightful Chinese mushrooms to choose from. This recipe contains multiple ingredients, half of which form the rich sweet and sour sauce.

Preparation Time: 30 Minutes
Serves: Four

1 1/2	cups	Polished rice, rinsed
3	cups	Water
Sauce:		
1/2	pound	Tofu, cut in 1 inch cubes
1/2	Tbs	Soy sauce, low sodium
1/4	cup	White wine
1/4	cup	Rice vinegar
1/4	cup	Ketchup
1/4	cup	Water
1/4	cup	Sugar
2	tsp	Corn starch
Sauté:		
1	medium	Onion, diced
2	Tbs	Ginger root, diced
2	tsp	Canola oil
2	medium	Carrots
1	medium	Red bell pepper
1	medium	Green bell pepper
2	cups	Mushrooms, sliced
2	cup	Broccoli, sliced thinly
16	ounces	Baby corn, canned (2 cups)
12	ounces	Pineapple chunks (1 1/2 cups)
2	cups	Frozen peas
1/2	cup	Cashews

Begin steaming rice, See "COOKING RICE" on page 236.

In a bowl, combine soy sauce, wine, vinegar, ketchup, water, sugar, and corn starch. Add tofu, set aside to marinate. (You can do this the day before and refrigerate, as the longer it marinates, the better it tastes.)

Sauté onion and ginger root 2-3 minutes in oil until onion softens. Cut carrots and peppers into long thin strips. Add mushrooms, carrots, and broccoli and sauté another 2-3 minutes. Add bell pepper, baby corn, pineapple with its juice, and marinated tofu. Cover and simmer for 5 minutes. Lastly, add frozen peas and cashews and simmer another 2 minutes. Serve over rice and enjoy!

Per Serving:	Calories:	674
	Saturated Fat:	2.5 grams
	Total Fat:	14.1 grams
	Vitamin C:	145% RDA
	Fiber:	10 grams

Fat (MUFA) 9%
Fat (other) 9%
Carbo's 69%
Protein 13%

SICHUAN EGGPLANT
WITH CASHEWS, PEPPERS AND BROCCOLI

Sichuan (also spelled szechwan) cooking originates in a region in China that relies on garlic, red pepper, leeks, ginger, and vinegar to flavor its cuisine. Their dishes are frequently spicy hot. This dish uses these flavors to enhance eggplant, broccoli, and cashews. You can serve this with rice or noodles.

Preparation Time: 20 Minutes
Simmer Time: 5 Minutes
Serves: Six

1/2	Tbs	Miso paste
1/2	cup	Hot water
1/2	pound	Tofu, cut in 1/2 inch cubes
1 1/2	tsp	Chili-Garlic paste
2	Tbs	Rice vinegar
1	Tbs	Chopped ginger root
1	Tbs	Soy sauce, low sodium
3	medium	Japanese eggplants, (or 1 regular)
2	medium	Leeks, diced
2	cups	Broccoli flowerets, sliced
2	medium	Red bell peppers, sliced in thin strips
1	tsp	Canola oil
3/4	cup	Cashews, chopped

Serve with:

18	ounces	Soba noodles

Garnish with: Thinly cut strips of green leak stems.

Dissolve miso in hot water. Marinate tofu in chili paste, vinegar, ginger root, soy sauce, and water/miso stock. You can marinate it all day refrigerated to improve the flavor.

Meanwhile, slice eggplant lengthwise into finger sized pieces. Place in microwave (or steam) for 5-6 minutes to precook. Bring a pot of water to boil for noodles.

Cut leeks in half lengthwise, then slice finely, cutting into first 1-2 inches of green. Slice broccoli and red bell pepper into long thin strips. Sauté vegetables for 1-2 minutes in oil. Add cashews, eggplant, and marinated tofu sauce, and simmer covered for 5-6 minutes.

Add noodles to boiling water and follow directions on package.

Place noodles on a large serving dish. Pour over stir fry and garnish with leek trimmings.

Per Serving:		
	Calories:	425
	Saturated Fat:	1.6 grams
	Total Fat:	9.0 grams
	Fiber:	10.4 grams
	Vitamin C:	162% RDA
	Fat%:	18%
	Protein%:	16%

STIR FRY WITH CASHEWS

This is an easy recipe, something you can make on the spur of the moment. Ad lib with the vegetable ingredients and use what you have available. Chili pastes vary greatly in how spicy they can be, so you need to adjust the amount according to your taste.

Preparation Time: 30 Minutes
Serves: Six

3	cups	Rice, polished
5	cups	Water
Sauce:		
1	Tbs	Corn starch
3	Tbs	Cold water
1	cup	Hot water
1	Tbs	Miso
1	Tbs	Soy sauce, low sodium
1	Tbs	Rice vinegar
1-2	tsp	Chili paste
Stir Fry:		
6	medium	Garlic cloves, diced
2	Tbs	Ginger root, diced
1	tsp	Canola oil
4	medium	Carrots, sliced into thin strips
2	cups	Broccoli, sliced into long thin strips
2	medium	Red bell peppers, sliced into thin strips
1	cup	Frozen peas
3/4	cup	Cashews, chopped
2	cups	Bok choy, chopped
2	cups	Kale, chopped

Steam rice, See "COOKING RICE" on page 236.

Dissolve corn starch in cold water. Set aside. In a separate bowl, dissolve miso in hot water and add soy sauce, vinegar, and chili paste. Set aside.

Sauté garlic and ginger in oil for 1 minute. Add carrots and sauté on medium heat for 2-3 minutes, stirring occasionally. Add broccoli and bell peppers, and heat another 2 minutes.

Meanwhile, combine corn starch and miso bowls, mix and add to sauté.

Add peas, cashews, bok choy, and kale to stir fry and simmer for 2-3 minutes, stirring occasionally.

Serve over cooked rice.

Per Serving:

Calories:	518
Saturated Fat:	1.9 grams
Total Fat:	10 grams
Vitamin C:	185% RDA
Fiber:	6.5 grams

Fat (other) 6%

Fat (MUFA) 9%

Carbo's 74%

Protein 11%

STIR FRY WITH BLACK BEAN SAUCE

This is an easy yet satisfying meal. Adjust chili paste to taste. If you don't have chili paste, substitute with chili pepper flakes or cayenne pepper, using half the amount.

Preparation & Cooking Time: 25-35 Minutes
Serves Four

2	cups	Rice, polished

Sauce:

2	Tbs	Cold water
1	tsp	Corn starch
2	tsp	Miso paste
1/2	cup	Hot water
2	tsp	Soy sauce, low sodium
1	Tbs	Sugar
1/2-2	tsp	Chili paste
1	Tbs	Rice vinegar
1/2	pound	Tofu, rinsed

Stir Fry:

2	medium	Japanese eggplants
4	medium	Garlic cloves, diced
1	Tbs	Ginger root, diced
3	medium	Carrots, sliced in thin strips
2	Tbs	Canola oil
15	ounces	Black beans
2	cups	Bok choy, chopped
3	cups	Broccoli, sliced
1	cup	Snow peas

Begin steaming rice, See "COOKING RICE" on page 236.

Dissolve corn starch in cold water in a small bowl and set aside.

In a separate bowl, dissolve miso paste in the hot water. Add soy sauce, sugar, chili paste, and vinegar. Stir in corn starch solution and add tofu, cut into 1/2 inch cubes. Set aside.

Cut eggplants lengthwise into quartered strips, then cut into finger length pieces. Place in microwave or steamer for 5 minutes to cook.

Sauté garlic and ginger root with the carrots for 3-4 minutes on medium heat with oil. Add bok choy, broccoli, snow peas, and eggplant. Heat another 2-3 minutes.

Lastly add sauce and beans, cover, and simmer for 3-4 minutes. I prefer to cook the beans myself for this dish (rather than using canned), leaving them slightly chewy. Don't overcook beans.

Serve with steamed rice.

Per Serving:	Calories:	628
	Saturated Fat:	0.9 grams
	Total Fat:	5.9 grams
	Fiber:	18 grams
	Vitamin C:	125% RDA

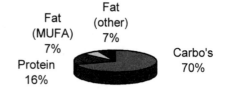

Fat (MUFA) 7%
Fat (other) 7%
Protein 16%
Carbo's 70%

BROCCOLI, SHIITAKES AND TOFU STIR FRY

This dish has a delicate flavor and aroma. Shiitake and oyster mushrooms add to the flavor, but any mushroom will do.

Preparation Time: 20 Minutes (plus 20 minutes for brown rice)
Simmer Time: 5 Minutes
Serves: Four

1 1/2	cups	**Brown rice**

Sauce:

1/2	pound	**Tofu, cut in 1/2 inch cubes**
1	Tbs	**Soy sauce,** low sodium
2	Tbs	**Sake (or white wine)**
1	Tbs	**Corn starch**
2	Tbs	**Cold water**
1/2	cup	**Hot water**
1/2	Tbs	**Miso**
1	Tbs	**Rice vinegar**

Stir Fry:

4	medium	**Garlic cloves, diced**
1	Tbs	**Ginger root, diced**
1	tsp	**Canola oil**
2	cups	**Shiitake &/or oyster mushrooms, sliced**
3	medium	**Carrots, cut into long, thin strips**
2	cups	**Broccoli, cut into long thin strips**

Begin steaming rice, See "COOKING RICE" on page 236.

Combine soy sauce and sake, and mix with cubed tofu. Set aside.

Dissolve cornstarch in cold water and set aside. In a separate cup, dissolve miso in hot water and vinegar. Combine tofu, miso, and cornstarch solutions.

Sauté garlic and ginger in oil for 1 minute on medium heat. Add mushrooms and carrots. Heat another 3 minutes, stirring occasionally. Add broccoli, and stir occasionally for 2 minutes.

Add the tofu and liquid to the sauté. Cover and simmer for another 2 minutes, stirring occasionally.

Serve with steamed rice.

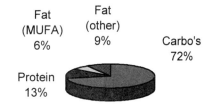

Fat (MUFA) 6%
Fat (other) 9%
Carbo's 72%
Protein 13%

Per Serving:		
	Calories:	405
	Saturated Fat:	0.7 grams
	Total Fat:	5.1 grams
	Vitamin C:	100% RDA
	Vitamin A:	327% RDA
	Fiber:	7.3 grams

ASIAN & MIDDLE EASTERN CUISINE

Southern Asia and the Middle East are home to the world's oldest civilizations and cuisines. The flavors vary greatly from India to Egypt, thanks to the large variety of spices, grains, and ingredients used.

INDIAN RICE

Indian rice is colorful and flavorful and goes well with curry dishes. I usually use basmati rice, although any type of rice will work.

Preparation Time: 10 Minutes
Simmering Time: 20-25 Minutes
Serves: Six

1	medium	Onion, diced
3	medium	Garlic cloves, diced
2	Tbs	Ginger root, diced
1	Tbs	Canola oil
1 1/2	cups	Basmati rice, rinsed
3	cups	Water
1/2	cup	Parsley, chopped
1/2	tsp	Cumin seeds
1/2	tsp	Paprika
1/2	cup	Raisins
1/2	cup	Frozen peas

In a large saucepan, sauté onion, garlic, and ginger root in oil for 3 minutes, until onion softens and turns yellow. Stir in rice and heat for 2 more minutes.

Add water and bring to a boil. Cover and simmer for 15-25 minutes, or until rice is tender, but slightly chewy.

Stir in remaining ingredients and cover for 3-5 more minutes before serving. You can also sauté the cumin seeds lightly until they become aromatic.

You can expand this into a main course by adding more veggies and garbanzo beans. For variety, add 1/4-1/2 cup of pistachios.

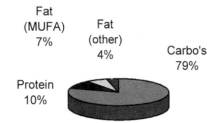

Fat (MUFA) 7%
Fat (other) 4%
Carbo's 79%
Protein 10%

Per Serving:	Calories:	241
	Saturated Fat;	0.2 grams
	Total Fat:	2.9 grams
	Fiber:	1.8 grams

RED PEPPER AND EGGPLANT CURRY

This is a colorful, delicious, and easy-to-make curry. Serve with Indian rice or regular rice for an easy dinner. If you have the time to make a fancy meal, consider adding Raita (yogurt salad), chutney and a lentil dish like dhal.

Preparation Time: 20 Minutes
Simmer Time: 10 Minutes
Serves: Six

1	medium	**Eggplant, cubed**
1	medium	**Potato, cubed**
2	medium	**Carrots, sliced**
6	medium	**Garlic cloves, diced**
3	Tbs	**Ginger root, diced**
1	medium	**Onion, diced**
3	Tbs	**Canola oil**
1/2	tsp	**Salt**
1	Tbs	**Curry powder**
1/8-1/2	tsp	**Cayenne pepper or chile powder, to taste**
2	tsp	**Corn starch**
1/4	cup	**Cold water**
1/4	cup	**Ketchup or tomato paste**
2	medium	**Bell peppers (red & green)**
1	cup	**Frozen peas**
1	cup	**Non-fat yogurt**
1/2	cup	**Cilantro, mint leaves, and/or parsley**
Garnish with		**Paprika and**
3	Tbs	**Pistachio nuts or sliced almonds**
Serve with:		
6	cups	**Cooked Indian or basmati rice**

Start rice, See "COOKING RICE" on page 236. Or, See "INDIAN RICE" on page 242.

Cut eggplant into 1/2 inch cubes and microwave, bake or steam for 6 minutes.

Cut potato into 1/2 inch cubes and sauté in oil on medium heat for 5 minutes, stirring occasionally. Meanwhile, cut a carrot lengthwise, then slice diagonally. Add carrot, garlic, ginger root, and onion and heat until onion begins to turn yellow, about 3 minutes. Add salt and curry spices with eggplant and sauté for 2-3 minutes. Dissolve corn starch into water, stir in tomato paste, and add to the curry. Simmer for 10 minutes.

Meanwhile, slice peppers into long, thin strips. Five minutes before serving, add peppers and frozen peas. Add cilantro and/or parsley 1-2 minutes before serving.

Take pan off the heat, wait 1 minute, then stir in yogurt. Garnish with paprika and nuts. Serve with rice.

Per Serving:	Calories:	473
	Saturated Fat:	1.0 grams
	Total Fat:	10 grams
	Fiber:	7.0 grams
	Vitamin C:	70% RDA
	Vitamin A:	144% RDA
	Fat%:	11%

INDIAN LENTILS (DHAL)

This makes an excellent side dish, and can be combined with rice and a side vegetable dish to form a complete meal. You can use most types of lentils, although we usually pick regular brown lentils for this dish.

Preparation Time: 10-15 Minutes
Simmer Time: 30-35 Minutes
Serves: Six

2	cups	**Lentils**
4	cups	**Warm water**
8	ounces	**Stewed tomatoes, chopped or puréed (1 cup)**

Add 3 teaspoons of curry powder to the lentils, or, follow the following directions with this mixture of spices:

1	Tbs	**Canola oil**
1/2	tsp	**Cardamom (seeds or powder)**
1	tsp	**Cumin seeds**
1	Whole	**Bay leaf**
2	Whole	**Cloves**
1	medium	**Cinnamon stick (whole)**
1/2	tsp	**Crushed red pepper**
1/2	tsp	**Turmeric powder**
1/2	tsp	**Cumin powder**

Bring lentils and water to a boil, and add stewed tomatoes. Reduce heat and simmer until tender, but not overly soft, about 25-45 minutes. (Cooking times vary with different lentils.)

Meanwhile, either add curry powder, or try the following:

Heat oil and curry spices for 1 minute on medium heat. Reduce heat and simmer for 2-3 minutes until fragrant, stirring occasionally. Remove from heat and add cooled curry spices to lentils and let them simmer together until lentils are done.

Serve with Indian rice, or use as a side dish to an Indian curry meal

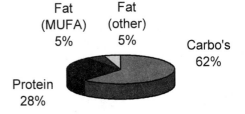

Fat (MUFA) 5%   Fat (other) 5%   Carbo's 62%   Protein 28%

Per Serving:	Calories:	257
	Saturated Fat:	0.3 grams
	Total Fat:	3.1 grams
	Fiber:	19.9 grams
	Zinc:	2.5 mg

FALAFEL

Falafel, tomatoes, lettuce, and yogurt make a great stuffing for pita bread. Add bean sprouts, avocado, or cucumber as you like.

Preparation Time: 20 Minutes
Sauté Time: 5 Minutes
Serves: Four

1/2	medium	**Sweet Onion, diced**
4	medium	**Garlic cloves, diced**
2	medium	**Carrots, diced**
2	Tbs	**Virgin olive oil**
1/8	tsp	**Salt**
1/2	tsp	**Cumin powder**
1/2	tsp	**Italian Herbs**
1	Slice	**Whole wheat bread, toasted and crumbled**
2	large	**Egg whites** (optional)
15	ounces	**Cooked garbanzo beans, rinsed and drained (2 cups)**
2	medium	**Tomatoes, chopped**
12	Tbs	**Mint leaves, minced** (optional)
1/3	cup	**Nonfat yogurt**
1	medium	**Lemon, juiced**
2	cups	**Bibb lettuce, chopped**
4	medium	**Pita bread, whole wheat, cut in half**

Sauté onion, garlic and carrots in 1 teaspoon of oil for 2-3 minutes on medium heat. Add salt, cumin and herbs and sauté another 1-2 minutes.

In a blender or food processor, combine breadcrumbs, egg whites, garbanzos and sauté mixture. Blend to form a chunky paste. (If you use canned beans, rinse well.) Form the mixture into eight flat patties.

In a frypan, heat 1 tablespoon of olive oil and sauté the patties. After 1-2 minutes, turn with a spatula and sauté other side. Repeat process with a second batch and remaining oil.

In a bowl, combine tomatoes, mint, yogurt and lemon juice and spoon into each pita pocket. Then, add lettuce and 2 patties into each pocket and serve.

Per Serving:		
	Calories:	487
	Saturated Fat:	1.6 grams
	Total Fat:	12 grams
	Vitamin C:	103% RDA
	Vitamin A:	216%

Fat (MUFA) 11%
Fat (other) 9%
Carbo's 63%
Protein 16%

SOUTHWEST AMERICAN CUISINE

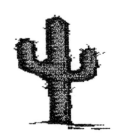

*D*ishes from the American Southwest are heavily influenced by Mexican and Native American cuisines. These dishes use beans, nuts, squash, corn, tomatoes, and of course, peppers. Vary the quantity of chili pepper to meet your taste. Stuffing vegetables with grains and spices is a popular tradition. Zucchini, squash, pumpkin, bell peppers, and tomatoes can all be stuffed and baked either as a side dish, or a complete meal.

Corn and beans remain important staples throughout Mexico and Central America. Spicy corn bread is fantastic with many bean dishes. As rice has infiltrated this regional cuisine, rice and bean dishes abound, too.

There are hundreds of pepper varieties. I have focused on bell peppers, which you'll find often in an average grocery store. Bell peppers change color as they ripen, going from green to either yellow, orange, or a vibrant red. Green peppers have a tart, strong flavor, while red peppers are more mild and sweet. Roasting peppers enriches and sweetens their taste. While many of these Southwestern recipes call for roasted peppers, you can always use unroasted peppers.

Chili pepper and cayenne pepper provide a vibrant, flavor to food. I have designed these recipes to be mild. Feel free to add more spice, but be sure to ask your guests for their preferences.

ROASTING PEPPERS

*R*oasted peppers go very well with Mexican and Latin dishes. They are sweet, delicious, and loaded with antioxidants.

Set oven on broil. Cut off pepper crown and scoop out seeds. (You can do a dozen peppers at a time and freeze what you don't use in individual packets for later use.)

Place peppers in a rimmed ovenproof pan or dish (to catch the pepper juice) on the top rack. Roast until skin browns, then turn. When all the sides are browned (about 12 minutes), remove from the oven.

Allow to cool a few minutes, and remove skin. Use immediately in your dish, or freeze and use later. You can chop peppers for stir fry, bake them in corn bread, or purée them for dip.

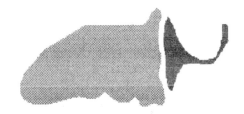

BURRITOS WITH BEANS, PEPPERS, & SALSA

This is a quick and easy meal, one my children and I enjoy greatly. It is colorful and satisfying.

Preparation: 15 Minutes
Serves: Four

3	*medium*	*Garlic cloves, diced*
1	*tsp*	*Olive oil*
2	*cups*	*Spinach, fresh and chopped*
8	*ounces*	*Sweet corn (1 cup), canned or frozen*
4	*ounces*	*Mild green chiles (1/2 cup)*
16	*ounces*	*Non-fat refried beans (2 cups)*
1/2	*cup*	*Nonfat cottage cheese*
1/2	*cup*	*Salsa (Ready-made or See "MEXICAN SALSA" on page 207.)*
8	*medium*	*Whole wheat tortillas*

Sauté garlic over moderate heat for 1-2 minutes in oil. Add spinach, corn, and peppers and continue to heat for 2 minutes. Add beans and simmer until bubbling. Stir in cottage cheese and salsa blending together for 1-2 minutes more.

Meanwhile, heat tortillas in a skillet, until they are soft and warm (about 10-15 seconds per side). Handle carefully.

Spoon a few tablespoons of bean mixture into the center of each heated tortilla, and roll into a burrito and serve.

For a side dish, serve with "LATIN RICE WITH TOMATOES & PEPPERS" on page 255.

Per Serving:	Calories:	390
	Saturated Fat:	0.6 grams
	Total Fat:	4.3 grams
	Fiber:	16.3 grams
	Vitamin C:	107% RDA

Fat (MUFA) 4%
Fat (other) 5%
Protein 20%
Carbo's 71%

Bean Photo

SQUASH STUFFED WITH
WILD RICE, PECANS AND VEGGIES

This is a colorful and delicious dish for the fall and winter. You can serve it for holiday meals, or just have it for dinner. You can use any type of squash. Butternut and acorn squash are easy to find in grocery stores. Serve as a colorful side dish, or a main course with a side salad.

Preparation Time: 20 Minutes
Baking and Cooking Time: 1 Hour
Serves: Six

1 1/2	cup	Wild rice
2	Tbs	Miso
3	medium	Squash, butternut
1	medium	Onion, diced
4	medium	Garlic cloves, diced
3	medium	Carrots, diced
1	Tbs	Virgin olive oil
1	tsp	Dried oregano
2	cups	Broccoli flowerets, sliced
1/2	cup	Pecans, chopped
2	medium	Tomatoes, chopped
1/2	cup	Cranberries (or blueberries)
Garnish with		**Parsley sprigs**

Preheat oven to 350° F. Begin cooking, see "COOKING RICE" on page 236

Meanwhile, cut squash in half lengthwise and scoop out seeds and stringy pulp. Place in oven, cut side down on an oven pan with edges. Bake for 30 minutes. Scoop out a depression for the stuffing and set aside to cool.

Sauté onion, garlic, and carrots in oil on medium heat for 3-4 minutes. Add oregano, broccoli, and pecans, cover and simmer for 4-6 minutes, until broccoli is tender, but still chewy. Mix in cranberries and set aside.

When rice is cooked, drain well. Combine simmered vegetables with rice and juice from baked squash.

Fill cut squash with rice and vegetable mixture. Bake for 10 minutes.

To serve, spoon remaining rice and veggie mixture onto each plate. Place a stuffed squash in the center of each plate and garnish with parsley sprigs.

Fat (MUFA) 12%
Fat (other) 7%
Carbo' 69%
Protein 12%

Per Serving:	Calories:	576
	Saturated Fat:	1.4 grams
	Total Fat:	9.9 grams
	Vitamin C:	203% RDA
	Vitamin A:	748% RDA

ENCHILADAS WITH ROASTED BELL PEPPERS

This is a mild version of enchiladas, using sweet bell peppers. Try this dish with a variety of pepper types for different flavors. Serve with rice.

Preparation Time: 20-30 Minutes
Baking Time: 20 Minutes
Serves: Six

Sauce:

2	medium	**Red bell peppers**
1	medium	**Onion, diced**
4	medium	**Garlic cloves, diced**
2	tsp	**Virgin olive oil**
1	tsp	**Dried oregano**
1	tsp	**Crushed red pepper**
1/2	tsp	**Cumin seeds**
1	large	**Tomato, chopped**
15	ounces	**Stewed tomatoes, puréed (2 cups)**
8	ounces	**Corn kernels (1 cup)**
1/4	cup	**Cilantro, chopped**
12	medium	**Corn tortillas**
1	cup	**Low-fat Monterrey Jack cheese, grated**

Enchilada Filling:

15	ounces	**Non-fat refried beans (2 cups)**
1	medium	**Red bell pepper**
1/2	cup	**Non-fat cheese, grated**
1/4	cup	**Pecans, chopped**

Roast peppers and chop; see "ROASTING PEPPERS" on page 246.

Preheat oven to 375° F. Sauté onion and garlic for 2 minutes in oil over medium heat, stirring occasionally. Add oregano, crushed pepper, and cumin. Heat another minute. Add tomato, stewed tomatoes, corn, cilantro and 2/3 of bell peppers and let simmer for 10-15 minutes.

To make filling, combine beans, remaining bell pepper, cheese, and pecans and heat until cheese has melted and beans bubble lightly.

In a hot skillet, warm each tortilla until soft. Spread some filling in each tortilla and roll into a burrito.

Pour half the sauce into a 9x12 inch oven-proof dish, and arrange rolled tortillas on it. Pour on remaining sauce and sprinkle cheese on top.

Bake 10 minutes, and garnish with sprigs of cilantro before serving.

Per Serving:

Calories:	490
Saturated Fat:	1.4 grams
Total Fat:	9.0 grams
Fiber:	9.3 grams
Vitamin C:	127%

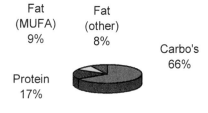

Fat (MUFA) 9%
Fat (other) 8%
Carbo's 66%
Protein 17%

BLACK BEAN CHILI
WITH PEPPERS & LIME

*L*ime juice and beans go well together, especially added to peppers and chili. You can substitute one medium onion for the leeks. Serve with corn bread or rice.

Preparation Time: 10-15 Minutes
Simmering Time: 20-30 Minutes
Serves: Four

6	medium	Garlic cloves, diced
2	medium	Leeks, diced
2	medium	Carrots, chopped
2	Tbs	Virgin olive oil
1	tsp	Oregano
1	tsp	Cumin powder
8	ounces	Green chiles, diced canned, (1 cup)
1	tsp	Crushed red pepper
30	ounces	Black beans, cooked and rinsed (4 cups)
1	Tbs	Miso
1	cup	Hot water
3	Tbs	Tomato paste
2-3	medium	Limes, juiced
1/2	cup	Cilantro, chopped

Garnish with: 4 Tbs non-fat sour cream and 1/2 cup of cilantro, chopped

In a large saucepan, sauté garlic, leeks and carrots in oil for 2 minutes over medium heat. Add oregano, cumin, chiles, and chili pepper flakes and simmer for 5 minutes. Add beans.

Dissolve miso in hot water and tomato paste and add to beans. Let simmer for another 20-25 minutes.

Two minutes before serving, add lime juice and half the cilantro.

Garnish with remaining cilantro and a spoonful of non-fat sour cream (or non-fat yogurt) over each serving. Serve with corn bread, see "CORN BREAD" on page 251.

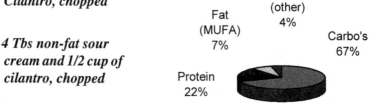

Fat (other) 4%
Fat (MUFA) 7%
Carbo's 67%
Protein 22%

Per Serving:		
	Calories:	450
	Saturated Fat:	0.9 grams
	Total Fat:	5.7 grams
	Vitamin C:	318% RDA
	Vitamin A:	215% RDA
	Fiber:	24 grams!

CORN BREAD

*P*eppers and corn kernels add a wonderful flavor to corn bread. Serve corn bread with chili or other bean dishes. Use bell peppers if you don't like chili spice.

Preparation Time: 10 Minutes
Baking Time: 40-45 Minutes
Serves: Eight Slices for Eight People

1	*cup*	*Cornmeal*
1	*cup*	*Pastry whole wheat flour*
4	*tsp*	*Baking powder*
1/2	*tsp*	*Salt*
3	*Tbs*	*Sugar*
2	*large*	*Egg whites, lightly beaten*
1	*cup*	*Non-fat milk*
1	*Tbs*	*Canola oil*
8	*ounces*	*Green chiles, diced and cooked (1 cup)*
8	*ounces*	*Corn kernels (1 cup), fresh, canned or frozen*

Preheat oven to 400° F.

Combine dry ingredients in a bowl. Blend wet ingredients in a separate bowl. Mix the wet and dry parts together.

Spray a non-stick pan with canola oil. Pour batter into it and bake 40-45 minutes, until the top is golden and a toothpick comes out dry. Remove from oven, let cool a few minutes, and serve.

Per Serving:		
	Calories:	187
	Saturated Fat:	0.4 grams
	Total Fat:	3.0 grams
	Fiber:	4.2 grams
	Vitamin C:	45%

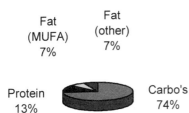

Fat (MUFA) 7%
Fat (other) 7%
Protein 13%
Carbo's 74%

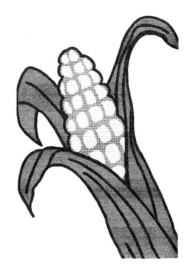

WILD RICE WITH
KALE, PECANS AND KIDNEY BEANS

This is an easy and filling meal. Substitute cabbage or broccoli if you can't find kale. Optionally, add sliced mushrooms with the garlic.

Preparation Time: 15 Minutes
Cooking Time: 50 Minutes (including rice)
Serves: Four

4	cups	**Cooked wild rice**	Start cooking wild rice, see "COOKING RICE" on page 236.
4	medium	**Garlic cloves, diced**	When rice is done, sauté garlic and herbs in oil for 1 minute. Add kale and beans, and sauté another 2 minutes.
1	tsp	**Italian Herbs**	
1	Tbs	**Virgin olive oil**	
6	cups	**Kale, sliced**	Add tomatoes, soy sauce, pecans, and cooked rice. Cover and simmer for 2-3 minutes. Don't overcook kale and tomatoes, saving shape and color.
15	ounces	**Cooked kidney beans**	
3	medium	**Tomatoes, cut in thin wedges**	
1 1/2	Tbs	**Soy sauce, low sodium**	Season with lime juice, garnish with parsley sprigs.
1/4	cup	**Pecans, chopped**	
1	medium	**Lime, squeezed**	
Garnish with:		**Parsley sprigs**	

Per Serving:

Calories:	426
Saturated Fat:	1.2 grams
Total Fat:	10.2 grams
Vitamin C:	232% RDA
Vitamin A:	191% RDA
Fiber:	11 grams

Fat (MUFA) 9%
Fat (other) 10%
Carbo's 63%
Protein 18%

TUCSON PASTA

This pasta, flavored with ingredients from the Southwest, reminds me of my years in Tucson. It is quick and easy to prepare and has a zesty flavor. I like it with fresh pasta, but any pasta will do. Look for flat ribbon pastas, with tomato, basil, or spinach flavors.

Preparation Time: 20 Minutes
Serves: Six

2	medium	**Bell peppers (different colors)**
6	medium	**Garlic cloves**
1	medium	**Onion**
2	medium	**Tomatoes, chopped**
18	ounces	**Fresh pasta (2 1/2 cups)**
1	Tbs	**Virgin olive oil**
1/4	tsp	**Salt**
1/2	tsp	**Paprika**
1/8-1/4	tsp	**Cayenne Pepper (optional)**
1	cup	**White beans, cooked and rinsed**
15	ounces	**Sweet corn (2 cups), frozen or canned**
1	cup	**Greens (spinach, chard, or other)**
1/4	cup	**Cilantro, chopped**

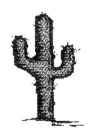

Roast peppers, see "ROASTING PEPPERS" on page 246. Roast whole onion and garlic in the same pan for 12 minutes. After 5 minutes, add chopped tomatoes to roast. Set aside to cool.

Meanwhile, bring water to a boil, with a dash of oil and salt. When boiling briskly, add pasta and cook until *al dente*.

Dice garlic and onion and sauté with salt in oil for 1 minute on medium heat. Add paprika, cayenne, rinsed beans, corn, roasted peppers, chopped greens, and tomatoes and heat for another 2-3 minutes, stirring occasionally.

When pasta is cooked, rinse and place on a serving plate. Mix half the cilantro with sauce. To serve, pour sauce over pasta, and garnish with remaining cilantro.

Fat (MUFA) 7%
Fat (other) 7%
Protein 13%
Carbo's 74%

Per Serving:		
	Calories:	480
	Saturated Fat:	0.9 grams
	Total Fat:	6.2 gram
	Vitamin C:	119% RDA

VEGGIE SLOPPY JOES

This is an easy, tasty recipe that my children enjoy. Serve with a salad or side of veggies to make a complete meal.

Preparation Time: 15 Minutes
Serves: Six

1	small	Onion, diced
4	medium	Garlic cloves, diced
2	tsp	Canola oil
1	medium	Red bell pepper, diced
12	ounces	Tomato sauce
1	Tbs	Chili powder
1	Tbs	Soy sauce, low sodium
1	Tbs	Brown sugar
15	ounces	Black beans, cooked
15	ounces	Pinto beans, cooked
1/4	cup	Pecans, chopped
6	medium	Whole wheat buns
6	Leaves	Lettuce

Sauté onion and garlic over medium heat with oil for 2-3 minutes. Add bell pepper and heat another minute. Stir in tomato sauce, chili powder, soy sauce, and brown sugar. Heat until bubbling, then reduce heat to simmer.

Rinse beans and add to mixture and continue to simmer another 3-5 minutes. Remove from heat and stir in pecans.

Toast or heat buns, serve bean mixture and top with a lettuce leaf.

Optionally, add fresh, chopped cilantro and corn kernels with pecans.

Per Serving:	Calories:	540
	Saturated Fat:	1.0 gram
	Total Fat:	7.4 grams
	Fiber:	26 grams

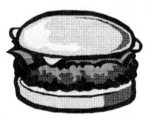

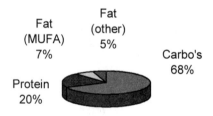

Fat (MUFA) 7%
Fat (other) 5%
Carbo's 68%
Protein 20%

LATIN RICE WITH
TOMATOES & PEPPERS

This is a rice dish we like to serve with Mexican and Latin American food. It's very colorful, and packed with nutrients. Use it as a side dish, or add black or pinto beans to serve as a main course. You can use basmati rice in place of brown rice, but rinse the basmati rice first and note that it cooks faster. I like kale in this dish, with its lacy shape and firm texture, but any type of greens will do.

Preparation Time: 15 Minutes
Simmering Time: 40 Minutes (20 minutes with basmati rice)
Serves: A Side Dish for Six (or a meal with beans for four)

1	medium	Onion, diced
4	medium	Garlic cloves, diced
1	tsp	Olive oil
1	tsp	Paprika
1/4	tsp	Salt
8	ounces	Sweet corn (1 cup)
1 1/2	cups	Brown rice
3	cups	Warm water
1	medium	Red bell pepper, sliced
2	medium	Tomatoes, chopped (or 14 ounces of drained canned tomatoes)
1/4	cup	Cilantro, chopped
1	cup	Greens, chopped (kale, spinach, or chard)
4	Tbs	Low-fat cheddar cheese, grated (optional)

Sauté onion and garlic in oil with paprika and salt over medium heat for 2-3 minutes, until onion starts to turn soft and yellow. Add corn and brown rice and sauté for another minute.

Add water and bring to a boil. Cover and simmer for 40 minutes until rice is nearly tender.

Stir in bell pepper, tomatoes, cilantro and greens. Sprinkle grated cheese on top (optional) and continue to simmer for 5-10 minutes. Remove from heat and serve.

Per Serving:	Calories:	136
	Saturated Fat:	0.6 grams
	Total Fat:	2.7 grams

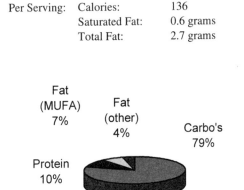

Fat (MUFA) 7%
Fat (other) 4%
Carbo's 79%
Protein 10%

SOUTHWESTERN TABOOLEH

This is a fun dish to make, featuring a Middle Eastern grain dish flavored with southwestern ingredients. As this is a light meal, offer hummus or guacamole dips as a starter.

Preparation Time: 20 Minutes
Serves: Six

2 ½	cups	**Water**
1	Tbs	**Miso**
2	cups	**Bulgur wheat**

Saute:

1	medium	**Onion, diced**
3	medium	**Garlic cloves, diced**
1/2	tsp	**Italian Herbs**
2	cups	**Oyster mushrooms, sliced**
2	tsp	**Virgin olive oil**
1	medium	**Red bell pepper, sliced**
15	ounces	**Pinto beans, cooked (2 cups)**

Add:

1 ½	cups	**Parsley, finely chopped**
1/2	cup	**Cilantro, chopped**
2	medium	**Tomatoes, chopped**
3	medium	**Lemons, juiced**
1/3	cup	**Pecans, chopped**

Garnish with:

1/2	small	**Avocado, sliced thinly**
Sprigs		**Parsley**

Bring water to a boil. Add miso and stir to dissolve. Add bulgur wheat, remove from heat. Stir occasionally.

Sauté onion, garlic, herbs, and mushrooms in oil on medium heat for 2 minutes. Add bell pepper and rinsed pinto beans and heat another 1-2 minutes. Remove from heat.

After bulgur wheat has absorbed liquid, about 20 minutes, mix in the sauté.

Add parsley, cilantro, tomatoes, lemon juice, and pecans and stir. Serve warm or chilled in a large salad bowl, or on a large serving plate covered with fresh leafy lettuce. Garnish with avocado slices and sprigs of parsley.

Per Serving:	Calories	455
	Saturated Fat:	1.4 grams
	Total Fat:	11.2 grams
	Fiber:	20 grams
	Vitamin C:	184% RDA
	Vitamin A:	109% RDA

Fat (MUFA) 12% Fat (other) 8% Carbo's 65%

Protein 15%

NACHOS

This dish is an easy-to-make party treat, or can provide a nutritious, low-fat meal that's fun to eat.

Preparation Time: 10 Minutes
Baking Time: Seven Minutes
Serves: Six

14	ounces	*Non-fat tortilla chips*
6	ounces	*Nonfat cheese, Monterrey Jack, grated (1 cup)*
4	medium	*Garlic cloves, diced*
1/2	tsp	*Italian Herbs*
3	tsp	*Virgin olive oil*
2	medium	*Red and green bell peppers, chopped*
15	ounces	*Refried beans, nonfat (2 cups)*
1/2	cup	*Cilantro*
1	cup	*Salsa*
15	ounces	*Corn kernels (1 cup)*
2	medium	*Tomatoes, chopped*
1	medium	*Lime, juiced, optional*

Preheat oven to 375° F. Pour chips into 2 oven pans or dishes for nachos. Spray each chip dish for 1-2 seconds with oil, stir chips and spray each dish for another 1-2 seconds. Grate cheese in a separate bowl and set aside.

Sauté garlic, herbs, peppers in 1 teaspoon of oil for 2 minutes on medium heat. Add beans and cilantro, reduce heat to low, and heat another 2 minutes.

Pour half of salsa and half the beans over chips and mix gently. Then, pour on remaining salsa, bean mixture, corn, and tomatoes. Sprinkle on grated cheese. Squeeze on lime juice and put in oven for seven minutes; don't over bake chips. Serve immediately.

Per Serving		
	Calories:	520
	Saturated Fat:	1.1 grams
	Total Fat:	7.1 grams
	Vitamin C:	93% RDA
	Fiber:	9.5 grams

Fat (MUFA) 5%
Fat (other) 6%
Carbo's 73%
Protein 16%

DESSERTS

Dessert provides the finishing touches to a meal. It doesn't have to be overly complex, sweet, or fatty; rather, it should satisfy. Dessert can be as simple as papaya with a splash of lime, or on a special occasion, as elegant as crêpes suzette.

MOCCA ICING

I like this icing for cakes and muffins. It works nicely as a dip for fruit, or to dribble over ice milk and frozen yogurt.

Makes enough for (1) nine inch, two-layer cake

1/2	cup	**Semisweet chocolate**
1/4	cup	**Coffee, brewed**
1/3	cup	**Sugar**
1/8	tsp	**Salt**
2	tsp	**Canola oil**

Melt chocolate in a double boiler. In a separate saucepan, heat coffee with sugar and salt. When chocolate is melted and coffee is near bubbling, mix. Add canola oil. Stir and remove from heat to cool.

As an icing, spread when cooled but still slightly warm.

As a fruit dipping, dip fruit when warm, then set fruit on a clean surface to cool and harden. Keep dipped fruit refrigerated until you serve.

CHOCOLATE-RASPBERRY ICING

I like this icing with my chocolate cake recipe, My boys and I also love to dip fresh raspberries and other fruit into this rich, flavorful coating.

1/2	cup	**Semisweet chocolate**
1/2	cup	**Raspberry sauce (see"RASPBERRY SAUCE" on page 209)**
1	tsp	**Canola oil**

Melt chocolate in a double boiler. Stir occasionally. Once melted, stir in canola oil. Meanwhile, make raspberry sauce, but do <u>not</u> add the corn starch or the lemon.

Slowly stir 1/2 the raspberry sauce into the chocolate. Let cool. Spread as an icing, or dip fruit in while still warm and let cool and harden before serving.

CHOCOLATE CAKE
WITH RASPBERRY SAUCE

This is a delicious, yet low-fat chocolate cake. Splurge and use quality chocolate. You can substitute blackberries for raspberries. The yam adds moisture to the cake.

Preparation Time: 25 Minutes
Baking Time: 45 Minutes
Serves: Twelve

2	cups	**Whole wheat pastry flour**
2	cups	**Sugar**
3/4	cup	**Cocoa powder**
2	tsp	**Baking Powder**
1/2	tsp	**Salt**
6	large	**Egg whites**
1/4	cup	**Canola oil**
1	cup	**White wine**
1	tsp	**Vanilla extract**
1	medium	**Yam, cooked & puréed**
Use		**Raspberry Sauce**
Topping:		**Raspberry chocolate Icing**
Garnish with:		**12 Whole berries &**
1/8	**Ounce**	**Chocolate shavings**

Preheat oven to 375° F. Lightly spray two non-stick, 9-inch cake pans with canola oil and dust with flour. Microwave the yam (about 6-8 minutes), remove the skin, and mash it into a purée.

Combine dry ingredients well. In a separate bowl, combine wet ingredients with mashed yam. Mix dry and wet parts together. Divide batter into the two baking pans. Bake for 45 minutes, or until inserted toothpick comes out dry.

Make "RASPBERRY SAUCE" on page 209. Thicken with non-fat sour cream.

Make either "CHOCOLATE-RASPBERRY ICING" on page 258 or make "MOCCA ICING" on page 258.

Cool pans on a rack for 10 minutes. Turn cake layers out and cool thoroughly. Place one layer on a serving plate and pour 1/2 of berry sauce on it. Add second layer, and cover the cake with icing. Place choice berries on cake. Use a potato peeler to garnish top of cake with chocolate shavings.

Fat (MUFA) 13%
Fat (PUFA) 7%
Carbo's 73%
Protein 7%

Per Serving:	Calories:	347
	Saturated Fat:	2.2 grams
	Total Fat:	8.1 grams
	Fiber:	6.4 grams
	Vitamin A:	44% RDA

PINEAPPLE-CARROT CAKE

This is a great snack, or it can be served as dessert. Chop the nuts and dried fruit coarsely, leaving chewy pieces within the cake.

Preparation Time: 15-20 Minutes
Baking Time: 55 Minutes
Serves: Eight

1	*tsp*	*Canola oil*
2	*large*	*Egg whites*
1 1/4	*cups*	*Brown sugar*
1	*tsp*	*Vanilla extract*
1	*cup*	*Carrots, grated*
1/2	*cup*	*Pineapple chunks, chopped*
1/2	*cup*	*Pecans, coarsely chopped*
1	*cup*	*Dried fruit (raisins, apricots, peaches, etc.) coarsely chopped*
1 1/2	*cups*	*Whole wheat pastry flour*
1	*tsp*	*Baking powder*
1	*tsp*	*Cinnamon*
1/2	*tsp*	*Allspice or ground cloves*

Preheat oven to 375° F. Spray a 9x5x3 loaf pan with oil, dust with flour.

In a bowl, mix oil, egg whites and sugar together. Then add vanilla, carrots, pineapple, pecans, and dried fruit. Add remaining ingredients and mix all into batter.

Pour batter into loaf pan. Bake until toothpick inserted comes out clean (about 50 minutes). Place pan on rack to cool for 5-10 minutes, then remove from pan.

Per Serving:	Calories:	291
	Saturated Fat:	0.6 grams
	Total Fat:	6.8 grams
	Fiber:	4.0 grams

Fat (MUFA) 13%   Fat (other) 6%   Carbo's 74%

Protein 7%

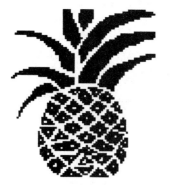

CRÊPES SUZETTE

This is a spectacular, delicious desert. The crêpes and sauce can be made in advance to cut serving time to 10 minutes. Serve with friends for a party or special event.

Preparation time: 45 Minutes
Serves: Six

Crêpes:

1/2	cup	**Whole wheat flour**
1/2	cup	**All purpose flour**
1	cup	**Non-fat milk**
2	tsp	**Canola oil**
1	tsp	**Grated orange peel**
1/4	tsp	**Salt**
1/4	cup	**Water**
3	large	**Egg whites**

Orange Sauce:

3	medium	**Oranges, juiced & finely grated rind**
1/3	cup	**Sugar**
1	Tbs	**Canola oil**
4	Tbs	**Orange marmalade**
2	Tbs	**Grand Marnier (or 1 tsp orange extract, & skip the flambé)**

Flambé:

4	Tbs	**Grand Marnier**

Per Serving:	Calories:	295
	Saturated Fat:	0.4 grams
	Total Fat:	5.3 grams
	Vitamin C:	66% RDA
	Fat%	18%

Crêpes: Mix flour, milk, orange peel, salt, water, and egg whites well. Heat a crêpe pan or a small non-stick skillet. (If you need to grease the pan, brush on 1/8 tsp or less of canola oil, or spray the pan with canola oil before pouring crêpe batter.) Pour 1/8 cup of batter into a hot pan on medium heat and tip pan to spread batter. Cook crêpes until golden, about 20-30 seconds for each side. (The first 1-2 crêpes are the hardest, because they stick to the unevenly heated pan.) Batter makes 12-14 crêpes.

Orange Sauce: Mix sauce ingredients in a bowl. Grate rind prior to juicing.

Just before serving: Heat orange sauce in a pan until bubbling, then dip crêpes into sauce. Using tongs, fold crêpes in half twice to form triangles as you place crêpes on a warm serving dish. Pour remaining heated sauce over crêpes. Heat remaining Grand Marnier in a pan until it *just starts* to bubble. Don't boil off the alcohol or it will not flambé.

To serve, light the heated Grand Marnier and pour immediately over the warm crêpes. Flames will last only a few seconds, but the flambé fragrance will remain.

BLUEBERRY & PORT FROZEN YOGURT

This is one of my favorite desserts. It is quick, easy, and delicious. Berry yogurt is tart unless you add extra sugar. You can easily substitute blueberries for blackberries, raspberries, or other fruit. The alcohol in the port helps prevent the yogurt from freezing rock hard, and the port adds a wonderful flavor. We use a pre-frozen "Donvier" Ice Cream Maker, but any ice cream maker will work. Or you can simply put it in the freezer for 3-5 hours to make a "slurry." A little canola oil makes the frozen yogurt texture creamier.

Preparation Time: 10 Minutes, plus 15 minutes for the ice cream to set
(This depends on your ice cream maker.)
Serves: Eight

32	ounces	**Non-fat plain yogurt (4 cups)**
2	cups	**Frozen berries**
1/2	cup	**Sugar**
4	Tbs	**Port**
2	Tbs	**Canola oil (optional)**

Pour yogurt, sugar, and port into a blender and blend. Add 1 cup of berries and blend until it is smooth. Then add the second cup and purée until berries are blended, with little chunks of fruit remaining.

Pour into ice cream maker. (Or place in the freezer 3-5 hours before serving if you don't have an ice cream maker.)

Per serving:	Calories:	135
(Without	Saturated Fat:	0.1 grams
Oil)	Total Fat:	0.4 grams

Per Serving:	Calories:	203
(With Oil)	Saturated Fat:	0.4 grams
	Total Fat:	3.9 grams

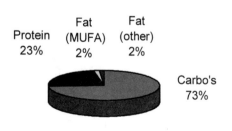

Protein 23% Fat (MUFA) 2% Fat (other) 2% Carbo's 73%

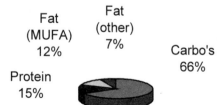

Fat (MUFA) 12% Fat (other) 7% Carbo's 66% Protein 15%

PINEAPPLE & ORANGE SORBET WITH GRAND MARNIER

This is a light dessert and easy to make. Add frozen berries to modify the flavor and color. The egg whites make the sorbet creamier and lighter; you can omit them if you wish.

Preparation Time: 10 Minutes
Makes: 5 Cups
Setting Time: 15 Minutes in a machine to 5 hours in the freezer.

2	cups	*Frozen pineapple chunks*
1	cup	*Frozen banana or frozen berries*
2	cups	*Orange juice*
2	large	*Egg whites (optional) **
3	Tbs	*Grand Marnier Liqueur*

Put frozen fruit, juice, and liqueur, into a food processor or a blender and purée until smooth.

Beat egg whites until slightly foamy, and mix with fruit and juice.

Follow the instructions for your ice cream maker. Or, place in the freezer for 3-5 hours to harden. Serve when thick, yet soft.

* Caution: There is always some risk of infectious diarrhea if you choose to eat uncooked egg products. It helps to wash the egg shells in soapy water before breaking the shell, but some risk may remain.

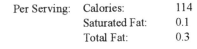

Per Serving:	Calories:	114
	Saturated Fat:	0.1
	Total Fat:	0.3

Percent Energy from Fat:	3%
Percent Energy from Protein:	9%
Percent Energy from Carbos:	88%

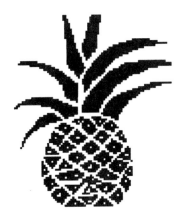

MANGO FROZEN YOGURT

This is a delicate and light dessert, especially satisfying after a spicy, curry meal. You can substitute any orange flavored liqueur for Grand Marnier, or skip the alcohol and add orange extract instead. Without the alcohol, make only what you will eat at once, as extra freezer time makes the yogurt very hard. The canola oil makes the yogurt creamier, without the saturated fat from cream.

Preparation Time: 10 Minutes,
Setting Time: 10-15 Minutes in a ice cream maker, or 5 hours in the freezer
Serves: Eight

2	*medium*	*Mangos*
2	*cups*	*Non-fat yogurt*
1/3	*cup*	*Sugar*
1/8	*tsp*	*Salt*
1	*Tbs*	*Canola oil, (optional)*
1/2	*tsp*	*Vanilla extract*
1	*Tbs*	*Grand Marnier, (optional)*

Slice fruit away from mango seed and skin.

Pour yogurt, sugar, salt, oil (optional), vanilla and liqueur into a blender and purée. Add half mango and blend until smooth. Then, add the other half of the mango and blend briefly, so chunks of mango remain in the yogurt.

Pour mixture into an ice cream maker. Or, place in the freezer for 3-5 hours to harden.

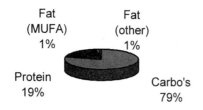

Fat (MUFA) 1%
Fat (other) 1%
Protein 19%
Carbo's 79%

Per Serving: **(With oil)**	Calories:	99.3
	Saturated Fat:	0.2 grams
	Total Fat:	1.9 grams
	Fat%:	17%

Per Serving **(No oil)**	Calories:	84
	Saturated Fat:	0.1 grams
	Total Fat:	0.2 grams
	Fat%:	1.7%

RICE PUDDING
WITH ALMONDS & KAHLUA

This rich, flavorful treat accompanies Indian food well. You can also serve it for breakfast. Plan for this dessert anytime by cooking extra rice for dinner.

Preparation Time: 10 Minutes
Baking Time: 40 Minutes
Serves: Four

2	cups	**Steamed rice**
1	cup	**Non-fat milk**
1/2	cup	**Raisins or dried dates**
1/3	cup	**Almond slices**
2	Tbs	**Kahlua (coffee liqueur), optional**
1/4	cup	**Brown sugar**
1	medium	**Banana, mashed**
1	large	**Egg white**
1/8	tsp	**Cinnamon, ground**
1/8	tsp	**Cardamom, ground**
Garnish with:		**Dash of Cinnamon and almond slivers**

Preheat oven to 350° F.

Mix ingredients together in a baking dish.

Place in the oven for 40 minutes. Let cool for 5-10 minutes and serve, or chill and serve cold later.

Garnish with a dash of cinnamon and almond slivers.

Per Serving;	Calories:	374
	Saturated Fat:	0.8 grams
	Total Fat:	7 grams
	Fat%:	17%
	Protein%:	10%
	Carbo's%:	73%

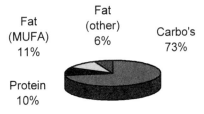

Fat (MUFA) 11%
Fat (other) 6%
Carbo's 73%
Protein 10%

RHUBARB & BLUEBERRY CRUMBLE

This delicious dish is easy to make. Substitute any type of berry for blueberries. You can also serve this for a special brunch.

Preparation Time: 10 Minutes
Baking Time: 20 Minutes
Serves: Six

1/2	cup	**Water**
1/4	cup	**Sugar**
4	cups	**Rhubarb, cut in 3/4 inch slices**
2	tsp	**Corn starch**
2	tsp	**Cold water**
2	cups	**Blueberries, frozen or fresh**
1 1/2	cups	**Low-fat granola (No more than 30% of calories from fat)**

Preheat oven to 375° F.

In a saucepan, combine water and sugar to rhubarb and bring to a boil. Lower heat and simmer for 5 minutes.

Dissolve corn starch in cold water and stir into rhubarb sauce.

Pour into a pie plate and mix in the blueberries. Sprinkle granola on top. (Avoid mixing the granola in with the sauce, or it looses its crunch.) Bake for 20 minutes. Serve hot.

To make in advance, you can bake the blueberries and rhubarb, but don't add the granola until ready to serve (or it will turn soggy). Pan-heat the granola or heat in oven and sprinkle over berries and rhubarb prior to serving.

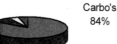

Fat (MUFA) 4%
Fat (other) 4%
Protein 8%
Carbo's 84%

Per Serving:		
	Calories:	110
	Saturated Fat:	0 grams
	Total Fat:	1.1 grams
	Fiber:	3.9 grams

BEVERAGES

*A*t times a special drink makes a meal better. Some drinks are wonderful as a snack. Mix fruit with either milk, yogurt, or juice in a blender and enjoy wonderful drinks. Here are some of my favorites.

BANANA-BLUEBERRY LASSI

A lassi is a fruit and yogurt drink. It makes a great snack, and I like it as a refreshing and filling dessert. Play with the flavors by changing fruit combinations.

Preparation Time: Two Minutes
Serves: Four (makes 4 cups)

1	cup	*Non-fat yogurt*
1	cup	*Non-fat milk (soy or dairy)*
1	cup	*Frozen blueberries*
1	medium	*Banana, ripe*
3-4	Tbs	*Honey*

Mix ingredients in a blender and serve immediately.

Per Serving:	Calories:	147
	Saturated Fat:	0.2 grams
	Total Fat:	0.6 grams
	Fat%:	3.5%

MANGO LASSI

Another great fruit and yogurt drink. Drink it as a snack, or a dessert.

Preparation Time: 5 Minutes
Serves: Four (makes 4 cups)

2	medium	*Mangos, chilled*
3	cups	*Non-fat yogurt*
2	Tbs	*Honey*

Remove mango pulp from seed and skin. Place in a blender with yogurt and honey and blend. Serve immediately.

Per Serving:

	Calories:	194
	Saturated Fat:	0.3 grams
	Total Fat:	0.6 grams
	Vitamin C:	50% RDA
	Fat%:	2.6%

CHAPTER 11   *APPENDIX*

NUTRIENT SUPPLEMENTS

SHOULD WE TAKE INDIVIDUAL VITAMIN SUPPPLEMENTS?

*E*very day, patients come to my office loaded with bags of vitamin supplements, asking for my advice. Even my medical colleagues send me e-mails asking for the newest and latest information on vitamins.

When considering nutrient supplements, the most important factor to first address is that they remain *SUPPLEMENTAL* to a healthy diet. Supplements were never intended to replace healthful foods. Study after study proves that nutrient rich foods are superior to supplements in enhancing health. Assuming you have found your own optimal diet, let's explore the most common vitamins and nutrients used to improve health.

Vitamin E

Vitamin E remains the most promising single antioxidant supplement. First, it appears to be safe in doses up to 200-400 international units daily. Second, unlike many other antioxidants, it is very difficult to consume Vitamin E in large doses without eating huge portions of fat. Third, Vitamin E does protect cells from oxidative damage. Lastly, Vitamin E trials have shown decreased rates of deaths and heart attacks in smokers.

Part of the confusion surrounding the effectiveness of vitamin E comes from the media overstating the results of uncontrolled trials. For example, look at two large research trials that showed a limited benefit in nurses and doctors who chose to take antioxidant supplements. These people were also less obese, smoked less, had lower blood pressure, exercised more, and ate better than a group that chose not to take

Vitamin E. There is little surprise that these studies and these people with healthy lifestyles had lower heart attack rates and lower cancer rates. Yet, vitamin salespeople and the press labeled these studies "proof" that Vitamin E supplements can save lives. In contrast, many scientists stated that there was an "association" between good health and Vitamin E, but there was no proof that Vitamin E supplements could save lives. Thus, we need to be careful interpreting these studies or we create confusion.

On the positive side, a small trial randomized one hundred people at high risk for strokes to receive either aspirin or aspirin and Vitamin E. They found a decreased rate of strokes in the Vitamin E group. These results are promising but will need more review.

Vitamin E is a special antioxidant that also decreases platelet stickiness in the blood stream. When platelets stick together, they form clots, blocking blood flow. Vitamin E appears to improve health both by acting as an antioxidant and by improving circulation.

High doses of Vitamin E have also been shown to *slow the progression* of Alzheimer's dementia.

Again on the positive side, a recent Finnish study with over 22,000 people found that *smokers* decreased their risk of developing angina (chest pain) by 9% after taking 50 mg per day of Vitamin E over 4.7 years. If you smoke, you are much better off quitting tobacco than continuing to smoke and taking Vitamin E!!! If you continue to smoke, I recommend that you discuss taking Vitamin E as a supplement (400 IU per day) with your medical provider.

Most recently, the CHAOS (Cambridge Heart Antioxidant Study) randomized 2,002 people (over half of whom had never smoked) with proven coronary artery disease to receive Vitamin E supplements or placebos. They were then followed for three years. The group taking Vitamin E had significantly fewer heart attacks: for every 38 people treated, one heart attack was prevented. But the Vitamin E group also had a non-significant increase in death rates, with one extra death for every 103 people treated. (Non-significant implies that the study size was too small to be sure of the results.)

We need more information on the best dosage and whom to treat before suggesting that everyone start taking Vitamin E. As of 1997, it remains unclear (unproven) if non-smokers without heart disease gain anything from taking Vitamin E supplements.

Compare the *CHAOS study using Vitamin E* with Renaud's and de Lorgeril's study of *a Mediterranean diet*. In the Vitamin E supplement study, one heart attack was prevented for every 38 people taking supplements. In the Mediterranean diet study, only 12 people had to try the diet to prevent one heart attack or cardiac related death. To me, the bottom line remains, lifestyle changes are more effective and safer than pills!

Considering the potential benefit we could gain from Vitamin E supplements, the minimal benefit noted in trials to date is surprising and disappointing. I would have predicted the supplements to be far more effective than we have seen. However, just as we have failed to identify the best types and combinations of carotenoids, I believe we have yet to identify the best types of Vitamin E, and what other nutrients should be given with it.

Vitamin E exists in many forms in natural food sources. In some chemical reactions for example, gamma forms of Vitamin E appear more powerful than alpha forms (an alpha form is the normal Vitamin E capsule sold). Dietary sources of Vitamin E already provide a vast array of Vitamin E types, as well as other antioxidants that work in synergy to improve our health. Hence, mixed Vitamin E supplements may in the future be more effective than what is currently available.

Vitamin C

There are no randomized clinical studies that support the theory that Vitamin C supplements can decrease death rates. Yet, several studies have shown that *foods* containing rich sources of Vitamin C do decrease death rates from strokes, heart attacks and cancer.

Vitamin C supplements *have* been shown to shorten the course of a cold when taken at the onset of respiratory symptoms. They might also help prevent cataracts. Vitamin C supplements appear very safe in doses up to 1000 mg to 2000 mg per day.

Surprisingly, the most common cause of scurvy (Vitamin C deficiency) in the United States occurs when people suddenly stop their high dose Vitamin C supplements; because their tissues are accustomed to eliminating high quantities of Vitamin C) (They become deficient when normal doses are resumed.) The bottom line for high dose (more than 1 gram daily) supplement takers is: if you cut back on your dosage, do so slowly over 1-2 months.

Folic Acid

Inadequate intake of folic acid increases the risk of birth defects and is associated with increased heart and circulation problems. Folic acid (also called folate) does not appear to affect cholesterol levels nor does it act as an antioxidant. However, plaque formation in arteries is higher when folic acid levels are low. This means that if we don't eat enough folic acid, this deficiency may increase our risks of coronary artery disease and peripheral vascular disease. (the loss of circulation in your arms and legs from blocked arteries.)

Green leafy vegetables, orange juice, and legumes (beans) are good sources of folic acid. (See Table 36 for folic acid content in foods.) Make sure you eat at least 0.4 mg (400 mcg = .4 mg) of folic acid daily, or take a supplement. A diet that provides 0.4 mg daily would consist of 1/2 cup of beans, one glass of orange juice, one bowl of a whole grain cereal, and 1-2 servings of green leafy vegetables. Or, you could eat one bowl of folic acid fortified cereal, like "Total" or "Product 19." We should all consume these highly nutritious food groups daily. The unfortunate reality is that most Americans don't.

TABLE 36. **Folic acid content in a variety of foods.**

FOOD	Folic Acid Content (mcg)
Total Cereal (3/4 cup)	400
Brewer's yeast (1 Tbs.)	313
Lentils cooked (1/2 cup)	179
Instant Oatmeal (1 packet)	150
Pinto beans (1/2 cup)	145
Garbanzo beans (1/2 cup)	145
Spinach cooked (1/2 cup)	131
Kidney beans (1/2 cup)	115
Asparagus (5 spears)	110
Orange Juice, concentrate (1 cup)	109
Spinach, Raw (1 cup)	109
Most breakfast cereals (1 cup)	100
Wheat germ, toasted (1/4 cup)	100
Orange juice, not concentrate (1 cup)	90
Romaine lettuce (1 cup)	76
Split peas (1/2 cup)	64
Peas or Brussels sprouts (1/2 cup)	47
Beets cooked (1/2 cup)	45
Broccoli cooked (1/2 cup)	39
Almonds	17
Banana	22
Tofu	19
Whole wheat bread (1 slice)	14
Milk, low-fat	12

Besides decreasing rates of artery disease, folic acid helps prevent birth defects in pregnant women. To prevent birth defects of a baby's spine, you need 400 mcg per day of folic acid prior to getting pregnant. All women during childbearing years should ensure an adequate intake of folic acid. If in doubt, eat a supplemented cereal or take a multivitamin with extra folic acid daily.

Beta Carotene

In controlled studies, beta carotene supplements have been a large disappointment. Randomized trials using beta carotene fail to show a clear benefit in preventing heart disease or cancer. In the large Finnish trial conducted on smokers, people taking placebo (sugar pills) did better than the antioxidant supplement group in avoiding lung cancer. People taking beta-carotene had an 18% higher risk of lung cancer and an 11% increased risk of death from heart disease. Unless more studies with beta carotene supplements are performed, this information states strongly *not* to use beta carotene as a supplement.

In contrast, studies in the United States and Europe show that people who consume abundant carotenoids through diet have lower risks of heart attacks, strokes, and cancer. The benefits noted with increased dietary antioxidants (especially dietary carotenoids) remain greater than with any of the vitamin supplement studies to date.

Beta carotene supplements flourished initially because studies showed that eating foods with beta carotene improved our health. However, beta carotene supplements have been found to alter the absorption of most carotenoids in food, changing our carotenoid balance.

Vitamin Supplement Summary

In summary, as of 1997 scientific trials on antioxidant supplements have failed to show a convincing benefit to their use in healthy people, and appear far less successful than studies of populations that use antioxidant-rich foods. So far, Vitamin E supplements provide a benefit to smokers and might also benefit people with known coronary artery disease or strokes. Folic acid supplements seem very helpful to people with folic acid deficiencies and for all women at risk of pregnancy. Vitamin C supplements shorten the duration of a cold. Beta carotene supplements given alone or with Vitamin E appear to be harmful.

I see the chemical reactions within us working in a delicate balance, much like an orchestra playing a piece by Mozart. Vitamin E itself plays a critical role in antioxidant balance, much like an orchestra's first violin. Simply adding more horns and clarinets in force will not improve the performance. The truth is, we do not yet know which antioxidants, in what proportions, are essential to reverse disease.

Healthy nutrition reflects the sum total of vitamins and nutrients that we consume. Good health grows from the *"synergy"* produced by these naturally occurring nutritional components. In contrast to antioxidant supplements, certain foods contain a balance of antioxidants. If you choose to take vitamin supplements, they will be far more effective if you ensure that they supplement your HEALTHY DIET.

WHAT ABOUT MINERAL DEFICIENCIES?

The mineral and vitamin producing industry has prospered as commercial farming depletes our soils. More people are taking supplements now than ever before. Yet eating five servings of whole grain products per day and seven or more servings of produce will markedly improve the mineral intake for the average American.

While a few areas of the country do have specific mineral shortages (like selenium), most areas don't. And as our current food supplies come from around the nation and often around the world, we normally don't worry about specific regional soil mineral shortages.

The best solution is to buy organic grains and organic produce. Organic crops aren't raised on fertilizers and usually have better mineral content. You can also cut out the added pesticides and hormones in these modern day agricultural products.

If you don't eat at least five servings of whole grains per day (preferably organic), I recommend you take a One-a-Day Vitamin as a mineral supplement. For more information on zinc and iron, see those sections starting with "ELEVEN MYTHS OF A VEGETARIAN DIET" on page 40.

Women may wish to add 500-800 mg of calcium daily. If you add calcium, combine it with a magnesium supplement. (For every 500 mg of calcium, add 250 mg of magnesium.) For more information on calcium, review the "Increased Bone Strength" section starting on page 17.

Magnesium

Many nutritional experts believe that magnesium deficiencies are common. Good food sources include green leafy vegetables, whole grains, and legumes. (Something many people miss!)

Magnesium is important in many ways:

- It provides a calming effect during stress.
- It lowers blood pressure.
- It helps muscles relax after activity.

During times of stress, you lose excess magnesium in the urine. People suffering from chronic stress sometimes report feeling calmer and more energetic with magnesium supplements.

ANTIOXIDANT VITAMIN & MINERAL DOSAGES

If you choose to take an antioxidant supplement, use common sense and stick with recommended and safe doses. In particular, excess mineral supplements can be severely toxic. Zinc, vanadium, and selenium *in excess* can produce major health problems.

Mineral and Vitamin Dosages

TABLE 37. For people taking antioxidants and minerals, here are the dosages suggested by national experts in the field for Vitamin E, Vitamin C, Zinc, Selenium, Copper, Chromium, and Magnesium.

Vitamin E	200-800 International Units (I.U.) per day. Vitamin E acts as an anti-coagulant and slows clotting. People taking coumadin or ASA as an anticoagulant should talk with their medical providers before adding Vitamin E as a supplement.
Vitamin C	500-1500 mg per day. Vitamin C can also be used to fight colds, with 1000 mg 4 times per day.
Zinc	15 mg per day, or, take a One-a-Day Vitamin with zinc. You can find zinc in fortified cereals like Total and Product 19. Diabetics are commonly zinc deficient and need zinc supplements. Zinc can also be used to fight a cold. A study at the Cleveland Clinic showed that taking zinc lozenges (13.3 mg of zinc every 2 hours while awake until symptoms resolved) had only 4 1/2 days instead of 7 1/2 days of symptoms. However, zinc-treated people had more nausea and bad taste.
Antioxidant Minerals	Trace minerals like selenium (adults need 50-100 mcg per day), copper (1-3 mcg per day), chromium (100-200 mcg per day), and magnesium (300-500 mg per day).

I am not ready to recommend that everyone jump on the antioxidant and vitamin supplement bandwagon. If you choose to take supplements, pick those in doses recommended for Vitamins C, Vitamin E, zinc, and folic acid. At worst, these vitamins appear harmless. At best, they may prove to be very beneficial. If you take carotenoid or flavonoid supplements, look for brands that offer a balanced and combined approach. Unfortunately, nobody knows what the best balance is.

I can think of reasons for healthy people to consider taking antioxidant supplements sporadically. There is strong evidence to support taking antioxidant supplements for a cold. On the other hand, the evidence for pollution exposure and overuse activities remains promising but theoretical.

- If you develop a cold, zinc, Vitamin C supplements, and Echinacea herbal teas all decrease the duration of your symptoms if you start them at the onset of your complaints.
- If you're exposed to pollution, (exhaust from cars and trucks, or gas powered tools, or if you spend an evening with cigarette smokers) consider Vitamin C 1000 mg and Vitamin E 400 IU before and after exposure.
- If you overexert, and you anticipate sore muscles later, consider Vitamin C 1000 mg and Vitamin E 400 IU before and after these stressful activities.

NATURAL SUPPLEMENTS

Natural supplements provide an array of nutrients packed inside a concentrated elixir or extract. The theoretical advantage is that you get all the natural agents working together. Garlic and ginger both act as potent natural antioxidants and can be eaten as food or bought in concentrated forms. (See "GARLIC" on page 100 and "GINGER" on page 102.)

Flavonoid Supplements

Flavonoids are found in many fruits and vegetables. Yet, a few sources are readily obtained only through supplements, (like ginkgo and milk thistle). They are commonly sold as combined flavonoids, or they can be bought individually. For example, you can buy all the flavonoids in Table 40 in one extract (from AMNI). Or, you can buy a single extract, like milk thistle extract in health food stores. The flavonoids in milk thistle extract are believed to help liver disease, and appear to reduce inflammation in people with chronic hepatitis.

Ginkgo biloba

Ginkgo biloba comes from an ancient Chinese tree. The Chinese have used its leaf extract for over 1,000 years. Ginkgo holds tremendous potential as an antioxidant booster. Unlike taking Vitamin E or Vitamin C supplements, ginkgo provides the synergy of many beneficial compounds working together.

TABLE 38. Common Flavonoids: Adapted with permission from Advanced Medical Nutrition, Inc.

PLANT SOURCE	FLAVONOID CLASS
Berries	Anthocyanins
Ginkgo	Biflavones
Green tea	Catechins and Flavones
Grape skin	Flavones and Anthocyanins
Citrus peel	Flavanones
Milk thistle	Silymarin
Pine bark	Pycnogenol

Ginkgo leaf extracts are packed with flavonoids, reported to extinguish the most potent free radicals. The European medical community has recognized ginkgo as an important medicinal agent for over a decade and ginkgo remains a leading over-the-counter medicine in European pharmacies.

Importantly, ginkgo protects our nervous system from free radical damage. The most intriguing use of ginkgo is in elderly people with memory loss. Although advertising adds herald its efficacy, in clinical studies it has only provided limited benefits to people with dementia. Don't mistake this as a "cure" for memory loss; rather, view ginkgo as a treatment that provides some benefit to people with memory dysfunction. In single dose studies, it has not been shown to improve memory in healthy people.

Other clinical trials have successfully used ginkgo to treat depression and to help patients after a stroke. The potential uses for ginkgo are still being explored.

Like Vitamin E, ginkgo reduces the oxidation of LDL cholesterol and could offer benefits in preventing heart attacks and strokes. Unfortunately, similar to Vitamin E, long-term ginkgo use does have side effects. In particular, both Vitamin E supplements and ginkgo extracts can cause serious bleeding problems when used long-term and in large doses.

In choosing the appropriate dosage, most clinical trials used 30 mg to 40 mg of ginkgo extract (such as ginkobene) three times daily. Higher doses are not recommended until their safety has been studied long-term.

MELATONIN

Melatonin is one of the best-selling over-the-counter pills on the market. Many of my patients and medical colleagues ask what I think of it.

Melatonin is a hormone normally produced in the brain by the pineal gland. Recent studies have shown it to be very helpful for insomnia, jet lag, and for people with sleep disorders. No studies have assessed its long-term safety, but for short-term use, it is safe, effective, and shy of side effects if you need an occasional good night's sleep.

It is currently being studied to treat dementia and other neurologic disorders. In addition to its role as a hormone, it acts as an antioxidant and could hold promise for preventing and treating Alzheimer's dementia and Parkinson's disease. Some researchers are even studying its use as an immune stimulant to help treat cancer.

Because we don't know the long-term safety of using melatonin regularly, I'm not going to recommend that my patients start taking melatonin regularly. I am more reluctant to alter brain hormones long-term than I am to add garlic or gingko as antioxidant extracts. I suggest you follow the results of studies using melatonin closely, as they appear to offer great promise.

For sleeping problems, try 1-2 mg a few nights per week. For jet lag, you can try 2-3 mg before bedtime. For now, even if you have chronic insomnia, I don't suggest taking melatonin more than 2-4 nights per week.

GLUTAMINE SUPPLEMENTS

Glutamine is an important amino acid during times of physical stress. Glutamine requirements increase greatly during many illnesses. In Japan and China, it is used regularly to treat stomach ulcers, heartburn, and to treat Crohn's disease. For adults, glutamine powder (1 gram) is dissolved in water and taken three times per day. It is also prescribed by some providers to treat diarrhea. Like all protein powders, it can cause problems when taken in excess.

When glutamine supplements are combined with weight training exercise, they are reported to enhance building muscle mass and to stimulate growth hormone production. Unfortunately, this benefit is countered by increased blood sugar levels and the long-term side effects remain unknown.

ENZYME AND COENZYME SUPPLEMENTS

While vitamins are compounds that our bodies cannot produce (hence we must eat them), our bodies can produce enzymes. Enzymes enhance normal chemical reactions. A variety of enzyme supplements offer theoretical benefits (and are for sale as supplements), but only a few have been proven to work in clinical trials.

Coenzyme Q-10 functions as both an enzyme and an antioxidant. In the mitochondria (the energy generating powerplant in each cell) coenzyme Q-10 aids in transporting oxygen's electrons to produce energy. As this energy production also generates dangerous free radicals, coenzyme Q-10 also acts as an antioxidant, squelching these hot radicals on the spot. Decreased coenzyme - 10 activity results in poor energy production. Heart cells in particular show the first signs of decreased coenzyme Q-10 activity.

In a variety of randomized clinical trials in people with known heart failure or in people facing heart surgery, coenzyme Q-10 supplements improved cardiac function and strength. The average dosage in studies was 100 mg daily. We do not yet know the long-term implication of taking coenzyme Q-10 supplements.

MEDICAL FOODS

In contrast to the studies that have reviewed the efficacy of taking 1 or 2 antioxidant vitamin supplements at a time, a whole new field is opening that attempts to provide an array of nutrients in a balanced supplement. The term *"medical foods"* refers to powdered supplements enriched with essential minerals, fatty acids, vitamins, and combined with carbohydrates and proteins unlikely to cause allergic reactions. Medical foods are formulated to be consumed under physician supervision and address specific medical conditions. While medical food supplements appear promising, we lack large, controlled, clinical outcome studies that show that they work. We also presume that they do no harm.

Multisupplements For Chronically Ill Individuals

If you have a debilitating illness (such as Chronic Fatigue Syndrome, Alzheimer's disease or fibromyalgia), the risk of taking nutraceuticals appears small (other than high cost), whereas the benefit of getting better or even of slowing further loss in independence seems appealing.

When we consider people with chronic illnesses, we must emphasize functionality. Jeffrey Bland, Ph.D. executive director of HealthComm International, articulates this clearly and has helped to develop a field that focuses on "Functional Medicine."

Above all, Functional Medicine supports the concept that people want to maintain their independence and remain functional. Hypoallergenic (low allergy) diets and multi-supplements (such as UltraClear Sustain ℞) are key elements in this therapeutic approach. As Dr. Bland would say, "We need to address people's healthspans, not just their lifespans. We must also design programs that meet individual's needs, supporting their biochemical individuality."

We are just beginning to understand the biochemical process around Parkinson's disease, chronic fatigue syndrome, and other debilitating illnesses like fibromyalgia. Western medicine has little to offer these people in the way of effective therapy. As these diseases appear to be related to oxidative stress and nutrient deficiencies, nutraceutical and medical food therapy options become attractive.

FURTHER READING

As I've noted many times, we are all unique individuals. No one program can work for everyone. Several other different programs are tailored for specific groups of individuals. My foremost goal remains to help you achieve maximum well-being and health.

Below are a list of other nutritional programs. If the Antioxidant Diet Program did not meet your specific needs, consider these. A brief description is attached. Good health and bon appétit!

Jeffery Bland, Ph.D., THE 20 DAY REJUEVENATION DIET PROGRAM

For people with chronic medical illnesses, this book emphasizes an elimination diet. It avoids foods that commonly cause food allergies (dairy, wheat, corn, etc.) and adds an array of nutrient and vitamin supplements. This information would be very helpful for people with complicated food allergies or for those with illnesses related to oxidative stress.

John McDougall M.D., THE MCDOUGALL PROGRAM, 12 DAYS TO DYNAMIC HEALTH

This program uses an ultra low-fat cooking style (less than 10% of calories from fat). It is vegan, using no meats, dairy, or egg products. The program relies heavily on carbohydrates.

Dean Ornish M.D., EVERYDAY COOKING WITH DEAN ORNISH

This book uses ultra low-fat (less than 10% of calories from fat) foods, tasty recipes designed by nationally known chefs, and some recipes from his patients. The recipes are vegetarian, using non-fat dairy and egg whites. The program was designed for people with heart disease and to reduce cholesterol levels, but anyone can follow this program.

Barry Sears Ph.D., THE ZONE

This is a high-protein, low-calorie diet that promotes short-term weight loss. There are no studies to show that long-term weight loss occurs if you follow this program.

This book promotes eating extra protein, with the "theory" that carbohydrates can only be eaten when combined with a nearly equal amount of protein. The information is presented as fact, but has been tested in only a handful of patients and remains unpublished in the academic world.

The type of fat chosen remains important, emphasizing monounsaturated fats. This approach might be useful for people who feel poorly following high-carbohydrate diets.

SPECIAL DIABETIC NEEDS

People with diabetes have elevated blood sugar levels. There are two types of diabetes, Type I and Type II. Most people with diabetes have Type II diabetes (also called adult onset diabetes). In contrast to Type I diabetes where the body stops making insulin, in Type II diabetes their body produces insulin, but the insulin doesn't work effectively and sugar levels and insulin levels increase.

There is a growing body of evidence supporting the concept that Type II diabetics can slow their metabolism to conserve weight and energy more efficiently than average adults. Thus, they appear to have a genetic adaptability for surviving famines or for gaining and maintaining weight. Unfortunately, during times of caloric excess and inactivity, that genetic advantage becomes a disease inducing time-bomb.

Exercise and Diabetes

I believe that the first and most important therapy for Type II diabetes should be increased activity. Aerobic activity has been shown to:

- improve the effectiveness of insulin action.
- increase metabolism
- promote weight loss
- normalize blood sugar and cholesterol levels

It can take months for somebody "out-of-shape" to reach therapeutic levels of activity, but one hour or more of moderate activity daily (such as a brisk walk) offers the best initial prescription for this disease. (See "STARTING YOUR PERSONALIZED EXERCISE PROGRAM" on page 135.)

Many medical providers (often out of frustration) over-treat Type II diabetes with medications when diet and exercise deserve more attention. Patients with diabetes should discuss activity options and diet plans with their medical providers, who given the opportunity, are often happy to help. I encourage you to share the exercise material in Chapter Six with your provider so that together, you can "fine-tune" a program to meet your needs.

Nutrients and Diabetes

As diabetic control worsens, nutritional and exercise requirements increase. People with diabetes have unique nutritional needs.

The first goal should be to restore blood sugar levels to normal.[1] As blood sugar levels rise, oxidative stress increases and excess urination overexcretes important minerals like zinc, chromium, and magnesium. Furthermore, poor diabetic control produces abnormal chemical reactions and hormone changes that impose additional nutritional needs for diabetic patients.

To compensate for these problems provoked by elevated blood sugar levels, I recommend the following supplements for diabetics, especially for those with poor control. Always check with your own medical provider to ensure that these supplements meet your unique medical needs.

To Control blood sugar levels:

- Gradually reach 45-60 minutes of exercise daily. (See Chapter Six, Starting Your Antioxidant Exercise Program.)
- Eat two servings of soy products daily (such as soy hot dogs, soy pepperoni, tofu, soy milk, etc.)
- Avoid all high glycemic foods. (See Chapter Five, Glycemic Indexes.)

To improve your sensitivity to insulin:

- Chromium 100 micrograms daily (to prevent chromium deficiency)
- Add omega-3 fats to your diet regularly [2]
- Avoid polyunsaturated fats (corn oil, peanut oil, etc.)
- Exercise daily

To improve your antioxidant protective system take:

- Vitamin E 400 IU daily
- Vitamin C 500 mg daily
- Magnesium 250-500 mg daily
- A One-A-Day Multi-Vitamin containing B-12, zinc, and folic acid, (or) eat a fortified cereal like "Total" or "Product 19" daily.

---

1. A blood test, called the Hemoglobin A1C level (or HgbA1C) is the best measure of overall diabetic control. It is designed to measure blood sugar control averaged over 12 weeks. A HgbA1C less than 6.0 represents good control, 6-8 is borderline control, and greater than 8.0 represents poor control. Diabetics don't normally benefit from adding medications unless their HgbA1C exceeds 8.0. Lifestyle changes remain the first step in therapy, even for levels greater than 8.0.

2. Until HgbA1C levels return to normal, plant sources of Omega-3 fats appear less effective than seafood sources in helping to restore cholesterol and sugar levels to normal. Therefore, in uncontrolled diabetics, fatty fish (like salmon) served 2-3 times per week, or daily fish oil capsules appear to improve insulin sensitivity. If your HgbA1C levels are close to normal, 1-2 teaspoons of flax oil daily taken with juices or in food appears to improve insulin sensitivity in diabetics. Nuts, soy products, green leafy vegetables and canola oil are other good sources of omega-3 fats.

WEEKLY MEAL PLANS: WEEKS 2-4

(For week ONE, see pages 188-192.)

The following pages provide meal lists for weeks 2-4 of the 28-Day Antioxidant Diet Program. You can plunge in and follow them daily, or you can sample them at your own speed.

The shopping lists following the meal plans will help you if you want to follow the daily program. The lists will help you follow the recipes without having to run back and forth from the store for missing items.

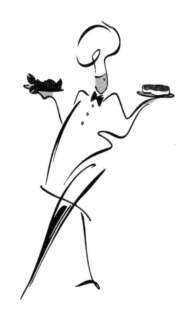

TABLE 39. Week Two Sample Recipes

DAY	Breakfast	Lunch	Snack	Dinner	Dessert
Mon	Coffee or tea, Whole wheat toast with marmalade & 1 tsp Almond spread. Orange juice	(Leftovers) Sweet & Sour Stir Fry & Cashews. Fresh fruit Water	Green tea	Non-fat chips with salsa & Bean Dip with Quesadillas. Sliced sweet potato. 1 Glass of wine or juice	Non-fat frozen yogurt with sliced fruit
Tues	Coffee or tea. Bowl of Total cereal with non-fat milk and raisins or frozen berries. Orange juice	(Fast Food Out) TACO BELL or TACO TIME: 2-3 light tacos. Water	Tea. 1 Piece of fruit	Pasta with basil, tomatoes, and artichoke hearts. Whole wheat bread. Green salad. 1 Glass of wine or water	Slice of melon Enjoy 1/2 ounce of fine chocolate
Wed	Coffee or tea. Bowl of oatmeal with fruit. Orange juice. Slice of melon	Left-over pasta with tomatoes, basil, and artichokes. Fruit Water	1 Pear and water	Sichuan Eggplant with cashews, peppers, broccoli. Rice Tea or water	Sorbet with sliced fruit
Thur	Coffee or tea. Whole wheat toast with almond butter & jam. Orange juice.	Whole wheat bread sandwiches with tomatoes, cucumber, mustard, & non-fat cheese. Fresh fruit. Water	Tea	Macaroni & Cheese with Veggies. Green Salad. Whole grain bread 1 Glass wine or water	Sorbet or Non-Fat yogurt with fresh fruit

TABLE 40. More, Week Two Sample Recipes

Fri	Coffee or tea. Bowl of Total cereal with non-fat milk, & fruit. Tomato Juice	Veggie burger with tomato slices & lettuce on a whole wheat bun. 1 Apple Water	1 apple and tea	Pizza with leeks, mushrooms, and roasted red peppers. Green salad. Wine or beverage	Frozen non-fat yogurt and fresh or frozen black-berries
Sat	Coffee or tea Whole rye toast with almond butter & marmalade. Orange Juice	DINING OUT	Trail Mix	Eggplant Lasagna. Steamed broccoli. Whole wheat bread. Green Salad. Wine or other beverage	Chocolate Cake with Blackberry Sauce
Sun	Coffee or Tea

Waffles with fruit

Grapefruit juice | Citrus and Spinach Salad Toast with Tomato sauce, Non-Fat Cheese, & Dill Weed Water | Bake Banana-Pecan Bread (for next week) | Raita Indian Rice Red Pepper & Eggplant Curry (Make extra for lunch) Tea, Water, or Wine | Banana-Pecan Bread with Non-Fat Yogurt |

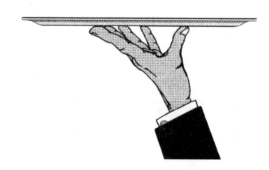

TABLE 41. Week Three Sample Recipes

DAY	Breakfast	Lunch	Snack	Dinner	Dessert
Mon	Coffee or tea. Whole wheat toast with almond butter & marmalade. Orange juice	Leftover lasagna. Fresh fruit	Green tea	Black Bean Chili with bell peppers & lime. Rice Water or 1 glass of wine	Non-fat frozen yogurt with sliced fruit
Tues	Coffee or tea. Bowl of Total cereal with non-fat milk and raisins and frozen blue-berries. Orange juice	(Leftovers) Indian Rice and Red Pepper & Eggplant Curry	Tea with Banana -Pecan Bread	Stir fry with cashews. Rice Tea or Wine	Rice Pudding with Almonds and Kahlua
Wed	Coffee Or Tea. Bowl of oatmeal with raisins. Orange juice.	(Leftover) Black bean chili. 1/4 Avocado. Fresh fruit Water		Southwestern Taboulleh. Water or 1 glass of wine	Sherbet. Sliced fruit
Thur	Coffee or tea. Whole wheat toast with almond butter & jam. Orange juice.	(Leftovers) Stir fry with cashews and rice	Tea. Banana -Pecan Bread	Miso Soup. Stir Fry with black bean sauce. Rice. Water, sake, or wine	Sliced fruit. Enjoy 1/2 ounce of "fine chocolate"
Fri	Coffee or tea. Bowl of Total cereal with non-fat milk, & raisins. Tomato Juice	Lunch Meeting: DINING OUT Pasta with sautéed veggies and pine nuts & olive oil. Green salad. Water	Tea. 1 Apple	Pizza in a Hurry. Green salad. Wine or beverage	Frozen non-fat yogurt

TABLE 42. More, Week Three Sample Recipes

Sat	Coffee or tea. Whole Rye toast with almond butter & Marmalade. Orange Juice	Leftover Stir Fry with Black Bean Sauce with Rice		Won Ton Soup. Mushroom, Ginger, & Broccoli Stir Fry. Rice Tea, Sake, or Wine	Blueberry and Port Frozen Yogurt
Sun	Coffee or tea. Waffles with fruit. Grapefruit juice	Garbanzo & Cauliflower Curry with Rice	Bake Wheat Bran Muffins with Apricots (for the week)	DINING OUT with friends	Soy milk with frozen cherries and orange juice

TABLE 43. Week Four Sample Recipes

DAY	Breakfast	Lunch	Snack	Dinner	Dessert
Mon	Coffee or tea. Whole wheat toast with almond butter & marmalade. Orange juice	(Leftovers) Mushroom & Broccoli Stir Fry. Rice. Tea or Water	Green tea. Muffins with Apricots	Spinach Soufflé. Steamed veggies. Whole wheat bread 1 Glass wine or water	Non-fat frozen yogurt. Sliced fruit
Tues	Coffee or tea. Bowl of Total cereal with non-fat milk and raisins and frozen blue-berries. Orange juice	Lunch Out	1 cup of tea, 1 piece of fruit	Falafel with Tomato, Lettuce, in Pita Bread. Latin Rice. 1 Glass wine or water (Make double portion for 2nd dinner with Latin rice this week)	Sorbet with fresh fruit

TABLE 44. Week Four Sample Recipes

Wed	Coffee or tea. Bowl of oatmeal with raisins. Orange juice.	Falafel Sandwich with sliced tomato and lettuce. Fresh fruit. Water	Green Tea	Hummus, sliced cucumbers, tomato, and lettuce in pocket bread.	Frozen yogurt. Fresh Fruit
Thur	Coffee or tea. Whole wheat toast with almond butter & jam. Orange juice.	Sandwich with avocado, hummus, tomato, and lettuce. Fresh fruit. Water	Tea with Muffins with Apricots	Nonfat chips with salsa. Enchiladas. with Latin Rice 1 Glass wine or water	Soy milk in blender with frozen or fresh cherries and orange juice
Fri	Coffee or tea. Bowl of Total cereal with non-fat milk, & raisins. Tomato Juice	Lunch Meeting: DINING OUT	Tea. 1 apple	Stuffed Squash with Wild Rice & Pecans. Steamed veggies. (Cook extra wild rice) 1 Glass wine or water	Sliced fruit. Enjoy 1/2 ounce of "fine chocolate"
Sat	Coffee or tea. French toast with fresh fruit. Juice	Sloppy Joe's with whole wheat buns. Green Salad. (Make extra for lunch next week) Water	Tea	Wild Rice with Kale, Almonds, and Mushrooms. Wine or Beverage	Rhubarb & Blueberry Crumble
Sun	Coffee or tea Oatmeal with raisins. Fresh fruit. Juice.	Nachos: with non-fat chips, non-fat bean dip, salsa, grated cheese, and Guacamole. Water	Roasted nuts	Tucson Pasta. Whole wheat bread. Green salad. 1 Glass wine or water (Make extra for lunch next week)	Home made frozen yogurt with blueberries and port

SHOPPING LISTS: WEEKS 1-4

This is a shopping list for 2 people eating adult sized portions. Double it for a family of four. You can copy this list and cross out what you have, or take the book to the store. I designed this list so that you can shop over the weekend for the week ahead.

STAPLES:

You will need the following:

- Soy sauce, look for low-sodium
- Miso (Japanese soybean paste that makes soup broth)
- Vegetable broth cubes for quick vegetable stock
- Vinegar, balsamic
- Vinegar, rice
- Canola oil
- Virgin olive oil (and/or extra virgin for salad dressings)
- Corn starch, baking powder
- Vanilla extract
- Salt
- Fine herbs, also called Herbes de Provence or Italian Herbs
- Ground cinnamon
- Ground cumin (and/or cumin seeds; you can substitute ground cumin when recipe calls for cumin seeds, but roasted cumin seeds taste fabulous in many dishes)
- Ground cayenne
- Ground curry powder or individual curry spices
- "Fine quality chocolate," a 4-8 ounce block should last one person 2-4 weeks.
- Fine mustard (such as Dijon)
- Chile sauce, or chile paste
- Sugar (white and brown)
- Cooking white wine (Chenin Blanc, or Chardonnay)
- Cooking port wine (optional)
- Marmalade (like orange-ginger)
- Jam (like raspberry, blackberry, etc.)
- Green Tea
- Rice (brown rice and/or polished oriental rice and/or Basmati or Texmati rice)

- Nut butter (almond butter, cashew butter, hazelnut butter, or pecan butter (sometimes you find them in health food stores). If you can't find these you can use peanut butter.
- Pasta (variety of shapes: like spirals, tubes, fettuccini, and regular spaghetti noodles)
- Nuts (if you buy in bulk, keep frozen in containers. Choose almonds, cashews, pecans, walnuts). If you don't have a machine or tool to slice almonds, consider buying them presliced in bulk.
- Whole wheat flour. Many recipes call for whole wheat pastry flour; you can substitute 1 cup whole wheat pastry flour for 1/2 cup whole wheat and 1/2 cup all purpose flour.
- Refried beans, nonfat
- Parmesan cheese for grating (or other nonfat cheese, or soy cheese)
- Snacks: Nonfat chips with low-fat bean dip and/or salsa, non-fat pretzels, Rye crisp crackers, dried fruit (like apricots)
- Canned beans (pintos, black beans, garbanzos)
- Frozen fruit and veggies
- Canned or frozen corn kernels

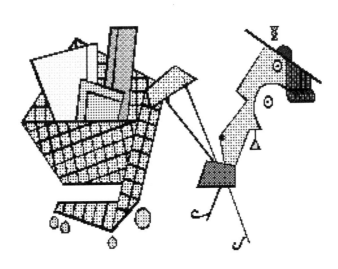

WEEK ONE: (Sunday afternoon through the following Sunday evening)

Check your supplies, and add what you don't have:

Produce:

12	Pieces	Fresh fruit for breakfast, snacks and desserts (apples, peaches, pears, melon)
4	Cups	Fresh or frozen fruit for cereals (berries, bananas, etc.)
3	Pounds	Tofu (3 blocks)
3	Heads	Garlic, nice and firm with large cloves
6	Medium	Onions
10	Cups	Broccoli
2	Medium	Lemons
2	Cups	Parsley
3	Med-Lg	Leeks
2	Cups	Celery
4	Medium	Red Bell Peppers
3	Medium	Green Bell Peppers
6	Cup	Mushrooms (for spaghetti sauce)
1	Medium	Zucchini squash
4	Medium	Tomatoes
2 1/2	Cups	Wild mushrooms (Shiitake, Porcini, Chanterelle, Portabellos, Oyster, etc.)
4	Medium	Shallots
1	Medium	Ginger root (Fresh meaning not dried and wrinkled,)
2	Medium	Japanese eggplants (or 1 medium regular eggplant)
7	Medium	Carrots
2	Cups	Green beans (or other green vegetable like asparagus, spinach, etc.)
4	Medium	Limes (or lemons)
1	Cup	Bok Choy (or other greens like cabbage, collard greens, or kale)
1	Cup	Cabbage (or can use other greens like bok choy, kale, or collard greens)
2	Medium	Potatoes, Russet
3	Medium	Beets, with greens

Grains

1	Loaf	Whole wheat bread (for sandwiches and toast)
1	Loaf	Whole grain bread (to warm in oven and serve with pasta)
1	Box	Total or Product 19 breakfast cereal
1	Box	Oatmeal (Buy enough for 1-2 servings per person twice per week for 1 month)
12	Ounces	Pasta, tubes for stuffing pasta with veggies and cheese
8	Ounces	Pasta, for spaghetti
12	Ounces	Pasta, fettuccini like (for peperonata)
2	Cups	Bulgur wheat (for taboulleh)
1 1/2	Cups	Brown rice or polished rice (already listed above under staples)

Condiments:

1	Cup	Dried fruit (dried apricots, apples, raisins, etc.)
1/2	Cup	Cashews
1/4	Cup	Walnuts chopped
1/2	Cup	Pecans, chopped

Dairy products:

1/2	Gallon	Non-fat milk, Buy cow's milk or a mix of calcium fortified rice milk, soy milk, and cow's milk.
1	Dozen	Eggs (free range if available)
1	Small block	Parmesan cheese (for grating), about 8-16 ounces, (optional; you can also use non-fat cheese)
2	Cups	Non-fat mozzarella cheese (for grating, or buy pre-grated)
2	Cups	Non-fat cottage cheese
32	Ounces	Non-fat plain yogurt for frozen yogurt (or buy pre-made frozen non-fat yogurt)

Canned Foods:

15	Ounce Can	Black beans
15	Ounce Can	Garbanzo beans
8	Ounce Can	White cooked beans
12 & 8	Ounce Cans	Pineapple chunks
16	Ounce Can	Baby corn
8	Ounce Can	Tomatoes
4	15 Ounce	Cans of tomatoes or buy 12 medium tomatoes for batch of tomato sauce

Beverages:

Green tea	1 bag/person/day
Tea	Herbal and/or black
Coffee	Optional
Red wine	Optional, 2-3 bottles for the week; 1 glass / person / day with a meal Seltzer, tonic water, other

Frozen foods:

2 1/2	Quarts	Citrus juice or vegetable juice (orange juice or grapefruit juice from frozen concentrate are great)
2	Cups	Frozen blueberries for frozen yogurt or buy premade, frozen non-fat yogurt and skip
		Sorbet or Sherbet: A flavor you like, 1-2 types for desserts
20	Ounces	Frozen snow peas, or buy fresh
1	Pack	Frozen veggie burgers (usually 8 veggie burgers/pack; 1 pack will last the month.)

WEEK TWO:

Produce:

8	Cups	Mixed salad greens
5	Cups	Broccoli
1 1/2	Cups	Parsley
1	Medium	Sweet potato
3	Medium	Onions
4	Medium	Tomatoes
4	Medium	Lemons
1	Cup	Cilantro leaves
2	Medium	Green bell peppers
4	Medium	Red bell peppers
10	Pieces	Fruit (apples, oranges, or 1/4 melon)
1	Medium	Cantaloupe (or 4 more pieces of fruit)
3	Medium	Bananas
1-2	Heads	Garlic
1	Medium	Cucumber
4	Medium	Carrots
1	Small-Med.	Fennel bulb (if you can't find, use 1 cup celery)
1	Pound	Tofu
2	Medium	Leeks
2	Cups	Fresh spinach leaves
1	Large	Grapefruit
1	Large	Orange
2	Medium	Japanese eggplants (or 1 more regular eggplant)
3	Medium	Eggplants
1	Medium	Potato, russet
	Medium	Yam
1/4	Cup	Mint leaves
2	Cups	Fresh berries (or frozen berries, or other fruit for breakfast cereals)

Grains:

1	Pack	Whole wheat tortillas (8-12 per pack)
1	Loaf	Whole grain bread for toast and sandwiches
16	Ounces	Pasta (any shape for pasta with basil and tomatoes)
12	Ounces	Lasagna noodles
1	Loaf	Whole grain dinner bread
1	Cup	Rice, Basmati (or Texmati or any kind)
8	Ounce	Soba noodles pack (Japanese section, or any pasta OK)
8	Ounces	Macaroni noodles

Condiments:

15	Ounce	Jar salsa, or check salsa recipe for ingredients
1	Bottle	Maple syrup (optional for breakfasts, or use jam, yogurt)
1/2	Cup	Raisins

1/3	Cup	Cashews

Canned Foods:

15	Ounce	Cans non-fat refried pinto beans (or cook and mash pintos)
8	Ounce	Can pineapple crushed (or chunks)
14	Ounces	Tomato sauce
4	Ounce	Can tomato paste

Dairy:

20	Ounces	Non-fat mozzarella cheese
8	Ounces	Reduced fat cheddar cheese (about 30-50% cal. from fat)
8-12	Ounces	Non-fat Monterey Jack cheese or other non-fat cheese
1/4	Cup	Non-fat sour cream (or non-fat cottage cheese)
32	Ounces	Non-fat plain yogurt to make frozen yogurt (or buy premade non-fat frozen yogurt)
16	Ounces	Non-fat plain yogurt
1/2	Gallon	Non-fat milk
6	Large	Eggs (or buy a dozen and save extras)
12-18	Ounces	Other non-fat or reduced fat cheese for slicing

Beverages:

Green tea	
Tea	Herbal and/or black
Coffee	Optional
Red wine	Optional, 2-3 bottles per week = 1 glass/person/day with meals
	Seltzer, tonic water, other

Frozen Foods:

Juice		Citrus or vegetable juice. Frozen concentrate OK. Buy enough to make 2 1/2 quarts
2	Cups	Frozen blackberries (pick or buy fresh if in season)
1/2	Gallon	Sherbet
24	Ounces	Peas
2	Cups	Frozen fruit (if you plan to make frozen yogurt)

The 28-Day Antioxidant Diet Program   293

WEEK THREE:

Produce:

3	Cups	Fresh salad greens
1-2	Medium	Bell peppers, for pizza (mixed colors)
2	Cups	Kale (or cabbage or other greens if you can't find kale)
1	Cup	Cilantro leaves
3	Medium	Limes
3	Medium	Bananas
2	Cups	Fresh fruit for breakfast, snacks, and desserts (apples, peaches, pears, 1/4 melon, etc.)
8	Pieces	Fresh fruit (apples, 1/4 melon, oranges, etc.)
2	Pounds	Tofu (firm)
1	Head	Garlic
3	Medium	Onions
2	Medium	Tomatoes
4	Leeks	(or 1-2 extra onions for black bean chili)
7	Cups	Broccoli
1	Cup	Parsley
2	Cups	Celery
1	Medium	Red bell peppers
2	Cups	Mushrooms, for pizza
6	Cups	Shiitake mushrooms (or other mushrooms). Canned in the Oriental food section are OK if you can't find fresh)
4	Medium	Shallots (or little green onions)
1	Medium	Ginger root, pick non-wrinkled & less branched
2	Medium	Japanese eggplants (or 1 regular eggplant)
10	Medium	Carrots
4	Cups	Bok Choy (or other greens like cabbage, collard greens, kale)
1	Medium	Potato, Russet
1	Medium	Yam
16-32	Ounces	Soy milk (calcium fortified if available, look for it near the tofu in the produce section)
1	Medium	Avocado

Grains:

1	Loaf	Whole grain bread for toast and sandwiches
12	Ounce Box	Total or Product 19 breakfast cereal
2	Cups	Bulgur wheat
6	Cups	Rice (or use from staples)
1	Cup	Basmati (or Texmati or any rice)
1	Pack	Won tons (about 10-20) 4 inches square

Canned Foods:

3	15 Ounce	Cans black beans (or cook yourself)
1	15 Ounce	Can kidney beans
4	Ounce Can	Pineapple chunks

Condiments:

1/2	Cup	Dried apricots
3/4	Cup	Cashews
1/3	Cup	Almond slices
1/2	Cup	Dried fruit

Dairy Products:

1/2	Gallon	Non-fat milk
6	Large	Eggs (you may have 6 left from last week)
1	Cup	Non-fat mozzarella cheese
32	Ounces	Non-fat plain yogurt for making frozen yogurt (or buy premade non-fat frozen yogurt)
1/2	Cup	Non-fat plain yogurt

Beverages:

Green tea
Tea   Herbal and/or black
Coffee   Optional
Red wine   Optional (2-3 bottles per week)
Seltzer, tonic water, etc.

Frozen Food:

		Citrus or vegetable juice. (Frozen concentrate OK, or buy fresh, jar, or canned) Enough to make 2 1/2 quarts)
16	Ounces	Frozen snow peas, or buy fresh
8	Ounces	Frozen cherries, for soy milkshakes
1	10-12 inch	Frozen pizza crust (or make a great crust from scratch out of the recipe section)

WEEK FOUR:

Produce:

8	Cups	Mixed salad greens
2	Cups	Broccoli
3	Cups	Parsley
6	Medium	Onions
12	Medium	Tomatoes
8	Medium	Lemons
1	Cup	Cilantro leaves
2	Medium	Green bell peppers
4	Medium	Red bell peppers
10	Pieces	Fruit (apples, oranges, 1/4 melon, 1 cup grapes)
1	Cup	Fresh or canned apricots, or peaches
2	Small	Butternut squash
7	Cups	Kale
1	Cup	Wild mushrooms (shiitake, oyster, or other. Canned OK too)
1/3	Cup	Fresh basil
2	Cups	Fresh or frozen rhubarb
1	Cup	Fresh or frozen blueberries
1	Head	Garlic
1	Medium	Cucumber
2	Medium	Carrots
1/2	Pound	Tofu
4	Cups	Green beans
1/4	Cup	Mint leaves
2	Cups	Fresh berries, fruit, or frozen fruit for breakfast cereals.
2	Medium	Avocados

Grains:

1	Loaf	Whole grain bread for toast and sandwiches
1	Pack	Whole wheat tortillas (8-12 per pack)
16	Ounces	Fresh pasta (for end of week, may buy later in the week)
1	Loaf	Whole grain dinner bread (for end of week, may buy later)
8		Whole wheat pita breads
3/4	Cup	Low fat granola (less than 30% of calories from fat)
3	Cups	Brown rice
16	Ounce bag	Non-fat corn tortilla chips
2	Cups	Wild rice

Condiments:

8	Ounces	Salsa, or make salsa and add recipe ingredients
1/2	Cup	Pecans
1/4	Cup	Almond slivers
12	Ounces	Tomato sauce (buy or make)

Canned Foods:

2	15 Ounce	Cans non-fat refried pinto beans (or cook and mash pintos)
15	Ounces	Stewed tomatoes
2	15 Ounce	Cans garbanzo beans
2	15 Ounce	Cans corn kernels
15	Ounce	Can black beans
15	Ounce	Can pinto beans
15	Ounce	Can white beans

Dairy Products:

16	Ounces	Non-fat mozzarella cheese
16	Ounces	Non-fat Monterey Jack or other reduced-fat cheese for enchiladas
32	Ounces	Non-fat plain yogurt to make frozen yogurt (or buy premade non-fat frozen yogurt)
1/2	Gallon	Non-fat milk
1	Dozen	Eggs (free range, if possible)
1	Cup	Egg substitute (like Egg Beaters
4	Ounces	Parmesan cheese (optional)

Beverages:

Green Tea	
Tea	Herbal and/or black
Coffee	Optional
Red wine	Optional
	Seltzer, tonic water, other

Frozen Foods:

		Citrus or vegetable juice: Frozen concentrate OK, but enough to make 2 1/2 quarts
1/2	Gallon	Sherbet
2	Cups	Frozen fruit (to make frozen yogurt)
1 1/2	Cups	Frozen chopped spinach

SELECTED BIBLIOGRAPHY

Alcohol and wine:

Bianchi C, et al., Alcohol consumption and the risk of acute myocardial infarction in women. *Journal of Epidemiology and Community Health* 1993;47:308-311.

Carnacini A, Arfelli G, Selected nutritional components of wine. *Alcologia* 1994;6:141-149.

Forman MR, et al., Effect of alcohol consumption on plasma carotenoid concentrations in premenopausal women: a controlled dietary study. *Am J Clin Nutr* 1995;62:131-135.

Fuhrman B, Lavy A, Aviram M, Consumption of red wine with meals reduces the susceptibility of human plasma and low-density lipoprotein to lipid peroxidation. *Am J Clin Nutr* 1995;61:549-554.

Gaziano JM, Buring JE, Breslow JL, et al., Moderate alcohol intake, increased levels of high-density lipoprotein and its subfractions, and decreased risk of myocardial infarction. *N Engl J Med* 1993;329:1829-34.

Gronbaek M, Deis A, Sorensen TIA, et al., Mortality associated with moderate intakes of wine, beer or spirits. *BMJ* 1995;310:1165-1169.

Klatsky AL, Armstrong MA, Friedman GD, Alcohol and Mortality. *Annals of Internal Medicine* 1992;117:646-654.

Renaud S, Lorgeril M, et al., Wine, alcohol, platelets, and the French paradox for coronary heart disease. *The Lancet* 1992;339:1523-1526.

Rimm EB, Ellison RC, Alcohol in the Mediterranean diet. *Am J Clin Nutr* 1995;61(suppl):1378S-1382S.

Weisse ME, Eberly B, Person DA, Wine as a digestive aid: comparative antimicrobial effects of bismuth salicylate and red and white wine. *BMJ* 1995;311:1657-1660.

Antioxidants and Oxidative Stress:

Meydani SN et al., Antioxidants and immune response in aged persons: overview of present evidence. *Am J Clin Nutr* 1995:62(suppl):1462S-76S.

Mangels AR et al., Carotenoid content of fruits and vegetables: An evaluation of analytic data. *J Am Diet Assoc.* 1993:93:284-296.

Reaven P, Dietry and pharmacologic regimens to reduce lipid peroxidation in non-insulin-dependent diabetes mellitus. *Am J Clin Nutr* 1995;62:1483S-9S.

Lea & Febiger, Modern Nutrition in Health and Disease, 1994, Eighth Edition, Volume 1, pgs 185-202 & 501-512.

Youngson R, The Antioxidant Health Plan: How to Beat the Effects of Free Radicals. 1994. *Thorsons, an Imprint of HarperCollins Publishers.*

Shigenaga MK, Hagen TM, Ames BN, Oxidative damage and mitochondrial decay in aging. *Proc. Natl. Acad. Sci. USA* Vol. 91, pp. 10771-107778, November 1994.

Dandona P, et al., Oxidative damage to DNA in deabetes mellitus. *The Lancet* 1996;347:444-445.

Wang H, Cao G, Prior RL, Total Antioxidant Capacity of Fruits. *J. Agri. Food Chem* 1996;44:701-705.

Wang H, Cao G, Prior RL, Oxygen Radical Absorbing Capacity of Anthocyanins. *J. Agri. Food Chem* 1997;45:304-309.

Cao G, Sofic E, Prior RL., Antioxidant Capacity of Tea and Common Vegetables *J. Agri. Food Chem* 1996;44:3426-3431.

Blood Pressure

Appel LJ, et al. (For the DASH collaborative research group), A Clinical Trial of the Effects of Dietary Patterns on Blood Pressure. *N Engl J Med* 1997;336:1117-24.

Bone Health and Osteoporosis:

Baran D, Sorensen A, Grimes J, et al., Dietary Modification with Dairy Products for Preventing Vertebral Bone Loss in Premenopausal Women: A Three-Year Prospective Study. *J Clin Endocrinol Metab* 1989;70:264-270.

Chapuy MC, Arlot ME, Duboeuf F, Vitamin D3 and Calcium to Prevent Hip Fractures in Elderly Women. *N Engl J Med* 1992;327:1637-1642.

Fleming KH, Heimbach JT, Consumption of Calcium in the U.S.: Food Sources and Intake Levels. *J. Nutr.* 1994;124:1426S-1430S.

Dawson-Hughes B, Calcium supplementation and bone loss: a review of controlled clinical trials. *Am J Clin Nutr* 1991;54:274S-280S.

Heaney RP, Protein intake and the calcium economy. *Journal of the American Dietetic Association* 1993;93:1259-1260.

Heaney RP, Nutritional Factors in Osteoporosis. *Annu. Rev. Nutr.* 1993;13:287-316.

Marsh AG, et al., Vegetarian lifestyle and bone mineral density. *Am J Clin Nutr* 1988;48:837-41.

Matkovic V, et al., Urinary calcium, sodium, and bone mass of young females. *Am J Clin Nutr* 1995;62:417-425.

National Institute of Health Consensus Panel, Optimal Calcium Intake. *JAMA* 1994;272:1942-1948.

Prentice A, Jarjou LMA, Cole TJ, et al., Calcium requirements of lactating Gambian mothers: effects of a calcium supplement on breast-milk calcium concentration, maternal bone mineral content, and urinary calcium excretion. *Am J Clin Nutr* 1995;62:58-67.

Recker RR, et al., Bone Gain in Young Adult Women. *JAMA* 1992;268:2403-2408.

Exon-Smith AN. The musculoskeletal system-bone aging and metabolic bone disease. In: Brocklehurst JC. *Textbook of Geriatric Medicine and Gerontology*. 3rd Ed. New York: Churchill Livingstone, 1985:758-759.

Cancer

Bal DG et al., Dietary Strategies for Cancer Prevention. *Cancer* 1993;72:1005-10.

Byers T and Guerrero N, Epidemiologic evidence for vitamin C and vitamin E in cancer prevention. *Am J Clin Nutr* 1995;62(suppl):1385S-92S.

Mackie BS, et al., Melanoma and Dietary Lipids. *Nutrition and Cancer* 1987;9:219-226.

Carotenoids:

Karstadt M, Schmidt S, Procter's Big Gamble, *Nutrition Action Health Letter* 1996; 23:4-7.

Byers T and Perry G, Dietary Carotenes, Vitamin C, and Vitamin E as Protective Antioxidants in Human Cancers. *Annu. Rev. Nutr.* 1992:12:139-159.

Liebman B, Just the carotenoid facts. *Nutrition Action Health Letter*, October 1994;21:12.

Mangels AR, et al., Carotenoid content of fruits and vegetables: An evaluation of analytic data. *Journal of the American Dietetic Association* 1993;93:284-296.

Kostic D, White, SW, Olson JA, Intestinal absorption, serum clearance, and interactions between lutein and B-carotene when administered to human adults in separate or combined oral doses. *Am J Clin Nutr* 1995;62:604-610.

Morris DL et al., Serum Carotenoids and Coronary Heart Disease. *JAMA* 1994;272:1439-1441.

Chocolate:

Denke MA, Grundy SM, Effects of fats high in stearic acid on lipid and lipoprotein concentrations in men. *Am J Clin Nutr* 1991;54:1036-1040.

Kris-Etherton PM, et al., The Role of Fatty Acid Saturation on Plasma Lipids, Lipoproteins, and Apolipoproteins: Effects of Whole Food Diets High in Cocoa Butter, Olive Oil, Soybean Oil, Dairy Butter, and Milk Chocolate on the Plasma Lipids of Young Men. *Metabolism* 1993;42:121-129.

Depression:

Hibbeln KR. Salem S. Dietary polyunsaturated fatty acids and depression: when cholesterol does not satisfy. *Am J Clin nutr* 1995;62:1-9.

Diet compliance success:

Barnard ND et al., Factors That Facilitate Compliance to Lower Fat Intake, *Arch Fam Med* 1995;4:153-158.

Barnard ND et al., Adherence and Acceptability of a Low-Fat, Vegetarian Diet Among Patients With Cardiac Disease, *J Cardiopulmanary Rehabil* 1992;12:423-431.

Environmental Impact:

Earth Save: Personal Food Choices... Global Results. 1996 Winter, Volume 6, Number 1.

Earth Save: Personal Food Choices... Global Results. 1995 Fall, Volume 6, Number 3.

Exercise:

Ginsburg GS, Agil A, O'Toole M, et al., Effects of a Single Bout of Ultraendurance Exercise on Lipid Levels and Susceptibility of Lipids to Peroxidation in Triathletes. *JAMA* 1996;276:221-225.

Skender ML, et al., Comparison of 2-year weight loss trends in behavioral treatments of obesity: Diet, exercise, and combination interventions. *Journal of the American Dietetic Association* 1996;96:342-346.

Ewbank PP, Darga LL, Lucas CP. Physical Activity as a Predictor of Weight Maintenance in Previously Obese Subjects. Obesity Research 1995;3:257-262.

Cooper KH. *Antioxidant Revolution.* Thomas Nelson Publishers, Nashville, 1994.

Lemon, Peter WR. Is Increased Dietary Protein Necessary or Benefiical for Individuals with a Physicially Active Lifestyle? *Nutrition Review* 1996;54:S169-S175.

Eye diseases:

Taylor AT et al., Relations among aging, antioxidant status, and cataract. *Am J Clin Nutr* 1995;62(suppl):1439S-47S.

Snodderly DM, Evidence for protection against age-related macular degeneration by carotenoids and antioxidant vitamins. *Am J Clin Nutr* 1995;62(suppl):1448S-61S.

Fats, Fatty Acids, Oils, and Lipids:

Abbey M et al., Oxidation of low-density liporoteins: intraindividual variability and the effect of dietary linoleate supplementation, *Am J Clin Nutr* 1993;57:391-398.

Aviram M and Eias K, Dietary Olive Oil Reduces Low-Density Lipoprotein Uptake by Macrophages and Decreases the Susceptibility of the Lipoprotein to Undergo Lipid Peroxidation, Ann Nutr Metab 1993;37:75-84.

Browner WS et al., What if Americans Ate Less Fat?, *JAMA*, 1991;265:3285-3291.

Louheranta AM, et al., Linoleic acid intake and susceptibility of very-low-density and low-density lipoproteins to oxidation in men. *Am J Clin Nutr* 1996;63:698-703.

Renaud S et al., Cretan Mediterranean diet for prevention of coronary heart disease, *Am J Clin Nutr* 1995; 61(suppl):1360S-13607S.

Renaud S et al., Influence of long-term diet modification on platelet function and composition in Moselle farmers, *Am J Clin Nutr* 1986:43:136-150.

Sears B, Lawren B. *Enter The Zone.* Regan Books, New York. 1995.

Sinclair AJ, et al., Diets Rich in Lean Beef Increase Arachidonic Acid and Long-Chain Omega-3 Poly-unsaturated Fatty Acid Levels in Plasma Phospholipids. *Lipids* 1994;29:337-343.

Fiber:

Anderson JW, et al., Hypocholesterolemic Effects of High-Fibre Diets Rich in Water-Soluble Plant Fibres. *Journal of the Canadian Dietetic Association* 1984;45:140-148.

Ripsin CM, Keenan JM, Jacobs DR, et al., Oat Products and Lipid Lowering: A Meta-analysis. *JAMA* 1992;267:3317-3325.

Wynder EL, Stellman SD, Zang EA, High Fiber Intake: Indicator of a Healthy Lifestyle. *JAMA* 1996;275:486-487.

Flavanoids

Hertog MGL, et al., Dietary antioxidant flavonoids and risk of coronary heart disease: the Zutphen Elderly Study. *Lancet* 1993;342:1007-11.

Knekt P, Jarvinen R, Reunanen A, Maatela J, Flavonoid intake and coronary mortality in Finland: a cohort study. *BMJ* 1996;312:478-481.

Garlic:

Dausch JB and Nixon DW, Garlic: A Review of Its Relationship to Malignant Disease, Preventive Medicine 1990;19:346-361.

Warshafsky S et al., Effect of Garlic on Total Serum Cholesterol, A Meta-analysis, Ann Intern Med. 1993;119:599-605.

Srivastava KC, Tyagi OD, Effects of a Garlic-Derived Principle (Ajoene) on Aggregation and Arachi-donic Acid Metabolism in Human Blood Platelets. Prostaglandins Leukotrienes and Essential Fatty Acids 1993;49:587-595, Longman Group UK Ltd.

Steiner M, Khan AH, Holbert, D, Lin RIS, A double-blind crossover study in moderately hypercholes-terolemic men that compared the effect of aged garlic extract and placebo administration on blood lipids. *Am J Clin Nutr* 1996;64:866-70.

Adler AJ, Holub BJ, Effect of garlic and fish-oil supplementation on serum lipid and lipoprotein concentrations in hypercholesterolemic men. *Am J Clin Nutr* 1997;65:445-50.

Ginger:

Paul Schulick, *Ginger: Common Spice and Wonder Drug.* Herbal Free Press Ltd. 1994.

Gingko:

Smith PF, et al., The neuroprotective properties of the Ginkgo biloba leaf: a review of the possible rela-tionship to platelet-activiting factor (PAF). *J Ethnopharmacol 1996 Mar;50:131-9.*

Kanowski S, et al., Proof of efficacy of the ginkgo biloba special extrat EGb 761 in outpatients suffering from mild to moderate primary degenerative dementia of the Alzheimer type or multi-infarct dementia. *Pharmacopsychiatry 1996 Mar;29(2):47-56.*

Maitra I, et al., Peroxyl radical scavenging activity of Ginkgo biloba extract EGb 761. *Biochem Pharmacol 1995 May 26;49(11):1649-55.*

Kose K, Dogan P, Lipoperoxidation induced by hydrogen peroxide in human erythrocyte membranes. Comparison of the antioxidant effect of Ginkgo biloba extract (EGb 761) with those of water-soluble and lipid-soluble antioxidants. *J Int Med Res 1995 Jan-Feb;23 (1):9-18.*

Glycemic indexes:

Miller JCB, Importance of glycemic index in diabetes. *Am J Clin Nutr* 1994;59(suppl):747S-752S.

Smith U, Carbohydrates, fat, and insulin action, *Am J Clin Nutr* 1994;59(suppl):686S-689S.

Jenkins DJA et al., Low glycemic index: lente carbohydrates and physiological effects of altered food frequency. *Am J Clin Nutr* 1994;59(suppl):706S-709S.

Rasmussen O et al., Differential effects of saturated and monounsaturated fat on blood glucose and insulin responses in subjects with non-insulin-dependent diabetes mellitus. *Am J Clin Nutr* 1996;63:249-53.

Jenkins DJA et al., Low glycemic response to traditionally processed wheat and rye products: bulgur and pumpernickel bread. *Am J Clin Nutr* 1986;43:516-520.

Parillo M et al., Different Glycaemic Responses to Pasta, Bread, and Potatoes in Diabetic Patients. Diabetic Medicine 1985;2:374-377.

Wolever TMS, The Glycemic Index. *World Rev Nutr Diet.* 1990:62:120-185.

Jenkins DJA et al., The Glycaemic Index of Foods Tested in Diabetic Patients: A New Basis for Carbohydrate Exchange Favoring the Use of Legumes. *Diabetaologia* 1983;24:257-264.

Salmeron J, et al. Dietary Fiber, Glycemic Load, and Risk of Non-Insulin-Dependent Diabetes Mellitus in Women. *JAMA* 1997;277:472-477.

Heart Disease and Diet:

Gramenzi et al., Association between certain foods and risk of acute myocardial infarction in women. *BMJ* 1990;300:771-773.

Kohlmeier et al., Epidemiologic evidence of a role of carotenoids in cardiovascular disease prevention. *Am J Clin Nutr* 1995;62(suppl):1370S-6S.

Ornish D, *Reversing Heart Disease* 1990; Ballantine Books

Rimm EB, Ascherio A, Giovannucci E, et al., Vegetable, Fruit, and Cereal Fiber Intake and risk of Coronary Heart Disease Among Men. *JAMA* 1996;275:447-451.

Ascherio A, Rimm EB, Giovannucci EL, Spiegelman D, Stampfer M, Willett WC, Dietary fat and risk of coronary heart disease in men: cohort follow up study in the United States. *BMJ* 1996;313:84-90.

Kidney stones:

Robertson WG et al., Should Recurrent Calcium Oxalate Stone Formers Become Vegetarians? *British Journal of Urology* 1979:51:427-431.

Mediterranean diets:

Willett WC et al., Mediterranean diet pyramid: a cultural model for healthy eating. *Am J Clin Nutr* 1995;61(suppl):1402S-1406S.

Verschuren WM M et al., Serum Total Cholesterol and Long-term Coronary Heart Disease Mortality in Different Cultures. *JAMA*, July12, 1995:274:131-136.

Dietary behavior change: the challenge of recasting the role of fruit and vegetables in the American diet. *Am J Clin Nutr* 1995;61(suppl):1397S-1401S.

Kushi SH et al. Health implication of Mediterranean diets in light of contemporary knowledge. Meat, wine, fats, and oils. *Am J Clin Nutr* 1995:61(suppl):1416S-1427S.

Mushrooms:

Weil A, *Boost Immunity with Medicinal Mushrooms*, Natural Health 1993; May/June:12-17.

Nuts:

Fraser GE, Sabate J, Beeson WL, Strahan TM. A Possible Protective Effect of Nut Consumption on Risk of Coroanry Heart Disease. *Arch Intern Med* 1992;152:1416-1424.

Sabate J, Fraser GE, Burke K, et al. Effects of Walnuts on Serum Lipid Levels and Blood Pressure in Normal Men. *N Engl J Med* 1993;328:603-7.

Kushi LH, Folsom AR, Prineas RJ, et al. Dietary Antioxidant Vitamins and Death from Coronary Heart Disease in Postmenopausal Women. *N Engl J Med* 1996;334:1156-62.

Dreher ML, Maher CV, Kearney P. The Traditional and Emerging Role of Nuts in Healthful Diets. *Nutrition Reviews* 1996;54:241-245.

Omega-3 (N-3) Fatty Acids:

De Lorgeril M, Renaud S, et al., Mediterranean alpha-linolenic acid rich diet in secondary prevention of coronary heart disease. *Lancet* 1994;343:1454-1459.

Mantzioris E, et al., Dietary substitution with an alpha linolenic acid-rich vegetable oil increases eicosapentaenoic acid concentrations in tissues. *Am J Clin Nutr* 1994;59:1304-1309.

Nettleton JA. Omega-3 Fatty acids: Comparison of plant and seafood sources in human nutrition. *J Am Diet Assoc.* 1991;91:331-337.

Garg ML, Clandinin MT. Alpha Linolenic Acid and Metabolism of Cholesterol and Long-Chain Fatty Acids. Nutrition 1992;8:208210.

Cunnane SC, et al. Nutritional attributes of traditional flaxseed in healthy young adults. *Am J Clin Nutr* 1994;61:62-68.

Hibbeln JR, Salem N. Dietary polyunsaturated fatty acids and depression: when cholesterol does not satisfy. *Am J Clin Nutr* 1995;62:1-9.

Kromhout D, Bosschieter EB, Coulander CL. The inverse relation between fish consumption and 20 year mortality from coronary heart disease. *N Engl J Med* 1985;312:1205-9.

Burr ML, et al. Effects of changes in fat, fish, and fibre intakes on death and myocardial reinfarctions: Diet And Reinfarction Trial (DART). *The Lancet* 1989;Sept 30:757-761.

Ascherio A, Rimm EB, Stampfer MJ, Giovannucci EL, Willett WC. Dietary intake of marine n-3 fatty acids, fish intake, and the risk of coronary disease among men. *N Engl J Med* 1995;332:977-82.

Sauerwald TU, et al., Effect of dietary alpha-linolenic acid intake on incorporation of docosahexaenoic and arachidonic acids into plasma phospholipids of term infants. *Lipids* 1996; 31:S131-S135.

Daviglus ML, et al., Fish Consumption and the 30-Year Risk of Fatal Myocardial Infarction. *N Engl J Med* 1997;336:1046-53.

Soy Products:

Anderson JW, Johnston BM, Cook-Newell ME, Meta-Analysis of the Effects of Soy Protein Intake on Serum Lipids. *N Engl J Med* 1995:333:276-82.

Jenkins DJA, Wong GS, Patten R, et al., Leguminous Seeds in the Dietary Management of Hyperlipidemia. *Am J Clin Nutr* 1983;38:567-573.

Murkies AL, Lombard C, Strauss BJG, et al., Dietary flour supplementation decreases post-menopausal hot flushes: Effect of soy and wheat. *Maturitas* 1995;21:189-195.

Strokes:

Gillman MW et al., Protective Effect of Fruits and Vegetables on Development of Stroke in Men. *JAMA*. 1995;273:1113-1117.

Trans Fatty Acids:

Mensink RP, Katn MB, Effect of dietary trans fatty acids on high-density and low-density lipoprotein cholesterol levels in health subjects. *N Engl J Med* 1990;323:439-435.

Willett W, Ascherio A, Response to the International Life Sciences Institute report on trans fatty acids. *Am J Clin Nutr* 1995;62:524-526.

Vegan diets:

Michael Klaper, M.D., *Vegan Nutrition: Pure and Simple*, 3rd Edition, 1994, Gentle World Inc.

John Robbins, Diet For A New America, 1987, *Stillpoint Publishing*, Walpole, NH

Neal Barnard, M.D., Eat Right, Live Longer. 1995, *Harmony Books*, New York.

Vegetarian diets:

American Dietetic Association, Position of The American Dietetic Association: Vegetarian diets. *Journal of the American Dietetic Association* 1993;93:1317-1319.

Fisher M, Levine PH, Weiner B, et al., The Effect of Vegetarian Diets on Plasma Lipid and Platelet Levels. *Arch Intern Med* 1986;146:1193-1197.

Hunt JR, Gallagher SK, Johnson LK, Lykken GI, High-versus low-meat diets: effects on zinc absorption, iron status, and calcium, copper, iron, magnesium, manganese, nitrogen, phosphorus, and zinc balance in postmenopausal women. *Am J Clin Nutr* 1995;62:621-32.

Kestin M, Rouse IL, Correll RA, Newstel PJ, Cardiovascular disease risk factors in free-living men: comparison of two prudent diets, one based on lactoovovegetarianism and the other allowing lean meat. *Am J Clin Nutr* 1989;50:280-287.

David Gabbe, *Why do Vegetarians Eat Like That?* 1994, Prime Imprints Ltd.

The National Institute of Nutrition (Canada), Risks and Benefits of Vegetarian Diets. *Nutrition Today* 1990; March/April:27-29.

Vitamin C:

Block G, Epidemiologic evidence regarding vitamin C and cancer. *Am J Clin Nutr* 1991;54:1310S-1314S.

Gale CR, Martyn CN, Winter PD, Cooper C, Vitamin C and risk of death from stroke and coronary heart disease in cohort of elderly people. *BMJ* 1995;310:1563-1566.

Vitamin E:

Stephens, NG, Parsons A, Schofield PM, et al., Randomised controlled trial of vitamin E in patients with coronary disease: Cambridge Heart Antioxidant Study (CHAOS). *The Lancet* 1996;347:781785.

Rapola JM, Virtamo J, Haukka JK, et al., Effect of Vitamin E and Beta Carotene on the Incidence of Angina Pectoris. *JAMA* 1996;275:693-698.

Meydani SN, et al., Vitamin E Supplementation and In Vivo Immune Response in Healthy Elderly Subjects. *JAMA* 1997;277:1380-1386.

Vitamin Supplements:

Bland J, Benum S. *The 20-Day Rejuvenation Diet Program.* Keats Publishing 1997.

Ulene A, Ulene V. *The Vitamin Strategy.* Ulysses Press, 1994.

Nutrition Action Health Letter. Center for Science in the Public Interest September 1995;22:5.

Weight Loss:

Kuczmarski RJ, Flegal KM, Compbell SM, Johnson CL, Increasing Prevalence of Overweight Among US Adults. *JAMA* 1994;272:205-211.

Ornish D, *Eat More, Weigh Less.* HarperPerennial 1993, A Division of HarperCollins Publishers

Zinc:

Aggett PJ, Comerford JG, Zinc and Human Health. *Nutrition Reviews* 1995;53:S16-S22.

Freeland-Graves J, Mineral adequacy of vegetarian diets. *Am J Clin Nutr* 1988;48:859-62.

Srikumar TS, et al., Trace element status in healthy subjects switching from a mixed to a lactovegetarian diet for 12 months. *Am J Clin Nutr* 1992;55:885-90.

Mossad SB, et al., Zinc lozenges for treating the common cold: a randomized, placebo-controlled study. *Annals Internal Medicine* July 15, 1996;125:81-8.

INDEX

For information on future books,
cooking and nutrition lessons, or to see
my *"Free Recipe of the Month,"* visit
my web site at: **www.drmasley.com**